Handbook

Amit Kumar · Kenneth Ouriel
Editors

Handbook
of Endovascular
Interventions

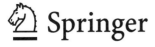 Springer

Editors
Amit Kumar, MD, FACS
Department of Surgery
Columbia University
New York, NY, USA

Kenneth Ouriel, MD, MBA,
  FACS, FACC
Syntactx
New York, NY, USA

ISBN 978-1-4614-5012-2   ISBN 978-1-4614-5013-9 (eBook)
DOI 10.1007/978-1-4614-5013-9
Springer New York Heidelberg Dordrecht London

Library of Congress Control Number: 2012950331

Printed on acid-free paper

Springer is part of Springer Science+Business Media (www.springer.com)

To my wife Natasha, and kids Tanishq, Vedha and Kush, who give me the strength and love to pursue my dreams

Preface

The field of endovascular treatment—be it in cardiology, interventional radiology, or vascular surgery—is a dynamic one. However, in this rapidly evolving field, the fundamentals remain the same. We are still taught to ensure that catheters are introduced over a wire, still taught never to lose control of the wire, etc. So while we are always looking for the next great tool on the horizon, one cannot use these new tools, without a sound understanding of the basics of endovascular treatment.

The purpose of this text is to provide basic principles and techniques of commonly performed endovascular interventions. We have endeavored not just to present one opinion, but by choosing a global field of authors, to reflect the everyday practice of the "world." There are other more comprehensive texts that delve into the details of any one procedure; however, this is the first text of its kind to be available to all practitioners of endovascular therapy, be they residents, fellows, or staff as well as nonmedical staff in the cath lab/interventional radiology suite/hybrid OR. Designed to be used as a day-to-day reference for any queries of "how to, when, and what ifs." To ensure that it is truly reflective of the questions we all sometimes have when thinking of the method to pursue, the chapters have been written by having a resident/fellow coauthor the chapter with a senior faculty member. This has been the defining principle for the book, from conception to completion—learning the technique from mentors, be it related to procedures or to authoring chapters or even the book.

New York, NY, USA
Amit Kumar, MD, FACS
Kenneth Ouriel, MD, MBA, FACS, FACC

Contents

Contributors

Andrei V. Alexandrov, M.D. Comprehensive Stroke Center, University of Alabama Hospital, Birmingham, AL, USA

Javier E. Anaya-Ayala, M.D. The Methodist Hospital Research Institute, The Methodist Hospital, Houston, TX, USA

Efthimios D. Avgerinos, M.D. Department of Vascular Surgery, Attikon University Hospital, Athens, Greece

Jean Bismuth, M.D. Division of Vascular Surgery, Department of Cardiovascular Surgery, The Methodist DeBakey Heart & Vascular Center, The Methodist Hospital, Houston, TX, USA

Haraldur Bjarnason, M.D. Divisions of Vascular and Interventional Radiology, Gonda Vascular Center, Mayo Clinic, Rochester, MN, USA

W. Austin Blevins, M.D. Kaiser Permanente Medical Group, Honolulu, HI, USA

Amman Bolia, M.D. Department of Imaging and Interventions, Leicester Royal Infirmary NHS Infirmary Square,, Leicester, UK

Marc Bosiers, M.D. Department of Vascular Surgery, A.Z. St. Blasius Hospital, Dendermonde, Belgium

Stefan Brew, M.B.Ch.B, M.Sc, M.H.B. (hons), FRANZCR Lysholm Department of Neuroradiology, National Hospital for Neurology and Neurosurgery, London, UK

Devang Butani, M.D. Department of Imaging Sciences, University of Rochester Medical Center, Rochester, NY, USA

Neal S. Cayne, M.D. Department of Surgery, NYU Lagone Medical Center, New York, NY, USA

C.I. Ochoa Chaar, M.D. Presbyterian University Hospital, Pittsburgh, PA, USA

Huiting Chen, M.D. Department of Surgery, University of Michigan Health System, Ann Arbor, MI, USA

Anthony J. Comerota, M.D., F.A.C.S., F.A.C.C. Jobst Vascular Institute, The Toledo Hospital, Toledo, OH, USA

Department of Surgery, University Of Michigan, Arbor, MI, USA

R. Clement Darling III, M.D. Institute for Vascular Health and Disease, Albany, NY, USA

Division of Vascular Surgery, Albany Medical Center Hospital, The Institute for Vascular Health and Disease, Albany, NY, USA

Alun Davies, M.D. Charing Cross Hospital, London, UK

Mark G. Davies, M.D., Ph.D., M.B.A. Department of Cardiovascular Surgery, The Methodist Hospital, Houston, TX, USA

Jean-Paul P.M. de Vries, M.D., Ph.D. Department of Vascular Surgery, St Antonius Hospital, Nieuwegein, The Netherlands

Koen Deloose, M.D. Department of Vascular Surgery, A.Z. St. Blasius Hospital, Dendermonde, Belgium

Marco Di Eusanio, M.D. Department of Cardiac Surgery, University of Bologna, Bologna, Italy

Jörg Ederle, Dr. med., Ph.D. Stroke Research Group, Institute of Neurology, University College London, London, UK

Guillermo A. Escobar, M.D. Section of Surgery, University of Michigan Health System, Ann Arbor, MI, USA

Vahid Etezadi, M.D. Baptist Cardiac & Vascular Institute, Miami, FL, USA

Dustin J. Fanciullo, M.D. Division of Vascular Surgery, University of Rochester, Rochester, NY, USA

Peter L. Faries, M.D. Department of Vascular Surgery, Mount Sinai Medical Center, New York, NY, USA

Rosella Fattori, M.D. Department of Cardiothoracovascular, University Hospital S. Orsola, Bologna, Italy

Roberto Ferraresi, M.D. Department of Cardiology, Instituto Clinico Citta Studi, Milan, Italy

Bram Fioole, M.D., Ph.D. Department of Vascular Surgery, St Antonius Hospital, Nieuwegein, The Netherlands

David Fiorella, M.D., Ph.D. Department of Neurological Surgery, Cerebrovascular Center, Stony Brook University Hospital, Stony Brook, NY, USA

Eric Fishman, M.D. Department of Vascular Surgery, Mount Sinai Medical Center, New York, NY, USA

Robert Fitridge, M.S. F.R.A.C.S. Department of Vascular Surgery, The Queen Elizabeth Hospital, University of Adelaide, Woodville, Australia

Jennifer Franke, M.D. Cardio Vascular Center Frankfurt, Frankfurt, Germany

Wendy Gaza, M.D. Stony Brook University Hospital, Stony Brook, NY, USA

David L. Gillespie, M.D. Division of Vascular Surgery, University of Rochester School of Medicine and Dentistry, Rochester, NY, USA

Michael Glasby, M.D. X-ray Department, Derby Royal Infirmary, Derby, UK

Peter Gloviczki, M.D. Vascular and Endovascular Surgery, Gonda Vascular Center, Mayo Clinic, Rochester, MN, USA

Manj Gohel, M.D. Charing Cross Hospital, London, UK

Christopher S.M. Hay, F.R.C.R. Royal Infirmary of Edinburgh, Little France, Edinburgh, UK

Peter K. Henke, M.D. Section of Vascular Surgery, University of Michigan Health System, Ann Arbor, MI, USA

Marius Hornung CardioVascular Center Frankfurt, Frankfurt, Germany

Charles Hubeny, M.D. Department of Imaging Sciences, University of Rochester Medical Center, Rochester, NY, USA

Karl Illig, M.D. Division of Vascular & Endovascular Surgery, University of South Florida, South Florida, FL, USA

Krassi Ivancev, M.D., F.R.C.S. Department of Radiology, Malmo University Hospital, Malmo, Sweden

Samir Kapadia, M.D. Sones Cardiac Catheterization Laboratory, Cleveland, OH, USA

Vikram S. Kashyap, M.D. Division of Vascular Surgery, University Hospitals Case Medical Center, Cleveland, OH, USA

Barry T. Katzen, M.D. Baptist Cardiac & Vascular Institute, Miami, FL, USA

Olaf Kaufman, M.D, Ph.D Divisions of Vascular and Interventional Radiology, Gonda Vascular Center, Mayo Clinic, Rochester, MN, USA

Thorarinn Kristmundsson, M.D. Vascular Center Malmo-Lund, Malmo University Hospital, Malmo, Sweden

Amit Kumar, M.D. Department of Surgery, Columbia University, New York, NY, USA

Neil G. Kumar, M.D. Division of Vascular Surgery, University of Rochester School of Medicine and Dentistry, Rochester, NY, USA

Evan Lau, M.D. Sones Cardiac Catheterization Laboratory, Cleveland Clinic, Cleveland, OH, USA

Justin S. Lee, M.D. Department of Radiology, Georgetown University Hospital, Washington, DC, USA

Wei Liang School of Medicine, Renji Hospital, Shanghai Jiaotong University, Shanghai, China

Christos D. Liapis, M.D. Department of Vascular Surgery, Attikon University Hospital, Athens, Greece

Peter H. Lin, M.D. Baylor College of Medicine, Houston, TX, USA

Christian B. Liu, M.D. Hospital Nossa Senhora das Graças, Curitiba, Brazil

Alan B. Lumsden, M.D. Department of Cardiovascular Surgery, The Methodist Hospital, Houston, TX, USA

Robyn A. Macsata, M.D., F.A.C.S. Department of Surgery, Veterans Affairs Medical Center, Washington, DC, USA

Michael S. Makaroun, M.D. Division of Vascular Surgery, Presbyterian University Hospital, Pittsburgh, PA, USA

Brian J. Manning, M.D., F.R.C.S.I. Multidisciplinary Endovascular Team, University College London and University College London Hospital, London, UK

Erich Minar, M.D. Department Angiology, Medical University of Vienna, Vienna, Austria

Renee C. Minjarez, M.D. Oregon Health Sciences University, Portland, OR, USA

Gregory L. Moneta, M.D. Division of Vascular Surgery, Oregon Health Sciences University, Portland, OR, USA

Barbara D. Moreira, M.D. University of Adelaide, Department of Vascular Surgery, The Queen Elisabeth Hospital Adelaide, Woodville, Australia

Ricardo C. Rocha Moreira, M.D., Ph.D. Department of Vascular Surgery Service, Hospital Universitario Cajuru da PUCPR, Curbitiba, PR, Brazil

Konstantinos G. Moulakakis, M.D. Department of Vascular Surgery, Red Cross Hospital, Athens, Greece

Jon G. Moss, M.R.C.P., F.R.C.R. Department of Interventional Radiology, North Glasgow University Hospitals, Glasgow, Scotland, UK

Eric Mowatt-Larssen, M.D. Department of Surgery, Duke University Health System, Durham, NC, USA

Deepak G. Nair, M.D. Sarasota Memorial Hospital, Sarasota, FL, USA

Allison C. Nauta, M.D. Georgetown University School of Medicine, Washington, DC, USA

Kenneth Ouriel, M.D. Syntactx, New York, NY, USA

Altin Palloshi, M.D. Clinical Cardiology-Heart Failure Unit, Istituto Scientifico-Universita Vita/Salute San Raffacle, Milan, Italy

Juan C. Parodi, M.D. Department of Vascular Surgery, Trinidad Hospital, Buenos Aires, Argentina

Joanna R. Powell, M.R.C.P., F.R.C.R. Department of Radiology, Glasgow Royal Infirmary, Glasgow, Scotland, UK

Timothy A. Resch, M.D., Ph.D. Vascular Center Malmo-Lund, Malmo University Hospital, Malmo, Sweden

Marc Ribo, M.D. Stroke Unit, Neurology Department, Hospital Universitari Vall d'Hebron, Ps. Vall d'Hebron, Spain

Sean P. Roddy, M.D. Department of Surgery, Albany Medical College, Institute for Vascular Health and Disease, Albany, NY, USA

Division of Vascular Surgery, Albany Medical Center Hospital, The Institute for Vascular Health and Disease, Albany, NY, USA

Marta Rubiera, M.D. Stroke Unit, Neurology Department, Hospital Universitari Vall d'Hebron, Ps. Vall d'Hebron, Spain

Russell H. Samson, M.D. Sarasota Memorial Hospital, Sarasota, FL, USA

Martin Schillinger, M.D. Department of Internal Medicine, Vienna Private Hospital, Vienna, Austria

Department Angiology, Medical University of Vienna, Vienna, Austria

Peter A. Schneider, M.D. Division of Vascular Therapy, Hawaii Permanente Medical Group, Kaiser Foundation Hospital,, Honolulu, HI, USA

Claudio Schönholz, M.D. Department of Radiology, Medical University of South Carolina, Charleston, SC, USA

Cynthia Shortell, M.D. Department of Surgery, Duke University Medical Center, Durham, NC, USA

Anton N. Sidawy, M.D., M.P.H. Georgetown University Medical Center,, Washington, DC, USA

Horst Sievert, M.D. Cardio Vascular Center Frankfurt, Frankfurt, Germany

James B. Spies, M.D., M.P.H. Department of Radiology, Georgetown University School of Medicine, Washington, DC, USA

Subhash Thakur, M.D. Jobst Vascular Institute, The Toledo Hospital, Toledo, OH, USA

S. Rao Vallabhaneni, M.D., F.R.C.S., E.B.S.Q. (Vasc) Royal Liverpool University Hospital, Liverpool, UK

Lina Vargas, M.D. Department of Vascular Surgery, Cleveland Clinic, Cleveland, OH, USA

Frank J. Veith, M.D. New York University Medical Center, New York, NY, USA

Martin Veller, M.D. Department of Vascular Surgery, University of Witwatersrand, Johannesburg, South Africa

Daynene Vykoukal, Ph.D. Department of Cardiovascular Surgery, Methodist DeBakey Heart & Vascular Center, The Methodist Hospital, Houston, TX, USA

Thomas W. Wakefield, M.D. Section of Vascular Surgery, University of Michigan Health System, Ann Arbor, MI, USA

David L. Waldman, M.D., Ph.D. Department of Imaging Science, University of Rochester Medical Center, Rochester, NY, USA

W. Richard Wilson, M.D. F.R.C.S. Department of Surgery, The Queen Elizabeth Hospital, University of Adelaide, Woodville, Australia

Jiwei Zhang, M.D. School of Medicine, Renji Hospital, Shanghai Jiaotong University, Shanghai, China

Chapter 1
Crossroads of Science and Therapy

Daynene Vykoukal and Mark G. Davies

Endovascular therapy now ranges across the spectrum of arterial and venous disease. This chapter will examine the changing basic science considerations relevant to endovascular therapy.

1 Arterial Biology

Vulnerable Plaque: The term "vulnerable plaque" is used to refer to the lesions that are prone to rupture and may cause life-threatening events such as acute coronary syndrome or stroke. Plaque rupture precipitates approximately 75% of all fatal coronary thrombi. Plaque rupture is a localized process within the plaque caused by degradation of a tiny fibrous cap, rather than by diffuse inflammation of the plaque. Rupture of a fibrous cap overlaying a vulnerable plaque is the

D. Vykoukal, Ph.D.
Department of Cardiovascular Surgery, Methodist DeBakey Heart & Vascular Center, The Methodist Hospital, Houston, TX, USA

M.G. Davies, M.D., Ph.D., M.B.A (✉)
Vascular Biology and Therapeutics Program,
The Methodist Hospital Research Institute, Houston, TX, USA

Department of Cardiovascular Surgery, Methodist DeBakey Heart & Vascular Center, The Methodist Hospital, Houston, TX, USA
e-mail: mdavies@tmhs.org

A. Kumar and K. Ouriel (eds.), *Handbook of Endovascular Interventions*,
DOI 10.1007/978-1-4614-5013-9_1,
© Springer Science+Business Media New York 2013

most common cause of coronary thrombosis. In up to 25% of cases, however, thrombosis may result from superficial erosion over a plaque. Plaques prone to rupture are characterized by a large lipid core and a thin fibrous cap, but plaques with erosion vary in size and composition. Inflammatory activity has been associated with plaque erosion and may have a role in the pathogenesis of endothelial damage. A plaque with a thin fibrous cap overlaying a large lipid core is at high risk for rupture. Influx of activated macrophages and T lymphocytes into the plaque follows, with subsequent elaboration of cytokines and matrix-degrading proteins, leading to a weakening of the connective-tissue framework of the plaque. Mechanical stresses may play an important role in plaque rupture. Irregularity of plaque shapes and the presence of a lipid core result in uneven distribution of wall tension along the arterial wall, with critical elevations at certain points. The thinner the fibrous cap, the less able it is to withstand chronic or progressive wall stress. Most fibrous caps have ruptured where the estimated circumferential stress is highest. Administration of statins leads to plaque stabilization by lowering lipids, decreasing inflammation, and stabilizing the extracellular matrix within the cap.

Distal embolization from the plaque has been identified as a significant issue in coronary, carotid, and renal interventions. Use of distal protection devices has reduced end-organ embolization in each of these beds. In the lower extremity, embolic signals have been noted during wire crossing, angioplasty, stent deployment, and atherectomy [1]. The frequency of embolization was greatest during stent deployment. Further data suggests that distal embolization may continue after the procedure, with embolic signals detected in the common femoral artery with Doppler ultrasound scanning in patients with iliac artery stenosis both before and soon after iliac percutaneous transluminal angioplasty (PTA), despite preangioplasty aspirin and intra-angioplasty heparin therapies. The occurrences of embolic signals were particularly frequent in the 2 h after angioplasty [2]. In a single-center prospective registry (PROTECT), macro-embolization occurred in 55% of patients. Clinically significant ($\geq$2 mm in diameter) macrodebris was found in 45% of patients [3]. In the PROTECT study and in a second smaller case series study, superficial femoral and popliteal artery atherectomy was associated with retrieved debris in the filter in all atherectomy cases [3, 4]. When the captured particles in embolic filters were examined, the particles were found to consist primarily of platelets and fibrin conglomerates, trapped erythrocytes, inflammatory cells, and extracellular matrix. Increased lesion length, increased reference vessel diameter, acute thromboses, and total occlusions have been positively correlated with higher amounts of captured particles ($p < 0.05$). However, by multivariate analysis, it appears that declotting procedures were the only independent predictor of increased embolic burden in the study [5]. The criteria for embolic protection device placement in the PROTECT registry and by implication the criteria for distal embolization were (1) moderate or severe calcification of any length, (2) total occlusions of any length, (3) a filling defect, (4) irregular (ulcerated) lesions at least 30 mm in length, (5) smooth, nonulcerated lesions at least 50 mm in length. In this study, distal embolization appeared to occur more frequently in females, current smokers with critical limb ischemia, and more complex procedures in single occlusive lesions, which are 3–10 cm in length and needed more than a simple angioplasty. The current dataset would validate calcification, total occlusion, and length parameters as risks for distal embolization. It is important to note that approximately two-thirds of the patients had an endovascular intervention to treat their distal embolization but that the more proximal the embolic event, the more likely that the patient underwent open embolectomy, particularly if the popliteal artery was compromised, which likely reflected the acute ischemic symptoms that occurred upon distal embolization and failure of initial therapy to reopen the occluded vessel. Distal embolization was associated with a greater likelihood of a major amputation but this finding can be confounded by the fact that the patients initially presented with critical ischemia, complex lesions, and poor distal runoff.

Response to injury of angioplasty and stent placement. To understand the benefits and potential problems of stent grafting, a fundamental understanding of the response to the injury of angioplasty, stent implantation, and PTFE healing is necessary. Angioplasty is a controlled injury to the vessel wall. The injury leads to a healing response in the intima and media, which involves a program of cell apoptosis, cell migration, cell proliferation, and extracellular matrix deposition [6–11]. Bone marrow cells can contribute to the pathogenesis of lesion formation after mechanical vascular injury by deposition on and inward migration from the luminal surface or invasion from the adventitia [12–14]. Following endothelial denudation of the femoral artery [14], the cellularity of the medial layer decreases as a result of acute onset of vascular smooth muscle cell (VSMC) apoptosis. One week after the injury, bone marrow-derived cells attach to the luminal side of the injured vessels. In addition to the changes in the intima and media, there are substantial changes in the adventitia, with infiltration of cells termed "myofibroblasts" which are redifferentiated fibroblasts [15, 16]. The presence of myofibroblasts is common in wound healing and leads to contraction of the wound. Injured vessels may undergo chronic elastic recoil or negative remodeling, which results in loss of luminal dimensions without a further increase in neointimal area. The degree of intimal hyperplasia that develops in a vessel is dependent on the length and depth of the injury [17]. The length of the injury influences the duration of the re-endothelialization process.

If angioplasty fails to achieve adequate luminal increase, causes vessel dissection or results in abrupt occlusion, intravascular stents are placed. The biology of in-stent restenosis is different than that seen after balloon angioplasty [18]. The response of a vessel to a stent is dependent on the stent design, length, composition, delivery system, and deployment technique [19]. After balloon angioplasty, there is thrombus formation, intimal hyperplasia development, elastic recoil, and negative remodeling. In contrast, after stent placement, elastic recoil and negative remodeling are eliminated [20] and thrombus formation followed by intimal hyperplasia development are the main contributors to in-stent restenosis [21, 22]. Stent placement in a vessel results in both a generalized injury to the length of the vessel exposed as well as the more focal injuries at the areas of stent placement. Intravascular ultrasound has demonstrated that stents induce uneven injury along their length due to poor apposition [20]. After stent placement, the surface of the metal implanted into the vessel is covered within 5 s by a strongly adherent monolayer of protein and within 1 min the surface is covered by fine layers of proteins, predominantly fibrinogen [23]. The interstices between the stent wires are filled with thrombus and the adherence of platelets and leukocytes is enhanced by disturbance of the electrostatic equilibrium [24, 25]. The basic mechanisms of smooth muscle cell proliferation and migration after stent placement are the same as those after balloon injury [26]. The intimal hyperplasic process in a stent is more prolonged and robust than in a balloon-injured artery and is proportional to the depth of injury that the recipient vessel sustains [27] and the inflammatory response induced [28]. It can often be much more significant at the ends than in the body of the stent. In addition, the adventitial response is prolonged, with adventitial giant cell body formation being noted. Stents prevent chronic elastic recoil and cause progressive atrophy of the media [29]. The presence of a stent changes the dynamics of the vessel wall both at the site of implantation and distally by changing the flexibility of the entire vessel. The stresses on the stent have led to fractures of the stent and these fractures are increased by increased patient mobility.

2 Aneurysm Biology

Aortic aneurysm formation is associated with advanced age, male gender, cigarette smoking, atherosclerosis, hypertension, and genetic predisposition. In the normal aorta, there is a gradual reduction of the medial elastin fibers, reducing from 80 layers in the thoracic aorta to 30 in the infrarenal portion. There is also a thinning of collagen within the media and thickening of the intima in the distal aorta. This anatomic difference is the rational for suturing open aortic grafts as close to the renals as possible to remove all low collagen layer infrarenal aorta. Aortic aneurysm formation has been linked with various autoimmune diseases, including giant cell arteritis, systemic lupus erythematosus (SLE), Takayasu's arteritis, and antiphospholid syndrome. Similar to these autoimmune diseases, the risk of AAA perhaps is increased by certain genotypes concerning human leukocyte antigen class II molecules. Viral and *Chlamydia pneumoniae* infection may contribute to inflammatory aneurysm development. Hemodynamics also play a role in aneurysm formation due to the spatial and temporal variations in hemodynamic forces, the formation of regions of stasis, and the transition to turbulence that facilitate intraluminal thrombus formation, lipid deposition, and various inflammatory mechanisms.

Histologically, elastin fragmentation and degeneration are observed in the aneurysm wall. Increased turnover and loss of types I and III fibrillar collagens as well as excessive elastolysis caused by increased collagenase, elastase, and especially matrix metalloproteinase (MMP) expression probably underlie aortic dilation and rupture. Chronic transmural inflammation, destructive remodeling of the elastic media, and depletion of medial smooth muscle cells are hallmarks of the process. Immune-mediated processes involving acute phase reactants, IFN-γ-producing T cells, and proinflammatory cytokines play an important role especially in the initiation of aneurysms. They have been shown to have an association with aneurysm size and are conceivably produced by the aneurysmal tissue itself. In vitro studies reveal that IL-10, IL-6, and C-reactive protein are at higher circulating levels in abdominal aortic aneurysms compared to controls. There is decreased expression of multiple cytokines and chemokines as well as diminished leukocyte trafficking in female aortas compared with male aortas.

Cytokines regulate MMP, serine protease, and cathepsin expression. MMPs (MMP-1, -2, -3, -9, -12, and -13), serine proteases (tissue-type plasminogen activator [t-PA]; u-PA; plasmin; and neutrophil elastase), as well as cysteine proteases (cathepsin D, K, L, and S) all localize in aneurysm walls at concentrations higher than those that occur in normal or stenotic atherosclerotic arteries. Endothelial cells, smooth muscle cells, fibroblasts, or macrophages can all produce these proteinases. CD40 ligation on inflammatory and vessel wall cells induces MMPs as well as neutrophil elastase expression and release from human vascular endothelial cells and monocyte/macrophages.

Growth and rupture of aortic aneurysm have been shown to result from increased collagen turnover as evidenced by increased type I collagen degradation products within the wall of aortic aneurysms. Collagen turnover critically depends on specific collagenases that cleave the triple helical region of fibrillar collagen. The study of the pathogenesis of aortic aneurysm has focused on its collagenolytic properties and degradation of the extracellular matrix. The extracellular matrix contains embedded vascular endothelial growth factor and transforming growth factor-beta, both responsible for maintenance of the extracellular matrix. These factors are downregulated by MMPs. Both MMP-2 and MMP-9 expose a cryptic epitope that inhibits angiogenesis and can control the inflammatory response through the modification of pro-inflammatory cytokines, chemokines, and shedding of membrane receptors.

3   Venous Biology

The pathophysiology of venous dermal pathology in chronic venous disease (CVD) is reflective of a complex interplay that involves sustained venous hypertension, inflammation, cytokine and MMP activation, and altered cellular function. Persistent venous hypertension leads to an inflammatory response by leukocytes, which in turn initiates a cascade of cytokine activity. Endothelial expression of specific adhesion molecules recruits leukocytes, and diapedesis of these cells into the dermal microvasculature promotes an inflammatory response with activation of cytokines and proteinases. Severe lipodermatosclerosis and healed ulcers contained significant numbers of mast cells around arterioles and post capillary venules, whereas in active ulcers macrophages were predominant in postcapillary venules. Fibroblasts were the most abundant cell type in all biopsies evaluated regardless of severity of disease, and no differences in inter-endothelial junction widths were observed. TGF-β appears to be the driving cytokine in the fibrotic response, while ulcer wound fluid contains MMPs, interleukin-1, and tumor necrosis factor-α that alter normal wound healing. Alterations in cell-cycle regulatory proteins in venous ulcer fibroblasts are consistent with a senescent phenotype, preventing satisfactory cell mediated wound healing. The extracellular matrix acts as a substrate for keratinocyte migration, thereby facilitating surface coverage in both acute and chronic wounds. Alterations in extracellular matrix alter wound healing responses. Ultimately, the persistent inflammatory-proteinase activity leads to advanced chronic venous insufficiency (CVI) and ulcer formation

4 Thrombosis Biology

The endothelium has a primary role in the regulation of intravascular coagulation by four separate but related mechanisms: participation in and separation of procoagulant pathways, inhibition of procoagulant proteins, production of thromboregulating compounds, and regulation of fibrinolysis. The basic barrier function of the endothelium separates intravascular coagulation factors (Factor VIIa) from Tissue Factor in the subendothelium and also prevents exposure of platelets to the pro-aggregating constituents of the subendothelium such as collagen and vWF. In addition to the passive barrier function, endothelial cells actively inhibit procoagulant proteins with the protein C pathway, an autoregulatory pathway that involves Protein C, Protein S, and thrombomodulin. Protein C is activated by thrombin, and Protein Ca inactivates Factor Va and VIIIa. Protein C activation by thrombin is enhanced by thrombomodulin, an endothelial cell protein, and the activity of Protein Ca is potentiated by a second endothelial derived peptide, Protein S. Protein S promotes Protein Ca interaction with Factor Va and VIIIa. Protein Ca also increases endothelial cell fibrinolytic activity by complexing with and decreasing the activity of the plasminogen activator inhibitory protein, PAI-1 and, thereby, increasing fibrinolysis. Finally, the endothelium also is a source of thromboregulating molecules (PGI_2 and TXA_2, NO and CO, surface ectonucleotidases, heparan sulfates), which may be defined as physiologic substances that modulate the early phases of thrombus formation. The endothelium participates in coagulation by producing a number of factors including high molecular weight kininogen (HMWK), Factor V, Factor VIII, and Tissue Factor. Tissue Factor, which is found mainly in subendothelium, is a procoagulant enzyme synthesized by the endothelium. Basal secretion of Tissue Factor is low compared to that of the underlying smooth muscle cells and fibroblasts. However, if the endothelial cells are stimulated or injured, they will increase Tissue Factor production by 10- to 40-fold. In the resting state, blood is actively maintained in a liquid form by endothelial cells and circulating plasma protein inhibitors such as antithrombin III and antitrypsin, which function to scavenge thrombin. In response to tissue injury, there is a loss of many natural anticoagulant mechanisms and initiation of a procoagulant response in a physiological attempt to exclude the injury and facilitate inflammation.

Primary hemostasis is a factor of platelet activation while secondary hemostasis is dependent on the coagulation cascades. Thrombosis is initiated when alterations in the properties of the vascular endothelium allow platelets to adhere to the endothelial cells or to the subendothelial connective tissue. Initial contact of a platelet under high flow conditions is mediated by the interaction of platelet glycoprotein Ib (GPIb complex) with vWF and under conditions of low flow by GPIa-IIa (VLA-2) and GPIc-IIa (VLA-5) complexes with collagen and fibronectin. Activated platelets release prepackaged platelet granule constituents (ADP from dense granules and fibrinogen from the alpha granules) after adhesion and undergo surface property changes which allow linkage to adjacent platelets, forming a platelet thrombus (a primary hemostatic plug). Within 45 s of platelet activation, the enzyme thrombin also is formed, allowing the local conversion of fibrinogen into fibrin and its adherence to and crosslinking of neighboring platelets through the GP IIb/IIIa integrin. A platelet-fibrin thrombus or a secondary hemostatic plug is formed that is more resistant to the shear stress of blood flow.

Traditionally, the serum-mediated initiation of fibrin formation has been divided into the intrinsic and extrinsic pathways of coagulation. The intrinsic pathway requires activation of Factor XII in association with high molecular weight kininogen and prekallikrein. The extrinsic pathway requires tissue factor to activate factor VII. The extrinsic pathway is responsible for the initiation of coagulation and the intrinsic factors are required for the growth and maintenance of clot formation once coagulation has begun. The current understanding of coagulation is that plasma containing factor VII must come in contact with tissue factor for the coagulation cascade to proceed. This forms a Tissue Factor-VIIa complex that converts factor X to Xa, which, in turn, leads to the conversion of prothrombin to thrombin, the focal point for the coagulation cascades that cleaves fibrinogen to form insoluble fibrin clot.

Fibrinolysis refers to the dissolution of the fibrin network that forms the supporting latticework of a thrombus. Formation of fibrin is a stimulus for activation of fibrinolysis. Plasminogen must be converted to plasmin for fibrinolysis to occur [30]. Plasminogen (glu-plasminogen) binds to endothelial cells and is converted to a form (lys-plasminogen) that is more efficiently activated. Plasmin degrades crosslinked fibrin, noncrosslinked fibrin, and fibrinogen. Degradation of noncrosslinked fibrin and fibrinogen results in the production of fibrin degradation products A, B, D, and E. Degradation of crosslinked fibrin is slower because of the presence of crosslinkages, which results in noncovalently bound fragments (DD and EE, the D-dimers). These latter fragments of fibrin can be considered markers of true fibrin degradation. Endothelial cells synthesize the plasminogen activators as single chain proteins and then secrete them. These single chain proteins then assemble into functional complexes and act as serine proteases. There are two forms of plasminogen activators (PA): the urokinase type (uPA) that activates plasminogen in the fluid phase, and tissue PA (tPA) that is most active when bound to fibrin [31, 32]. Normal endothelial cells express tPA. However, if stimulated by a variety of cytokines and other factors, they preferentially synthesize uPA and downregulate tPA synthesis. In addition to these two fibrinolytic enzymes, endothelial cells also secrete two PA inhibitors, PAI-1 and PAI-2. Both are serine protease inhibitors and form equimolar complexes with active uPA or tPA molecules. PAI-1 requires the presence of fibronectin in the extracellular matrix to maintain its active conformation and is therefore inactive outside the matrix. The thrombin–thrombomodulin pathway also is involved in the regulation of fibrinolysis. Thrombin Activatable Fibrinolysis Inhibitor (TAFI), a carboxypeptidase, is a plasma protein that is a substrate, like protein C, for the thrombin–thrombomodulin complex. TAFI$_a$ suppresses glu-plasminogen but not lys-plasminogen activation by tPA in the presence of a fibrin analogue that had been exposed to plasmin (clotted fragment X). Through the activation of Protein C and TAFI, the thrombin–thrombomodulin complexes can downregulate coagulation and fibrinolysis. Bleeding, the most serious complication of thrombolytic therapy with tissue-type plasminogen activator (t-PA), is thought to result from lysis of fibrin in hemostatic plugs and from the systemic lytic state caused by unopposed plasmin. One mechanism by which systemic plasmin can impair hemostasis is by partially degrading fibrinogen to fragment X, a high-molecular-weight clottable fibrinogen degradation product, which retains clottability but forms clots with reduced tensile strength that stimulate plasminogen activation by t-PA more than fibrin clots [33]. It accumulates after treatment with t-PA but not with t-PA given with alpha 2-antiplasmin. It does not accumulate with use of more fibrin-specific agents [34].

Thrombolysis is the pharmacological dissolution of fibrin thrombus by exogenously delivered agents. These agents form plasmin, which leads to the degradation of fibrin, fibrinogen, Factor V, and Factor VII. Plasminogen is found free in the circulation and within the thrombus, which allows for activation of plasmin within a thrombus by regional perfusion. Streptokinase binds plasminogen to form an active complex, which then activates another plasminogen to form plasmin. Use of streptokinase is associated with an increased incidence of complications such as allergic reactions or hemorrhages and has fallen out of favor. The success of urokinase was due to its nonantigenic properties and its direct activation of plasminogen without the formation of an intermediate complex. As a nonspecific activator, however, it can, in high doses, induce systemic fibrinolysis. r-tPA or alteplase is a recombinant version of the naturally occurring tPA protein; its activity is enhanced by the presence of fibrin. The final product is recombinant plasminogen activator rPA or reteplase. rPA is a recombinant derived mutant lacking the three nonproteolytic domains of r-tPA. A comparison of the efficacy, safety, and costs associated with catheter-directed thrombolysis (CDT) with urokinase (UK) and the recombinant agents alteplase (tissue plasminogen activator [TPA]) and reteplase (recombinant plasminogen activator [RPA]) in the treatment of symptomatic deep vein thrombosis (DVT) reveals that each of the agents is safe and effective, but that the new recombinant agents are significantly less expensive than urokinase [35].

First-generation thrombolytics (streptokinase and urokinase) have no fibrin binding capabilities and cause systemic plasminogen activation with concomitant destruction of hemostatic proteins [36]. A primary driving force behind the development of the second-generation plasminogen activator tissue plasminogen activator (tPA or alteplase) was its ability to bind to fibrin and target thrombolysis. Several third-generation thrombolytic agents have been developed [37]. They are either conjugates of plasminogen activators with monoclonal antibodies against fibrin, platelets, or thrombomodulin; mutants, variants, and hybrids of alteplase (reteplase, tenecteplase and pamiteplase) and prourokinase (amediplase); or new molecules of animal (vampire bat) or bacterial (*Staphylococcus aureus*) origin. These variations may lengthen the drug's half-life, increase resistance to plasma protease inhibitors, or cause more selective binding to fibrin. Compared with the second-generation agent (alteplase), third-generation thrombolytic agents such as monteplase, tenecteplase, reteplase, lanoteplase, pamiteplase, and staphylokinase result in a greater angiographic patency rate in patients with acute myocardial infarction, although, thus far, mortality rates have been similar for those few drugs that have been studied in large-scale trials. Bleeding risk, however, may be greater.

References

1. Lam RC, Shah S, Faries PL, McKinsey JF, Kent KC, Morrissey NJ. Incidence and clinical significance of distal embolization during percutaneous interventions involving the superficial femoral artery. J Vasc Surg. 2007;46(6): 1155–9.
2. Al-Hamali S, Baskerville P, Fraser S, Walters H, Markus HS. Detection of distal emboli in patients with peripheral arterial stenosis before and after iliac angioplasty: a prospective study. J Vasc Surg. 1999;29(2):345–51.
3. Shammas NW, Dippel EJ, Coiner D, Shammas GA, Jerin M, Kumar A. Preventing lower extremity distal embolization using embolic filter protection: results of the PROTECT registry. J Endovasc Ther. 2008;15(3):270–6.
4. Suri R, Wholey MH, Postoak D, Hagino RT, Toursarkissian B. Distal embolic protection during femoropopliteal atherectomy. Catheter Cardiovasc Interv. 2006;67(4):417–22.
5. Karnabatidis D, Katsanos K, Kagadis GC, Ravazoula P, Diamantopoulos A, Nikiforidis GC, et al. Distal embolism during percutaneous revascularization of infra-aortic arterial occlusive disease: an underestimated phenomenon. J Endovasc Ther. 2006;13(3):269–80.

6. Perlman HM, Krasinski L, Walsh K. Evidence for the rapid onset of apoptosis in medial smooth muscle cells after balloon injury. Circulation. 1997;95: 981–7.

7. Clowes AW, Reidy MA, Clowes MM. Kinetics of cellular proliferation after arterial injury. I: Smooth muscle cell growth in the absence of endothelium. Lab Invest. 1983;49:327–33.

8. Clowes AW, Schwartz SM. Significance of quiescent smooth muscle cell migration in the injured rat carotid artery. Circ Res. 1985;56:139–45.

9. Hanke H, Strohschneider T, Oberhoff M, Betz E, Karsch KR. Time course of smooth muscle cell proliferation in the intima and media of arteries following experimental angioplasty. Circ Res. 1990;67:651–9.

10. Majesky MW, Schwartz SM, Clowes MM, Clowes AW. Heparin regulates smooth muscle S phase entry in the injured rat carotid artery. Circ Res. 1987;61:296–300.

11. More RS, Rutty G, Underwood MJ, Brack MJ, Gershlick AH. Assessment of myointimal cellular kinetics in a model of angioplasty by means of proliferating cell nuclear antigen expression. Am Heart J. 1994;128:681–6.

12. Sata M, Saiura A, Kunisato A, Tojo A, Okada S, Tokuhisa T, et al. Hematopoietic stem cells differentiate into vascular cells that participate in the pathogenesis of atherosclerosis. Nat Med. 2002;8:403–9.

13. Sata M. Molecular strategies to treat vascular diseases. Circ J. 2003;67: 983–91.

14. Tanaka K, Sata M, Hirata Y, Nagai R. Diverse contribution of bone marrow cells to neointimal hyperplasia after mechanical vascular injuries. Circ Res. 2003;93:783–90.

15. Scott NA, Martin F, Simonet L, Dunn B, Ross CE, Wilcox JN. Contribution of adventitial myofibroblasts to vascular remodelling and lesion formation after experimental angioplasty in pig coronaries. FASEB J. 1995;9:A845. abstract.

16. Ferrer P, Valentine M, Jenkins-West T, Gale T, Gu K, Havens C, et al. Periadventitial changes in the balloon injured rat crotid artery. FASEB J. 1996;10:A618. abstract.

17. Sarembock IJ, LaVeau PJ, Sigal SL, Timms I, Sussman J, Haudenschild C, et al. Influence of inflation pressure and balloon size on the development of intimal hyperplasia after balloon angioplasty. A study in the atherosclerotic rabbit. Circulation. 1989;80:1029–40.

18. Cwikiel W. Restenosis after balloon angioplasty and/or stent insertion – origin and prevention. Acta Radiol. 2002;43:442–54.

19. Lowe HC, Oesterle SN, Khachigan LM. Coronary In stent restenosis: current status and future strategies. J Am Coll Cardiol. 2002;39(2):183–93.

20. Hoffman R, Mintz GS, Dussaillant RG, Popma JJ, Pichard AD, Satler LF, et al. Patterns and mechanisms of in stent restenosis: a serial intravascular ultrasound study. Circulation. 1996;94:1247–54.

21. Moreno PR, Palacios IF, Leon MN, Rhodes J, Fuster V, Fallon JT. Histopathologic comparison of human coronary in stent and post balloon angioplasty restenotic tissue. Am J Cardiol. 1999;84:462–6.

22. Virmani R, Farb A. Pathology of instent restenosis. Curr Opin Lipidol. 1999; 10:499–506.

23. Baier RE, Dutton RC. Initial events in interaction of blood with a foreign surface. J Biomed Mater Res. 1969;3:191.
24. Emneus H, Stenram U. Metal implants in the human body. Acta Orthop Scand. 1965;36:116.
25. Parsson H, Cwikiel W, Johansson K, Swartbol P, Norgren L. Deposition of platelets and neitrophils on porcine iliac arteries and angioplasty and Wallstent placement compared with angioplasty alone. Cardiovasc Intervent Radiol. 1994;17:190.
26. Bai H, Masuda J, Sawa Y, et al. Neointima formation after vascular stent implantation: spatial and chronological distribution of smooth muscle cell proliferation and phenotypic modulation. Arterioscler Thromb. 1994;14:1846.
27. Schwartz RS, Huber KC, Murphy JG, et al. Restenosis and the porportional neointimal response to coronary artery injury: results in a porcine model. J Am Coll Cardiol. 1992;19:267–74.
28. Kornowski R, Hong MK, Fermin OT, Bramwell O, Wu H, Leon MB. In-stent restenosis: contributions of inflammatory responses and arterial injury to neointima hyperplasia. J Am Coll Cardiol. 1998;31:224–30.
29. Sanada JL, Matsui O, Yoshikawa J, Matsuoka T. An experimental study of endovascular stenting with special reference to the effects on the aortic vasa vasorum. Cardiovasc Intervent Radiol. 1998;21:45.
30. Gertler JP, Abbott WM. Prothrombotic and fibrinolytic functions of normal and perturbed endothelium. J Surg Res. 1992;52:89–52.
31. Henkin K, Marcotte P, Yang H. The plasminogen-plasmin system. Prog Cardiovasc Dis. 1991;34:135–62.
32. Robbins K. The plasminogen-plasmin enzyme system. New York: Lippincott; 1995.
33. Schaefer AV, Leslie BA, Rischke JA, Stafford AR, Fredenburgh JC, Weitz JI. Incorporation of fragment X into fibrin clots renders them more susceptible to lysis by plasmin. Biochemistry. 2006;45(13):4257–65.
34. Weitz JI. Limited fibrin specificity of tissue-type plasminogen activator and its potential link to bleeding. J Vasc Interv Radiol. 1995;6(Pt 2 Suppl): 19S–23S.
35. Grunwald MR, Hofmann LV. Comparison of urokinase, alteplase, and reteplase for catheter-directed thrombolysis of deep venous thrombosis. J Vasc Interv Radiol. 2004;15(4):347–52.
36. Longstaff C, Williams S, Thelwell C. Fibrin binding and the regulation of plasminogen activators during thrombolytic therapy. Cardiovasc Hematol Agents Med Chem. 2008;6(3):212–23.
37. Verstraete M. Third-generation thrombolytic drugs. Am J Med. 2000;109(1): 52–8.

Chapter 2
Computerized Registry
for Endovascular Interventions

Russell H. Samson and Deepak G. Nair

1 What Is a Computerized Vascular Registry?

A vascular registry is a clinical and research tool based on the
collected clinical data of patients treated by an individual or group of
vascular specialists. In its simplest form, this may be a box of index
cards upon which are written data such as the patient's name, age,
date of surgery, and procedure performed. When analyzed at a later
stage the specialist could determine patient volume for a given time
period, average age, and most frequently performed procedures. Such
a database is referred to as a *flat* database. Such databases can become
extremely complex with thousands of data points recorded including
variables such as risk factors, medications, techniques (e.g., stents
used, procedure time), etc. Under such circumstances the use of the
computer becomes a significant time saver. A computerized database
offers many conveniences that will speed up data entry and retrieval
and also add the benefit of assuring uniformity of data collection. For
example, entry of a specific procedure can be achieved by clicking on
a drop-down menu which lists alphabetically all the many hundred

R.H. Samson, M.D. (✉) • D.G. Nair, M.D.
Sarasota Memorial Hospital, 5741 Bee Ridge Road, Sarasota, FL 34233, USA
e-mail: rsamson@veinarteries.com

A. Kumar and K. Ouriel (eds.), *Handbook of Endovascular Interventions*,   15
DOI 10.1007/978-1-4614-5013-9_2,
© Springer Science+Business Media New York 2013

procedures that the vascular specialist may perform. By typing in the first letter of the procedure the cursor will be taken directly to the relevant group of procedures allowing a single mouse click to insert what may be a very complex procedure. This will also prevent the user from using different phraseology for the procedure that may at a later stage complicate data retrieval. As an example one may refer to a procedure as a "femoropopliteal stent graft" or a "stent graft—femoropopliteal" and these two would be seen as differing procedures when in fact they are the same.

2 Why Should One Have a Registry?

A question often asked is why the specialist or hospital should invest time or money in a registry? The simple answer is that a registry is a clinical tool that may be as important to that physician as textbooks or journals. The database not only provides information on one's own practice patterns but, most importantly, it offers a constantly updated evaluation of one's results, complications, and successes. These can be compared to national or regional norms. Based on this information one can adjust techniques, modify indications, and hopefully improve outcome over time. Furthermore, in a litigious age where informed consent has become paramount, one can appropriately inform one's patients about risk based on one's own statistics. Further, a registry gets more useful as one's practice matures since it will provide more relevant data as the database increases in size.

3 Local Societal, National, and International Registries

By pooling one's data with other regional, national, and international databases information such as prevalence of disease and practice patterns can be readily obtained. The larger numbers that such combined registries offer increases the statistical relevance of data and allows the evaluation of rare diseases or uncommon complications. Several countries have taken the lead in establishing such regional or national vascular registries including the Swedish and Finnish Vascular Registries and the Melbourne Vascular Surgical Association Audit in Australia. The American Venous Forum has established a venous registry and the American Vascular Foundation has set up a carotid endarterectomy (CEA) and carotid stenting (CAS) registry. The latter is endorsed by the Society of Interventional Radiology. The American College of Cardiology has established a similar database (the CARE® registry). Both meet all requirements for reimbursement of CAS as listed by the Center for Medicare and Medicaid Services (CMS). The web-based data forms are easy to use and take just minutes to complete. Confidential benchmarking reports are available to compare site-specific CAS/CEA risk factors and complication rates to other institutions. The registries support multiple users with unique usernames and passwords.

The Society of Interventional Radiology has also developed a database (HI-IQ® or Health and Inventory Information for Quality) that functions not only as a registry but also a software program to document all functions of the interventional suite and radiology department. This includes such parameters as inventory control, patient scheduling, and follow-up. The program can also function as an electronic medical record for the interventional radiology (IR) department recording all aspects of the patient's progress through that facility. There are similar commercial software programs that will also accomplish the registry feature as well as inventory control, suite management, scheduling, etc. Some of these will function in IR departments as well as cath labs and surgical operating rooms and will not only record IR procedures but also cardiac interventions as well as cardiac and vascular surgery (e.g., ApolloLX® by LumedX®, Seattle Washington).

The requirements of the relevant national database should be taken into consideration when defining the fields required for a personal database. This will facilitate merging or integrating the two databases at a later stage. The Society for Vascular Surgery in the Unites States has defined terms for standardized reporting of procedures and outcomes in most areas of vascular and endovascular interventions. References for these reporting standards are listed in the reference section of this chapter. Adaptation of these terms for fields should promote uniformity in reporting.

4   What Is the Difference Between a Flat and a Relational Database?

Computers offer an added advantage in that they easily allow creation of what are known as relational databases whereby two flat databases can be relationally combined to offer extended information. If one wanted to store follow-up data about a patient's vascular procedure using the flat index card handwritten format, one would probably have to use a separate index card with follow-up information. In order to make sure that it was not filed in the wrong place, the user would of necessity have to once again enter some salient patient demographic data such as the patient's name and identity number and would have to update the patient's age for the date of the follow-up. On the other hand, a relational database would set up a new screen of information about the follow-up and tie all the previous information together based on one key identifying data point such as identity number. The computer could automatically update information such as age at follow-up and duration of procedure patency.

The major benefit of a computerized database will be achieved when one needs to retrieve data. Sifting through thousands of index cards with hundreds of different data points can be extremely tedious and prone to error. On the other hand, a computerized relational registry can be "mined" for data often in an instant allowing for the production of data output in multiple formats including spreadsheet tables and life-table graphs.

5   What Are Fields and Which Ones Are Commonly Required?

Some concepts need to be defined in order to fully benefit from a computerized registry. The data points that the user wants to store are entered into *fields*. An example of a field would be a label marked "Gender" where one would choose from appropriate entries "male" or "female." A field entry can be entered by choosing from a list of choices in a drop-down list or by entering the text or numerical directly. In general, the latter technique is not preferred since typing errors can lead to mistaken data. The computer would consider the procedure "aort*o*gram" as being different from "aort*a*gram." The collection of related fields on the screen is referred to as a *form*. An example would be a form to collect patient demographics such as name, age, sex, address, insurance carrier, etc. A *query* is a question one asks of the database. An example in its simplest form would be "what is the average age of all my patients?" However, this could be as complex as "what is the 5 year patency of all infrainguinal self-expanding nitinol stents in male patients with type 2 diabetes and hypertension?" The resultant life-table graph or table would be considered a *report*.

5.1 Examples of Disease-Specific Fields

As will be described below, there are national registries some of which are disease or procedure specific. For example, a registry dealing with comparisons between carotid stenting and carotid endarterectomy will require numerous fields pertaining to the underlying carotid pathology as well as the techniques involved in treating the patient and the lesion. Accordingly these databases will utilize some general fields that are common to most databases such as patient's age, gender, hospital, performing physician's first and last names, etc. Then disease specific fields will be required such as lesion location, calcification, percent stenosis, peak systolic velocity from the carotid duplex, and aortic arch type. Associated diseases also need to be entered such as diabetes (insulin dependent or diet controlled), New York Heart Classification of cardiac risk, smoking history, etc. Procedure-specific fields may include stent manufacturer, stent length, stent design (open or closed), type of embolic device used, cross clamp time for CEA, shunt used or not, type of anesthesia, etc. Complications are also important such as stroke, transient ischemic attack, cranial nerve injury, hematoma, etc. Common fields for tracking endovascular aortic aneurysm therapy include aneurysm size; length of the normal aortic neck, aortic neck angle; distance from the lowest renal to the aortic bifurcation; endograft used; endoleak (present –yes/no; type 1–4, etc.). Infrainguinal endovascular interventions can be tracked using the following field examples: TASC classification of the lesion, stent name, pre- and postangioplasty stenosis, lesion calcification, complications (dissection, hematoma, false aneurysm, arteriovenous fistula, etc.)

A venous registry may require fields such as CEAP classification, saphenous vein diameter, laser ablation joules used, complications of treatment (burns, neuropathy, phlebitis, pulmonary embolism), etc.

6 Setting Up One's Own Registry: Design Considerations

Computer software is available to form the basis for these databases. Such software is referred to as "Database Management Systems." Examples include Microsoft Access® (Microsoft Corp., Redmond, Ca) and FoxPro® (Microsoft Corp., Redmond, Ca).

An obvious benefit of establishing one's own registry is that it can be customized specifically to one's own desires and requirements. However, to be truly functional a significant amount of time and money will be required for its design since a poorly constructed database will not function or provide erroneous information. This will not only prove frustrating but also costly in terms of wasted financial resources and time. Accordingly, before building the database the specialist should define all the fields that will be required and set up all relevant relationships. It will be helpful to evaluate some of the current societal registries to see what fields are commonly used. This will be especially important if one is planning to later import the data into one of the national databases. Often it will help to identify the most common queries that will be used since this will help identify the fields that will be necessary. It should also be understood that relational databases can become very complex and need careful advance planning. Poorly designed forms and data input design can lead to the aphorism "garbage in, garbage out." Vascular registries can be especially complex if one needs to establish queries such as assisted and secondary patency life tables.

Further, the best-constructed registry for the most well-intentioned user will be useless if the database is not maintained. Unfortunately this is an all too common occurrence. Such failure can be traced to design faults as well as human frailty. It is a common error by many designers to include every data point that they can think of even if these will have little clinical relevance. Databases that are too large will require too much time and effort to enter all the data.

Registries, including some commercial ones, have been available for many years. Varying in expense, capabilities, and ease of use commercial registries may be difficult to evaluate. It is recommended that the potential user evaluate a working copy of the software. Certain key functions should be available. The program must be able to let the user define and add fields preferably in a manner that will appear on the monitor screen as a drop-down allowing mouse-click selection rather than requiring text entry. This will lessen the possibility of typographical error. Similarly, it should have an ample selection of predefined reports yet allow the user to add their own reports to query the database. Programs that require the software developer to write the query or generate the report should be avoided unless this can be achieved in a timely and inexpensive fashion. Since a significant amount of time and energy will be required to enter data, it is imperative that the vendor be stable and able to commit to long-term support. The software should also support networking between computers in the same location and preferably even in differing areas of the city. Some may be web accessible.

7 Maintaining a Registry

The benefit of a vascular registry is its ability to track outcome over time. Knowledge about what type of procedures we are performing may be interesting, but the database will only become a clinical tool when it provides information about patency, stroke rates, and long-term morbidity or success. This requires a dedication to data entry. Similarly, erroneous data will also negate the benefit of the registry. A registry that is not well maintained will ultimately prove valueless.

Tools have been developed by most commercial registries to facilitate data entry. These include printed forms available in the operating room or clinic that can be completed at that site and then entered into the computer by a different computer entry person at a later stage. Computers can also be strategically placed in the operating room or clinic so that the surgeon can enter the data immediately. Personal Digital Assistants (PDAs) can be used by some registries instead of paper forms or computers. A benefit of these devices is that

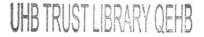

fields added on the main program computer will automatically be included on the PDA. Paper forms need to be reprinted every time a new field is added.

No matter which method is used, there has to be a commitment to data entry. Ideally the primary or performing physician should enter the data. In a university setting a qualified resident or fellow may substitute. A research nurse who is well versed in the specialty may also be a suitable data entry person. Assigning data collection to an untrained or uninformed person who has to rely on chart review will lead to invalid data input. Such persons can, however, be used to transfer data from paper forms into the computer, but even here data errors can occur.

The most difficult area for data input occurs with patient follow-up. Often this is not done by the performing physician but rather a resident or nurse. In a busy clinic, time to complete data entry may be limited. Accordingly, some programs will include a vascular laboratory module that links the reporting of the vascular lab study to the registry database such that the technologist can update the follow-up at the time of the vascular laboratory study. Patients lost to follow-up will also negate the value of long-term data. Accordingly, commercial programs should provide a report that identifies patients that have not been seen for follow-up so that they can be recalled.

8   Utilizing the Registry

Data in the registry is useless unless it can be queried for information. It can be argued that until data is utilized, information does not exist. Accordingly it is imperative that extracting information be easily accomplished. Commercial programs should have constructed pre-programmed reports that will answer most clinical questions. Examples would be life-table curves for patency, stroke rate, and mortality. Well-constructed reports should allow the user to define what fields need to be included in the search. For example, one should be able to narrow down the report to performing physician, hospital, stent manufacturer, lesion length, and any other variable that is required. Frequent use will facilitate an understanding of the program and the benefits of the information.

8.1 Information That Can be Gleaned from the Registry Includes

(a) *Patients who have not been followed-up*: This is especially important for patients who have had stents where inadequate follow-up can lead to stent occlusion and limb loss. This is also of paramount importance for aortic endografts where failure to diagnose an endoleak with aneurysm expansion can lead to rupture and death.

(b) *Comparison of competitive techniques*: This becomes important in evaluating new procedures such as CEA versus CAS, or femoro-popliteal bypass versus angioplasty.

(c) *Comparison of equipment or devices*: such as different carotid stents or embolic protection devices.

(d) *Complication rates*: such as stroke, amputation, renal failure, hematoma, dissection following angioplasty, etc.

(e) *Practice management information*: In these times of diminished reimbursement, practice management information may be critical to running a viable practice or department. A registry can provide information such as referral volume and patient demographics. Patient tracking will assure that patients will not be lost. Some commercial programs will also generate form letters to these patients reminding them of the importance of follow-up care. Marketing opportunities may develop when exemplary results can be documented. Similarly, substandard results should stimulate an improvement in technique that may result in improved patient volume.

9 The Ten Commandments of Computerized Databases: Do's and Don'ts

(a) Learn the software before entering patients. It is advisable to be aware of all the features of the software before entering definitive patient data. Accordingly, it is mandatory that one reads the instruction manual that comes with the package. Many users have jumped right in without doing this only to find that their valuable data is not functional. Before entering the first patient's data, most programs will require some basic information to be entered. This will usually include such information as names of involved physicians and assistants, hospitals referring physicians and demographics about the practice. In order to become well versed in the program, try entering some test patient data using easily identifiable imaginary patient names. Then use the "delete-patient" feature before entering actual patient data.

(b) If you are making your own database plan ahead for as many variables as possible and try to estimate all the questions you may want the database to answer

(c) Always back up the program. Data should be backed up daily. Most programs will have a backup facility included with the software. Ideally a copy of the data should be maintained away from the facility as well. This can be done by copying the data to a storage medium such as a compact disc that can be kept off-site. There are also data storage areas that can be accessed for a fee through the Internet.

(d) Try to live with the software that you buy and avoid customization if possible. When the software company updates their product or brings out a new version, customized features may not be supported. On the other hand, some programs will allow the user to add fields to collect data or information that the programmers may not have thought of. For example, one may want to collect information about patients' cholesterol. These are called user-defined fields and will be supported by future upgrades. The ability to add such fields without assistance from programmers is a very valuable benefit offered by such software. However, before adding such a field always think about what your goal is in seeking this added information and make sure you define in advance the choices that can be entered into the field. If only free form text can be entered always double check spelling, since just one letter misspelled will prevent that data from being retrieved at a later date.

(e) Keep up with the latest versions. Changes in government coding of procedures and indications and new research advances are constantly changing the data environment. Out of date software can result in useless information.

(f) Get in the habit of entering the data directly into the computer rather than writing information down and then entering data at a later stage. This will prevent transcription errors from occurring.

(g) Use the short cuts that the program may offer. For example, some programs will allow an old follow-up to be copied to a new data form when a patient comes back for a follow-up visit. Then only new data or changes need be entered.

(h) Test the data early to make sure the database is supplying the correct information. Don't believe it just because it comes from a computer

(i) Remember the adage that "garbage in is garbage out." Proof your entries!

(j) Don't despair when you first start using these programs. They will become second nature with time.

References

1. Baker JD, Rutherford RB, Bernstein EF, Courbier R, Ernst CB, Kempczinski RF, Riles TS, Zarins CK. Suggested Standards for reports dealing with cerebrovascular disease. J Vasc Surg. 1988;8:721–9.
2. Johnston KW, Rutherford RB, Tilson MD, Shah DM, Hollier L, Stanley JC. Suggested standards for reporting on arterial aneurysms. J Vasc Surg. 1991;13:452–8.
3. Ahn SS, Rutherford RB, Becker GJ, Comerota AJ, Johnston KW, McClean GK, Seeger JM, String ST, White RA, Whittemore AD. Reporting standards for lower extremity arterial endovascular procedures. J Vasc Surg. 1993;17:1103–7.
4. Ahn SS, Rutherford RB, Johnston KW, May J, Veith FJ, Baker JD, Ernst CB, Moore WS. Reporting standards for infrarenal endovascular abdominal aorta aneurysm repair. J Vasc Surg. 1997;25:405–10.
5. Eklöf B, Rutherford RB, Bergan JJ, Carpentier PH, Gloviczki P, Kistner RL, Meissner MH, Moneta GL, Myers K, Padberg FT, Perrin M, Ruckley CV, Smith PC, Wakefield TW. American venous forum International Ad Hoc Committee for revision of the CEAP classification. J Vasc Surg. 2004;40: 1248–52.
6. AVA Vascular Registry. http://www.vascularweb.org/professionals/Vascular_ Registry/index.html
7. The CARE® registry. http://www.ncdr.com/webncdr/CarotidStent/Default.aspx

Chapter 3
Considerations in Evaluating Results of Endovascular Treatment

Vahid Etezadi and Barry T. Katzen

1   Need for Evaluation of One's Own Results

Self-assessment and quality improvement have always been important in medicine, but they are particularly pertinent in the field of endovascular therapy for the following reasons:

(a) Endovascular therapy is a rapidly evolving field. Although introduction of the new techniques and devices may produce better outcomes, this could be at the cost of increased complications because of a learning curve. Only an unbiased outcome analysis can provide the information to determine if overall quality of care is improved with new approaches.

(b) The endovascular approach, in many cases, is not the only available treatment even at a single medical center. Comparable data are mandatory to justify this approach against the preexisting care.

(c) Multiple specialties may perform identical procedures leading to competitions over turf and quality of care. Benchmarking one's practice against others can demonstrate those differences of care which determine what is excellence and what is mediocrity.

V. Etezadi, M.D. • B.T. Katzen, M.D. (✉)
Baptist Cardiac and Vascular Institute, 8900 N. Kendall Dr.,
Miami, FL 33176, USA
e-mail: barryk@baptisthealth.net

A. Kumar and K. Ouriel (eds.), *Handbook of Endovascular Interventions*,   27
DOI 10.1007/978-1-4614-5013-9_3,
© Springer Science+Business Media New York 2013

(d) There is a nationwide concern with medical errors, especially those which cause patient harm.

2 Patient Selection

The general applicability or external validity of an outcome report depends on the patient selection. Accurate and detailed description of the evaluated population is crucial to a clinician to determine whether his or her patient population would benefit from the treatment and make a meaningful comparison with other related studies. Here are some special points, in addition to the general principles, to consider when selecting patients for assessing an endovascular treatment:

- Specific indication for treatment should be clear and comparable among the patient population. For instance, the outcomes of varicose vein interventions for cosmetic reasons are not necessarily comparable with the ones performed for nonhealing ulcers.
- Evaluation technique, including imaging modalities used for pre- and post-procedure assessment, should be consistent.
- The patient population should be stratified for systemic comorbidities, severity of the disease, and any previously performed related interventions.
- Pretreatment preparation, type of anesthesia, operator experience, intraprocedural use of any medications or adjunctive devices or techniques, post-procedural analgesia, anticoagulation regime, follow-up intervals and methods should be comparable.
- In randomized studies, management in control group should be a standard, currently accepted method of management to allow the best evaluation of the potential role of the new endovascular technique.

3 Which Data Source to Pursue?

Publications in established and reputable journals are the best way to disseminate or find new information. The quality of the journal may be related to the publication source (a professional society for example), but rankings are available for each journal. The impact factor (IF) which is being reported annually is one of the commonly used ones. In addition, conferences and online forums are valuable resources for interactive education and sharing the information about the current practice and upcoming developments.

4 Parameters for Assessment of Endovascular Interventions (Tables 3.3–3.10)

(a) *Symptomatic improvement.* These refer to patient functional status and quality of life. Such evaluations are better to be quantified using validated criteria, such as venous disability score (VDS), walking impairment questionnaire, or other quality of life (QOL) questionnaires. However, due to their subjective nature, these parameters should generally be supplemented by objective measures of clinical improvement when used for assessing and comparing the outcomes.

(b) *Clinical parameters.* They are combinations of standard clinical categories with objective measurements which together define the impact of the treatment on a patient's quality or duration of life, or the clinical manifestations of the disease.

(c) *Disease parameters.* These are the individual characters of the disease which could be related to the anatomy (e.g., site, anatomy, length, and distribution) or its hemodynamic characters (e.g., pressure gradients and runoff) and should be classified accordingly.

(d) *Cost-benefit.* Assessment of cost-effectiveness of a treatment is important but often complicated. Focusing purely on charges could be misleading since they often arbitrarily set and may not accurately reflect the actual resources used for treatment. However, indirect measures related to cost can give some indications, for instance, cost of screening, anesthesia and equipments, procedure time, total days of hospitalization, complete recovery time, cost of treating comorbid conditions, and cost of follow-up. Ideally, the cumulative costs per patient for each treatment should be measured based on all of those factors.

5   Standardized Reporting Practices

(a) *Risk factors*

Risk factor is defined as any factor that can affect the incidence, clinical course, and outcome of a disease. When discussing the endovascular therapy, risk factor usually refers to any factor that could affect the treatment outcome. These risk factors should be recorded, graded, and compared based on the disease and the treatment. Cumulative risk factor scoring systems for some of the endovascular treatments have been suggested too. Table 3.1 shows an example of standardized grading scales for common risk factors recommended by the Society of Interventional radiologists (SIR).

(b) *Outcome*

1. *Success*: measurement of success depends on the outcomes criteria defined in the study design and is commonly evaluated with use of anatomic, hemodynamic, and clinical criteria.

    • *Anatomic success*: generally considered as improvement in the angiographic appearance.

    • *Hemodynamic success*: refers to objective evidences of improved flow across the treated area.

    • *Technical success*: has different definitions based on the procedure. In general, a procedure is considered to be technically successful when both hemodynamic and anatomic successes have been achieved.

    • *Clinical success*: refers to relief or improvement of the clinical parameters of the disease which affects the patient's quality or duration of life.

    • No matter which one of these criteria is being chosen as the end point of the study, in all of the above, the "improvement" must have a clear definition according to the recognized criteria. Some of these criteria have been presented under the disease-specific reporting section.

2. *Patency*: patency of an endovascular treatment is defined by the necessity of performing subsequent interventions on or at the margins of the treated vascular segment in order to maintain the function of the original procedure.

    • *Primary patency*: Uninterrupted function of the treatment without any interventions.

- *Primary assisted patency*: Adjunct interventions were necessary to maintain the uninterrupted function of the original treatment.
- *Secondary patency*: Adjunct interventions were necessary to restore the function of the original treatment.
- Patency reflects the anatomic and hemodynamic success of the procedure but not necessarily its clinical outcome. The modality used for assessing patency should be clear and consistent throughout the study.

(c) *Follow-up and complications*

1. Follow-up periods should generally be categorized as immediate (0–1 month), short term (1–12 months), and long term (>12 month).
2. Complications should be categorized, listed, and graded (Table 3.2).
3. Procedural mortality should be reported by using the 30-day limit unless it occurs during the same, but longer, hospitalization. Cumulative survival data, which include the late mortality, also have to be reported.
4. When it is possible, the mortality should be categorized into death due to:
   - Underlying disease
   - Delayed complication of the intervention
   - Unrelated factors

6 Disease-Specific Reporting Criteria (Tables 3.11–3.16)

The professional societies involved in endovascular treatment regularly publish reporting guidelines for the current interventions. Examples of criteria which have been suggested by the Society of Interventional Radiologists (SIR) for some of more common diseases or intervention have been listed below.

Table 3.1 SVS/ISCVS grading system for common risk factors[a]

Risk Factor	Grade	Complication
Diabetes	0	None
	1	Adult onset, diet controlled
	2	Adult onset, insulin controlled
	3	Juvenile onset
Tobacco use[a]	0	Never or none for last 10 years
	1	None current, but smoked in last 10 years
	2	Less than 1 pack/day[b]
	3	Greater than 1 pack/day
Hypertension	0	None[c]
	1	Easily controlled with single drug
	2	Controlled with two drugs
	3	Requires more than 2 drugs or uncontrolled
Hyperlipidemia	0	Cholesterol/triglycerides within normal limits for age
	1	Mild elevation, controlled by diet
	2	Types II, III, IV requiring strict diet control
	3	Requiring diet and drug control
Cardiac Status	0	Asymptomatic, normal ECG
	1	Asymptomatic, h/o MI _6 mo, or occult MI by ECG
	2	Stable angina, controlled ectopy, or asymptomatic arrhythmia, drug compensated CHF
	3	Unstable angina, symptomatic or poorly controlled ectopy/arrhythmia, poorly compensated CHF, MI within 6 months
Carotid Disease	0	No symptoms, bruit, or evidence of disease[d]
	1	Asymptomatic but evidence of disease
	2	Transient or temporary stroke
	3	Completed stroke with permanent neurologic deficit
Renal Status	0	No known renal disease, serum creatinine _1.5 mg/dL, creatinine clearance _50 mL/min
	1	Serum creatinine 1.5–3.0 mg/dL, creatinine clearance 30–50 mL/min
	2	Serum creatinine 3.0–6.0 mg/dL, creatinine clearance 15–30 mL/min
	3	Serum creatinine _6.0 mg/dL, creatinine clearance _15 mL/min, or on dialysis or with transplant

(continued)

Table 3.1 (continued)

Risk Factor	Grade	Complication
Pulmonary Status	0	Asymptomatic, normal CXR, PFT 20% of predicted
	1	Asymptomatic or mild dyspnea on exertion, mild CXR parenchymal changes, PFT 65–80% of predicted
	2	Between 1 and 3
	3	PFT: VC _1.85, FEV1 _1.2 L or _35% of predicted, Max. Vol. ventilation _28 L/min or _50% of predicted, PCO$_2$ _45 mm Hg, supplementary oxygen needed, pulmonary hypertension

Note. *ECG* electrocardiography, *MI* myocardial infarction, *CHF* congestive heart failure, *CXR* chest radiograph (x-ray), *PFT* pulmonary function test, *VC* vital capacity, *FEV1* forced expiratory volume in 1 s, PCO$_2$ partial pressure of carbon dioxide. Reprinted with permission from [7]

[a] 0 _ absent, none, negligible; 1 _ mild; 2 _ moderate; 3 _ severe
[b] Includes abstinence less than 1 year
[c] Cutoff point, diastolic pressure regularly above or below 90 mm Hg
[d] Determined by noninvasive test or arteriography

Table 3.2 Classification of complications by outcome

Minor complications
- No therapy, no sequela
- Minor therapy or minor sequela, includes unplanned overnight hospital admission for observation only (<24 h)

Major complications
- Requires major therapy or unplanned hospitalization (24–48 h)
- Requires major therapy, unplanned increase in the level of care, prolonged hospitalization (>48 h)
- Permanent adverse sequela
- Death

Data adapted from: SIR Reporting Standards for the Treatment of Acute Limb Ischemia with Use of Transluminal Removal of Arterial Thrombus. N Patel et al. J Vasc Interv Radiol 2003; 14:S453–S465

Table 3.3 Clinical categories of acute limb ischemia

Category	Description	Findings		Doppler signals	
		Sensory loss	Muscle weakness	Arterial	Venous
I. Viable	Not immediately threatened	None	None	Audible	Audible
II. Threatened					
(a) marginal	Salvageable if promptly treated	Minimal (toe) or none	None	Often inaudible	Audible
(b) immediately	Salvageable with immediate revascularization	More than toes, associated with rest pain	Mild, moderate	Usually inaudible	Audible
III. Irreversible[a]	Major tissue loss or permanent nerve damage Inevitable	Profound, anesthetic	Profound, paralysis (rigor)	Inaudible	Inaudible

[a]When presenting early, the differentiation between category IIb and III may be difficult

Data adapted from: Recommended standards for reports dealing with lower extremity ischemia: Revised version, Rotherford R et al. J Vasc Surg 1997;26:517–38

Table 3.4 Clinical categories of chronic limb ischemia

Grade	Category	Clinical description	Objective criteria
0	0	Asymptomatic, no hemodynamically significant occlusive disease	Normal results of treadmill*/stress
I	1	Mild claudication	Treadmill exercise completed, postexercise AP is greater than 50 mm Hg but more than 25 mm Hg less than normal
	2	Moderate claudication	Symptoms between those of categories 1 and 3
	3	Severe claudication	Treadmill exercise cannot be completed, postexercise Ap is less than 50 mm Hg
II	4	Ischemic rest pain	Resting AP of 40 mm Hg or less, flat or barely pulsatile ankle or metatarsal plethysmographic tracing, toe pressure less than 30 mm Hg
III	5	Minor tissue loss, nonhealing ulcer, focal gangrene with diffuse pedal ischemia	Resting AP of 60 mm Hg or less, ankle or metatarsal plethysmographic tracing flat or barely pulsatile, toe pressure less than 40 mm Hg
	6	Major tissue loss, extending above transmetatarsal level, functional foot no longer salvageable	Same as for category 5

Note.—AP ankle pressure
Five minutes at 2 mph on a 12° incline.
Data adapted from: Standards for evaluating and reporting the results of surgical and percutaneous therapy for peripheral arterial disease. J Vasc Interv Radiol 1991;2:169–174

Table 3.5 Definitions of success for endoluminal revascularization devices

I. **Technical**: Meets the criteria for both anatomic and homodynamic success in the immediate post-procedure periods

A. **Anatomic**: <30% final residual stenosis measured at the narrowest point of the vascular lumen
Continued anatomic: < 50% recurrent stenosis

B. **Hemodynamic**: ABI or thigh/brachial index improved by 1.0 or greater above baseline and not deteriorated by >0.15 from the maximum early post-procedure level, or pulse volume recording distal to the reconstruction maintained at 5 mm above the preoperative tracing (only for patients with incompressible vessels)

II. **Clinical**: Immediate improvement by at least 1 clinical category, sustained improvement by at least 1 clinical category, patients with tissue loss (categories 5 and 6) must move up at least 2 categories and reach the level of claudication to be considered improved

Data adapted from: Reporting Standards for Clinical Evaluation of New Peripheral Arterial Revascularization Devices. Saks et al. J Vasc interv Radiol 2003;14:S395–S404

Table 3.6 Definitions of improvement of lower limb arterial diseases

Grade	Definition
+3	Markedly improved. Symptoms are gone or markedly improved. ABI increased to >0.90
+2	Moderately improved. Still symptomatic but with improvement in lesion category.[a] ABI increased by >0.10 but not normalized
+1	Minimally improved. Categorical improvement in symptoms without significant ABI increase (0.10 or less) or vice versa (but not both)
0	No change. No categorical shift and less than 0.10 changes in ABI
−1	Mildly worse. Either worsening of symptoms or decrease in ABI of >0.10
−2	Moderate worsening. Deterioration of the patient's condition by one category or unexpected minor amputation
−3	Marked worsening. Deterioration of the patient's condition by more than one category or major amputation

[a]Categories refer to clinical categories in Table 3.2 and 3.3.
Data adapted from: Standards for evaluating and reporting the results of surgical and percutaneous therapy for peripheral arterial disease. J Vasc Interv Radiol 1991;2:169–174

Table 3.7 Reporting requirements and recommendations for endoluminal revascularization devices

Data	Required	Highly recommended	Recommended
Pretreatment evaluation[a]			
Risk factors/Comorbidities	X		
Measures of disease severity			
Stenosis of treated site	X		
Runoff grade	X		
Eccentricity			X
Noninvasive indices (ABI, TBI, PVR)	X		
Treadmill (claudicants)	X		
graded treadmill		X	
Functional status		X	
Quality of life		X	
Treatment description	X		
Posttreatment evaluation[a]			
Follow-up angiogram		X	
Technical success			
Anatomic			
Stenosis	X		
Luminal gain		X	
Hemodynamic			
Noninvasive (ABI, TBI, PVR)	X		
intravascular pressures		X	
Clinical success			
Improvement category	X		
Functional status		X	
Quality of life		X	
Treadmill (claudicants)	X		
Graded treadmill (claudicants)		X	
Separate life-tables for anatomic, hemodynamic, and clinical data	X		
Complications	X		
Compliance		X	
Costs			
Gross estimate (equipment, length of stay, ICU days, # encounters)		X	
Detailed			X

Note. *TBI* thigh/brachial index, *PVR* pulse volume recording, *ICU* intensive care unit

[a]Both binary and continuous data are required when appropriate.

Data adapted from: Reporting Standards for Clinical Evaluation of New Peripheral Arterial Revascularization Devices. Saks et al. J Vasc interv Radiol 2003;14:S395–S404

Table 3.8 Some of the definitions being used for reporting the outcome of aortic aneurysm repair

Primary outcome criteria

Prevention of: (1) aneurysm rupture; (2) death from aneurysm rupture; and (3) aneurysm-related death that may result from primary or secondary treatment.

Secondary outcome criteria

Assessment of markers that suggest a continuing or increasing risk of rupture, such as aneurysm enlargement or endoleak

Primary technical success

Successful introduction and deployment of the device in the absence of surgical conversion or mortality, type I or III endoleaks, or graft limb obstruction

Assisted primary success

Unplanned endovascular procedures were necessitated to achieve technical success

Secondary technical success

Unplanned surgical procedures were necessitated to achieve technical success

Clinical success

Successful deployment of the endovascular device at the intended location without death as a result of aneurysm-related treatment, type I or III endoleak, graft infection or thrombosis, aneurysm expansion (diameter ≥ 5 mm, or volume ≥ 5%), aneurysm rupture, or conversion to open repair

Primary clinical success

Clinical success without the need for an additional or secondary surgical or endovascular procedure

Assisted primary clinical success

Clinical success achieved with the use of an additional or secondary endovascular procedure

Secondary clinical success

Clinical success obtained with the use of an additional or secondary surgical procedure

Endoleak

Persistence of blood flow outside the lumen of the endoluminal graft but within the aneurysm sac, as determined by an imaging study

Endotension

Aneurysm enlargement after endovascular repair in the absence of a detectable endoleak

Device failure

The integrity of the endovascular device may be compromised at the time of deployment (*early device failure*) or at some late date after graft implantation (*late device failure*)

Table 3.9 Venous clinical severity score[a]

Attribute	Absent = 0	Mild = 1	Moderate = 2	Severe = 3
Pain	None	Occasional, not restricting activity or requiring analgesics	Daily, moderate activity limitation occasional analgesics	Daily, severe limiting activities or requiring regular use of analgesics
Varicose veins	None	Few, scattered branch varicose veins	Multiple: GSV varicose veins confined to calf or thigh	Extensive: thigh and calf or GSV and SSV distribution
Venous edema	None	Evening ankle only	Afternoon edema, above ankle	Morning edema above ankle and requiring activity change, elevation
Skin pigmentation	None or focal, low intensity (tan)	Diffuse, but limited in area and old (brown)	Diffuse over most of gaiter distribution (lower 1/3) or recent pigmentation (purple)	Wider distribution (above lower 1/3), recent pigmentation
Inflammation	None	Mild cellulitis, limited to marginal area around ulcer	Moderate cellulitis, involves most of gaiter area (lower 2/3)	Severe cellulites (lower 1/3 and above) or significant venous eczema
Indurations	None	Focal, circum- malleolar (<5 cm)	Medial or lateral, less than lower 1/3 of leg	Entire lower 1/3 of leg or more
Active ulcers, *n*	0	1	2	>2
Active ulceration duration	None	<3 months	>3 mo, <1 year	Not healed >1 year
Active ulcer, size	None	<2 cm diameter	2–6 cm diameter	>6-cm diameter
Compressive therapy	Not used or not compliant	Intermittent use of stockings	Wears elastic stockings most days	Full compliance: stockings + elevation

Note. — *GSV* Great saphenous vein, *SSV* small saphenous vein

[a] Data adapted from: Recommended reporting standards for endovenous ablation for the treatment of venous insufficiency: Joint Statement of the American Venous Forum and the Society of Interventional Radiology. S. Kundu et al. J Vasc Interv Radiol 2009; 20:S417–S424

Table 3.10 Venous disability score[a]

0	Asymptomatic
1	Symptomatic but able to carry out usual activities[b] without compressive therapy
2	Can carry out usual activities[b] only with compression and/or limb elevation
3	Unable to carry out usual activities[b] even with compression and/or limb elevation

[a] Data adapted from: Reporting Standards for Endovascular Treatment of Lower Extremity Deep Vein Thrombosis. S Vedantham et al. J Vasc Interv Radiol 2006; 17:417–434

[b] Usual activities _ patient's activities before onset of disability from venous disease

Table 3.11 Recommendations for reporting standards

	Required	Recommended
Pre-EVA evaluation (Sect. 1)		
Patient population	☑	☐
Age, gender, race	☑	☐
Clinical indication for EVA	☑	☐
Anatomic location of treated vein	☑	☐
CEAP staging	☑	☐
Clinical Severity Score	☐	☑
Study design		
Inclusion criteria	☑	☐
Exclusion criteria		☐
Comorbid diseases	☑	☐
Functional status and QOL	☐	☑
Pretreatment imaging	☑	☐
Primary reason for treatment	☑	☐
EVA description (Sect. 2)		
Pretreatment preparation	☐	☑
Method of vein access	☑	☐
Intraprocedural imaging	☑	☐
Device or chemical agent description	☑	☐
Device or chemical agent description	☑	☐
Energy source, duration	☑	☐
Total energy deposited, or dose of sclerosant	☑	☐
Adjunctive techniques	☑	☐

(continued)

Table 3.11 (continued)

	Required	Recommended
Anesthesia	☑	☐
Length and diameter of vein	☑	☐
Post-EVA evaluation (Sects. 3 and 4)		
Complications		
Immediate	☑	☐
30-day	☑	☐
Follow-up imaging at regular intervals	☑	☐
Follow-up of clinical status	☑	☐
QOL assessment	☐	☑
Uniform duration of follow-up	☐	☑
Need for additional procedures	☑	☐
Costs/cost-effectiveness	☐	☑
Primary outcome	☑	☐

EVA Endovenous ablation, *QOL* quality of life
Data adapted from: Recommended Reporting Standards for Endovenous Ablation for the Treatment of Venous Insufficiency: Joint Statement of the American Venous Forum and the Society of Interventional Radiology. Kundu et al. J Vasc Interv Radiol 2007; 18:1073–1080

7 Vena Caval Filter Placement

Table 3.12 Summary of reporting standards and level of recommendation[a]

	Required	Highly recommended	Recommended
Patient assessment	×		
Age	×		
Gender	×		
Underlying disease	×		
Anticoagulation use	×		
Deep vein thrombosis (diagnosed)	×		
Pulmonary embolism (diagnosed)	×		
Risk factors		×	
Indications for placement	×		

(continued)

Table 3.12 (continued)

	Required	Highly recommended	Recommended
Filter Placement			
IVC transverse diameter	×		
IVC/renal vein abnormality	×		
Spinal deformity		×	
Access site patency		×	
Device Assessment			
Device identification	×		
Guide wire use	×		
Reason for selection		×	
Intended duration of placement	×		
Procedural Assessment			
Physician specialty		×	
Physician level training		×	
Location of procedure			×
Type anesthesia		×	
Method IVC evaluation		×	
Insertion site		×	
Method of access		×	
Use of ultrasound		×	
Deployment site		×	
Technical success rate		×	
Clinical sequelae		×	
Follow-Up Assessment			
% patients followed	×		
Patient status	×		
Cause of death		×	
Time to death or failure		×	
Venous duplex		×	
Postphlebitic symptoms		×	
Anticoagulation	×		
Complication of anticoagulation	×		
Suspected/proven pulmonary embolism	×		

(continued)

Table 3.12 (continued)

	Required	Highly recommended	Recommended
Diagnosis of pulmonary embolism		×	
Treatment of pulmonary embolism			×
Filter stability	×		
IVC patency	×		
Method of determining patency	×		
Outcomes reported as raw numbers and %	×		
Source of data	×		

[a]Reprinted from: Recommended Reporting Standards for Vena Caval Filter Placement and Patient Follow-Up. The Participants in the Vena Caval Filter Consensus Conference. J Vasc Interv Radiol 2003; 14:S427–S432

Table 3.13 Reporting criteria for filter retrieval[a]

1. Anticoagulant medications: Specify type and duration of use
2. Implantation period
3. Filters not retrieved: Specify reasons
4. Site of venous access for retrieval
5. Imaging of vena cava prior to retrieval: Include imaging technique, position of filter and trapped emboli
6. Complication or technical difficulty during retrieval: Describe any additional equipment or techniques used
7. Imaging of vena cava following retrieval: Include imaging technique and evidence of vena caval injury

[a]Reprinted from: Reporting Standards for Inferior Vena Caval Filter Placement and Patient Follow-up:Supplement for Temporary and Retrievable/Optional Filters J Vasc Interv Radiol 2009; 20:S374–S376

8   Uterine Artery Embolization for Uterine Leiomyomata

Table 3.14   Uterine artery embolization reporting criteria

Potentially Relevant Patient Data
- Patient weight, oral contraceptive, and tobacco use
- Age of menstrual onset (menarche)
- Pregnancy history and outcome
- Previous pathologic evaluation, i.e, endometrial biopsy, hysteroscopy, and/or dilation and curettage
- Previous leiomyoma therapies
- Comorbid disease
- Follicle stimulating hormone (FSH) levels
- Hemoglobin levels
- Creatinine levels

Uterine and Fibroid Data
- Uterine size by physical examination
- Uterine and dominant fibroid size and/or volume
- Quantification of extent of fibroids:
  - single dominant, two to five fibroids, more than five fibroids
- Fibroid location within the uterus:
  - intramural, transmural, subserosal
  - pedunculated or broad-based

Symptom Severity
- Quality of life
- Pain severity
- Bulk symptoms
- Blood loss

Technique
- Operator(s) training and specialty
- Number of cases performed at institution(s) before starting the report
- Procedure duration
- Arterial access
- Catheters
- Embolic Materials:
  - type, size, amount
- Adjunct Therapies

(continued)

Table 3.14 (continued)

End point
- Anatomic: defined according to study design
- Hemodynamic: defined according to study design
- Clinical: defined according to study design

Complication
- Specified and categorized according to SIR criteria:
  - Early
  - Late

Data adapted from: Reporting Standards for Uterine Artery Embolization for the Treatment of Uterine Leiomyomata. S.C Goodwin et al. J Vasc Interv Radiol 2003; 14:S467–S476

9 Renal Artery Revascularization

Table 3.15 Definition of outcomes for renal artery revascularization

- *Angioplastic failure:*
  Elastic recoil or flow-limiting dissection resulting in >30% residual luminal narrowing
- *Primary stent placement*
  Stent placement without an initial attempt at balloon dilation
- *Restenosis*
  Stent placement for recurrent stenosis (>50% luminal narrowing) or recurrent translesional gradient after initially successful PTRA, with recurrent clinical symptomatology
- *Anatomic success*
  <30% residual stenosis after PTRA or stent placement
- *Hemodynamic success*
  Lowering of the translesional gradient to below the threshold established for intervention
- *Clinical outcomes*
  Hypertension
  Cure: diastolic blood pressure <90 mm Hg and systolic blood pressure <140 mm Hg, off antihypertensive medications.
  Improvement: diastolic blood pressure <90 mm Hg and/or systolic blood pressure <140 mm Hg on the same or reduced number of medications (or reduced number of defined daily doses as described by the World Health Organization) *or* a reduction in diastolic blood pressure by at least 15 mm Hg with the same or a reduced number of medications.
  Failure: no change or inability to meet these criteria for cure or improvement
  Benefit: cure or improvement

(continued)

Table 3.15 (continued)

<u>Renal function</u>
Improvement: increase in the absolute value of the estimated GFR after treatment by $\geq$(ETH)% compared to pretreatment values, or a $\geq$(ETH)% positive change in the slope of the GFR after treatment.
Stabilization: absolute value of the estimated GFR within$\pm$(ETH)% of pretreatment values, or a positive change (improved renal function) in the slope of GFR$<$(ETH)% after treatment. This is applicable only if $\alpha1<0$.
Failure: deterioration in estimated GFR after treatment by $\geq$(ETH) %, or a zero value or negative change in the slope of the GFR after treatment ($\alpha1\geq\alpha2$).
Benefit: improvement or stabilization

PTRA Percutaneous transluminal renal angioplasty, *GFR* Glumerular filtration rate, *ETH* threshold effect size, $\alpha1$: slope of GFR before treatment, $\alpha2$: slope of GFR after intervention

Data from: Guidelines for the Reporting of Renal Artery Revascularization in Clinical Trials. Rundback et al. J Vasc Interv Radiol 2003; 14:S477–S492

10　Transjugular Intrahepatic Portosystemic Shunts (TIPS)

Table 3.16 Outcome definitions for TIPS[a]

Technical Success
• Successful creation of a shunt between the hepatic vein and intrahepatic branch of the portal vein.
Hemodynamic Success
• Successful post-TIPS reduction of the portosystemic gradient below a threshold chosen for that study.
Clinical Success
• Interval of time during which the patient remains free of the symptoms alleviated by the TIPS

[a]Data from: Reporting Standards for Transjugular Intrahepatic Portosystemic Shunts. Haskal et al. J Vasc Interv Radiol 2003; 14:S419–S426

References

1. http://www.sir.org
2. http://www.americanheart.org
3. http://www.endovascular.org
4. http://www.vascularweb.org
5. Society of Interventional Radiology 2009 Standards' Division Guidelines Supplement. J Vasc Interv Radiol 2009; 20: Supplement
6. Sacks D, Bakal CW. Quality improvement for endovascular procedures. In: Ouriel K, Katzen BT, Rosenfield K, editors. Complications in endovascular therapy. NY: Taylor & Francis; 2006.

Chapter 4
Billing and Coding: Endovascular and Related Open Procedures

Sean P. Roddy and R. Clement Darling III

1 Coding: Why Do We Need This?

Patient care is the primary goal for every physician. That said, each practice has the ability to optimize billing, coding, and, ultimately, reimbursement without sacrificing quality outcomes. The correctness of the billing submission involved commonly leads to timely reimbursement by the insurance carrier. Conversely, the probability that a rejected claim will ever be paid to the physician decreases significantly each time a claim is denied. Therefore, all efforts should be centered on generating a claim that is without error, is medically appropriate, and describes the service correctly. This chapter is only a guideline for the physician since each insurance payer has their own rules and regulations.

Operative notes and angiography reports are, in essence, "billing receipts." What is stated within the transcribed document occurred whereas what is omitted did not. Therefore, the practitioner should focus extra effort to include each portion of a multiple step procedure, especially when complex endovascular therapies are performed.

S.P. Roddy, M.D. (✉) • R.C. Darling III, M.D.
Department of Surgery, Albany Medical College,
Institute for Vascular Health and Disease, Albany, NY, USA

Division of Vascular Surgery, Albany Medical Center Hospital,
The Institute for Vascular Health and Disease, Albany, NY, USA
e-mail: roddys@albanyvascular.com

A. Kumar and K. Ouriel (eds.), *Handbook of Endovascular Interventions*,
DOI 10.1007/978-1-4614-5013-9_4,
© Springer Science+Business Media New York 2013

Knowing the true definition of each CPT code as well as medical necessity requirements will greatly facilitate claim reimbursement.

2 Physician Payment Fundamentals

The International Classification of Diseases was created by the World Health Organization, is currently in its 9th Edition (ICD-9), and is updated annually on October 1st of each year. The first section is a numerical list of diseases presented as code numbers in a tabular form and the second section is an alphabetical index of the disease entries with corresponding diagnostic code numbers. Each ICD code consists of a three, four, or five digit number. It is important to report the most clinically appropriate description for a patient's given condition whenever possible. That said, there are instances where several diagnoses will all be medically suitable.

Procedure billing is taken from the Current Procedural Terminology (CPT) manual which is maintained and copyrighted by the American Medical Association who updates it annually, effective January 1st. It is a systematic listing of all procedures that are currently performed by health care providers. CPT codes are usually grouped into three general categories: evaluation and management (E&M) codes, surgical procedure codes, and radiologic codes.

(a) E&M codes are typically patient and practitioner interaction such as office visits, consultations, and hospital evaluations.

(b) Surgical procedure codes involve the work and care around the time of an operation termed a "global surgical package" (including all preoperative care, intra-procedural care, and postoperative care for a given time period). In most instances, that global period extends from the day before surgery to 90 days after the procedure. Minor surgery, however, may have a zero day global period (just the actual date of the procedure) or a ten day global period associated with it that extends from the day of surgery to 10 days after the procedure.

(c) All radiologic codes in CPT are further classified in one of three categories: catheter manipulations, imaging studies, and interventions. Endovascular billing uses all three and is termed "component coding." Catheter manipulations occur when vessels are traversed and selected most commonly via a femoral or brachial artery puncture. Imaging includes the interpretation of angiography in various vascular beds. Interventions include things such as embolization, angioplasty, stent placement, atherectomy, thrombolysis, intravascular foreign body retrieval, or endograft deployment.

In the Medicare system, the *Resource Based Relative Value Scale (RBRVS)* was created to help compare medical treatments and interventions across specialties. It involves a basic unit termed the *Relative Value Unit or RVU*. All CPT codes have a set amount of RVUs. The total RVUs in a claim are then multiplied by a conversion factor determined each year by congress. Each geographic area also has an index based on that region's cost of living. Payment is then rendered to the physician using the RBRVS formula.

When more than one CPT code is billed on the same session, the code designated the highest degree of work is paid in its entirety. All subsequent nonradiologic codes are paid at 50 % of their assigned work value. This decrease is termed the "multiple procedure discount." Imaging codes (i.e., codes that begin with the number 7) or vascular laboratory codes are not subject to this discount. Additionally, add-on codes are exempt from this fee reduction.

3 Hospital Outpatient Prospective Payment System

The Balanced Budget Act of 1997 established a new payment system for services provided in a hospital outpatient setting that was implemented in August 2000. Groups, termed Ambulatory Payment Classifications (APC), were created for facility reimbursement. Each category is similar both clinically and in terms of the utilized hospital resources. A payment rate is established each year for every APC. Hospitals may be paid for more than one APC for treatment of an individual patient.

4 Inpatient Payment System

The Social Security Act created a payment system under Part A of Medicare for hospital inpatient services. This has been termed the inpatient prospective payment system (IPPS). Patient care under the

IPPS is assigned into a diagnosis-related group (DRG). Each DRG has a reimbursement based on average hospital resources required to care for Medicare patients in that category. Approved teaching hospitals have additional payments through the indirect medical education (IME) adjustment. The funding is calculated using a ratio of residency positions to hospital beds for operating costs and a ratio of residency positions to the facility's average daily census for capital costs. The "disproportionate share hospital adjustment" allows a hospital with an excessive low-income population to receive an increase in Medicare payment. Some hospital admissions are "outliers" and pose an extraordinary burden of the facility. The IPPS has an add-on payment for such a situation which is designed to protect against substantial financial loss in these costly admissions.

5   Open Vascular Surgery Coding

Open revascularization is coded based on the inflow artery, outflow artery, and conduit. The bypass is classified as "vein," "other than vein," or "in situ vein." Endarterectomy of a vessel has its own set of codes based on anatomic location. Be aware that endarterectomy of the proximal or distal anastomosis is bundled with the reconstruction. Open aneurysm repair is reported using the artery treated. The description includes the wording "repair of aneurysm, pseudoaneurysm, or excision (partial or total) and graft insertion, with or without patch graft; for aneurysm and associated occlusive disease." In essence, all open repair techniques for a specific arterial aneurysm fall under one CPT code. CPT codes 35201–35286 describe vascular repair of traumatized vessels in specified anatomic locations.

6   Endovascular Surgery Coding

Coding for endovascular procedures is subject to component coding guidelines for the use of catheters, imaging, and intervention. *Catheterization* coding requires description in an operative record of the arterial entry site, vessels traversed within the body, and final resting point for the end of the catheter at the time of imaging. Nonselective implies that the puncture vessel itself is used for imaging or a catheter is advanced along the cannulated artery retrograde into the aorta. Selective catheterization occurs when a vessel is cannulated at an arterial branch point off a nonselected vessel, usually the aorta. The initial artery traversed off the aorta is termed first order. As further branching occurs within that vascular family, the arteries are designated second and then third order. When selective catheterizations occur below the diaphragm, CPT codes 36245, 36246, and 36247 describe first, second, and third order catheterizations, respectively. Work above the diaphragm is described by CPT codes 36215, 36216, and 36217 for first, second, and third order, respectively. *Imaging* includes image intensifier manipulation, table positioning, contrast injection, and interpretation of the angiography in a specific vascular bed. External carotid, renal, visceral, spinal, adrenal, and pelvic arteriography require a selective catheter placement. Coding such imaging with a nonselective catheterization would be inappropriate. The basic exam is included in more selective exams. The unilateral (75722) and bilateral (75724) renal arteriogram CPT codes include selective renal angiography as well as flush aortography. Therefore, a basic abdominal aortogram (75625) would never be coded at the same time as selective renal arteriography.

In previous years, many practices did a diagnostic angiogram and identified a lesion that could be treated using endovascular techniques. However, the therapeutic intervention was performed on a subsequent date of service. This allowed for payment on the angiography twice for the same clinical condition. To discourage this practice and to ensure that the Center for Medicare and Medicaid Services (CMS) would only pay once for angiography, version 10.3 of the National Correct Coding Initiative (CCI) created a policy on October 1, 2004 that bundled imaging with intervention. Therefore, one must dictate into the operative report if no prior angiography was done in a given clinical situation which then allows addition of the −59 modifier to the imaging codes for reimbursement.

The last piece of endovascular billing is the concept of intervention. This includes embolization, transluminal angioplasty, stent placement, atherectomy, thrombolysis, transcatheter foreign body retrieval, or endograft deployment. Most of these procedures are described through two CPT codes: one code which begins with a three and another code that begins with a seven. Coding for lower extremity arterial endovascular interventions has been revised for 2011 (Table 4.1).

Table 4.1 2011 lower extremity codes

Intervention vascular segment	Percutaneous transluminal angioplasty (PTA)	Atherectomy (with/without PTA)	Stent (with/without PTA)	Stent+Atherectomy (with/without PTA)
Iliac	37220	N/A	37221	N/A
Additional Ipsilateral Iliac	+37222	N/A	+37223	N/A
Femoropopliteal	37224	37225	37226	37227
Tibial/Peroneal	37228	37229	37230	37231
Additional Ipsilateral tibial/peroneal	+37232	+37233	+37234	+37235

Cervical carotid artery stenting with (37215) or without (37216) distal protection is special in that this represents a divergence from component coding. The work associated with catheter placement, selective imaging of the carotid arteries, placement of the stent, and use of a protection device are all bundled into one code.

7 Vascular Lab Coding

Noninvasive vascular lab testing can be broken down into four main categories: arterial physiologic, arterial ultrasound, venous physiologic, and venous ultrasound. Many insurance carriers consider certain specific diagnoses appropriate for payment within each category. One cannot just attach a procedure code to a payable diagnosis code. The clinical symptoms accompanying that diagnosis must be documented in the medical record.

Noninvasive arterial physiologic testing includes functional measurement procedures such as transcutaneous oxygen tension plethysmography ($TCPO_2$), segmental Doppler waveform analysis, or pulse volume recording (PVR). Use of a handheld Doppler by itself for determination of an ankle-brachial index is considered part of the physical exam and is not separately reportable. The CPT codes that describe studies in this category are all bilateral. Therefore, unilateral studies necessitate the −52 modifier (reduced services) and will usually require documentation.

Noninvasive arterial ultrasound testing has two designations: "complete bilateral" and "unilateral and/or limited." There is no documentation as to how much is required for a study to be defined as complete. A bilateral study that looks at only a few arteries in each leg (i.e., popliteal artery evaluation bilaterally for aneurysm) is "limited" despite both extremities being scanned. Cerebral imaging with extracranial carotid studies has similar designations as far as laterality and image requirements. Abdominal imaging is based on abdominal graft or artery imaging versus arterial inflow and venous outflow evaluation of the retroperitoneal organs. Hemodialysis access scanning is justified if documentation describes elevated venous pressure on dialysis, elevated recirculation times, low urea reduction rates, or the presence of a palpable "water hammer" pulse on examination but routine surveillance is prohibited by a national CMS coverage decision.

Noninvasive venous physiologic studies include air plethysmography (APG) and are coded as complete bilateral studies. Anything less requires the −52 modifier.

Noninvasive venous ultrasound studies also include "complete bilateral" and "unilateral and/or limited." Remember that "complete bilateral" requires evaluation of both deep and superficial veins such that bilateral vein mapping that does not include deep system imaging would be considered "unilateral and/or limited." Lastly, there is one code (G0365) introduced for evaluation of arterial inflow and venous outflow of patients who require dialysis access creation and who have never had a prior arteriovenous fistula/graft construction. This is a unilateral code that cannot be billed with a −50 modifier. However, once a patient has a failed access, reverting to the other venous codes is appropriate.

8   CTA and MRA Coding

The computed tomography that is required in most patients with arterial pathology includes an initial noncontrast examination as well as an arterial phase computed tomographic angiogram (CTA) with timed intravenous contrast injection and image postprocessing. Together, this evaluation is reported by CPT codes: 71275 in the chest, 74175 in the abdomen, and 72191 in the pelvis. It is not appropriate to separately code for the administration of contrast material. The American Medical Association has specifically published in 2007 "if reconstruction postprocessing is not done, it is not a CTA study."

Magnetic resonance imaging (MRA) follows similar billing patterns based on anatomic location: 70544 (head), 70547 (neck), 71555 (chest), 74185 (abdomen), 72198 (pelvis), and 73725 (lower extremity).

The majority of these examinations are interpreted by radiologists and then selectively "re-interpreted" by the vascular specialist. The "re-interpretation" is not reimbursable currently. An increasing number of centers owned by vascular surgeons have purchased CT scanning equipment for their office. This venture is limited by state and federal regulations as an in-office ancillary service. CTA and MRA fall under the Deficit Reduction Act (or DRA) for Medicare beneficiaries which reduces the technical payment in an office setting for certain radiologic studies to the lesser of the Hospital Outpatient Prospective Payment System and the Medicare Physician Fee Schedule.

9   Coding Conscious Sedation with Procedures

Reporting moderate (or conscious) sedation is based on the intra-service time and the age of the patient. When the physician who is performing the service is also overseeing the sedation, an independent trained observer (e.g., a nurse) is required. In the case where one performs diagnostic and/or therapeutic angiography, the first 30 min of care in patients age 5 years and older is described by CPT code 99144. Each additional 15 min of intra-service time is coded with the add-on description 99145. Remember that recovery time is specifically not included in intra-service time. CPT codes listed in Appendix G of the CPT manual specifically include the conscious sedation for the procedure description. Examples include tunneled dialysis catheter insertion (36558), hemodialysis catheterization and imaging (36147), and the percutaneous angioplasty codes (35470-6). Be aware that intra-service time for the physician requires face-to-face contact from the administration of the initial sedative to the "conclusion of personal contact."

10   Modifiers

Modifiers are always two digit numbers that can be appended to a claim. They describe circumstances which allow for full or partial payment in situations that would otherwise be denied as "global" or inclusive to another procedure. Examples include the −50 modifier (bilateral) and the −59 modifier (override a CCI edit). Radiology modifiers include the -TC (or technical component) and the −26 (or professional component) modifiers. When the equipment is owned by a practice in an office setting, no modifier is appended (termed "billing global"). If a test is performed in the hospital where the hospital owns the equipment, a physician would bill for the professional fee only using a −26 modifier.

11   Evaluation and Management (E&M) Coding

Patient evaluation is reported through E&M coding. A new patient is defined as someone who has not been seen within 3 years. The interaction is based on three components: history, physical examination, and medical decision making. The lowest level of any one of these three determines the billing intensity.

Inpatient and outpatient consultation by specialists have typically been reported to insurance carriers by CPT codes 9925X and 9924X, respectively. In the 2010 final Medicare Physician Fee Schedule published by CMS, these codes have been changed from status "A" to status "I." This change means that, when these code descriptions are submitted, payment will not longer be rendered whether processed as a primary or a secondary carrier. The initial hospital evaluation coding (CPT codes 9922X) is appropriate for all physicians on first encounter with the patient. The admitting physician of record will append modifier -AI for reporting and tracking purposes but not to alter reimbursement. The new patient office visit codes (CPT codes 9920X) are now appropriate for initial assessment. Follow-up office consultations for new problem in an established patient will no longer be reported using 9924X coding. Unfortunately, the established patient visit (9921X) is appropriate when a patient has been seen within the last three years.

References

1. 2010 Physicians' Professional ICD-9-CM International; classification of diseases, Vol 1&2. Salt Lake City: The Medical Management Institute, 2009.
2. Current Procedural Terminology cpt 2010 Professional Edition. Chicago: American Medical Association, 2009
3. The 2009 SIR Interventional radiology coding CD. Fairfax. Society of Interventional Radiology, 2009.

Chapter 5
Radiation Management: Patient and Physician

Charles Hubeny, Devang Butani, and David L. Waldman

1 Introduction

Ionizing radiation is a powerful tool that interventionalists use daily to diagnose and treat a variety of diseases. Since ionizing radiation potentially has deleterious effects for patients and those working in an angiographic suite several organizations advise on regulations for radiation protection. These rules are usually adopted by state and federal regulatory bodies. The International Commission of Radiological Units and Measurements (ICRU) and the National Committee on Radiological Protection and Measurements (NCRP) are the two most accepted agencies in the United States.

In addition to following dose limitations for occupational and nonoccupational exposure delineated by the ICRP and NCRP, patient dose should be limited by the *as low as reasonably achievable* (ALARA) principle. The interventionalist needs to make every reasonable effort to limit ionizing radiation exposure to the patient ensuring the benefits of the procedure outweigh the risks.

C. Hubeny, M.D. • D. Butani, M.D.
Department of Imaging Sciences, University of Rochester Medical Center, Rochester, NY, USA

D.L. Waldman, M.D., Ph.D. (✉)
Imaging Science, Department of Surgery, University of Rochester Medical Center, Rochester, NY, USA
e-mail: David_waldman@urmc.rochester.edu

A. Kumar and K. Ouriel (eds.), *Handbook of Endovascular Interventions*, 59
DOI 10.1007/978-1-4614-5013-9_5,
© Springer Science+Business Media New York 2013

2   Radiation

A. Radiation is defined simply as the transfer of energy through space or matter. In vascular interventional, X-rays are the principal form of ionizing radiation utilized for diagnostic and therapeutic procedures. X-rays are created in a vacuum tight X-ray tube where electrons are accelerated with high velocity from a cathode to collide with an anode made of tungsten. The maximum energy of an X-ray photon is determined by the maximum energy of the electron. For example, a 30 kV electron can only make X-rays with a maximum energy of 30 keV.

B. Two main types of radiation are created during this process:

   1. *Bremsstrahlung*: Continuous spectrum of X-ray photons is produced when incident electrons are slowed down while interacting with the electric fields of atoms. The difference in kinetic energy is emitted as an X-ray.

   2. *Characteristic radiation*: A discrete level of energy is emitted as an X-ray from ionization of the anode from the incident electrons. The energy is characteristic of the anode (usually tungsten).

C. Of the X-rays created, the nondiagnostic low energy X-rays are filtered away (usually with aluminum), decreasing the patient dose, leaving mostly diagnostic X-rays which contribute to the making of an image.

3   Interaction of Radiation with Tissue

A. X-rays have potential for transmission and absorption, which contribute to making an image, or scatter, which degrades the image. Scattered photons degrade an image. The two main interactions with tissues are:

   1. *Photoelectric effect*: The X-ray photon is absorbed by the inner electron shell (K-shell) resulting in ionization. The energy difference is emitted as an Auger election or radiation as an outer shell electron fills this vacancy. The probability of photoelectric effect absorption increases significantly with atomic number

and is highest as the X-ray photon energy just exceeds the K-shell binding energy (K-edge).

This principle is important in endovascular imaging as iodinated contrast is used to visualize otherwise less radiodense blood vessel at energies just above the K-edge of iodine, 33 keV.

2. *Compton scatter*: The X-ray photon interacts with a loosely bound outer shell electron causing the X-ray to be deflected with less energy. The energy difference is transferred to the ejected electron.

4   Radiation Effects

A. X-rays transfer energy to tissue mainly as heat but a smaller fraction is deposited through ionization. Ionization has potential to cause biological damage and most concerning are changes to DNA or RNA. This can occur by direct or indirect ionization.

Direct ionization: The interaction between photon and DNA/RNA molecule resulting in ionization and subsequent damage.

Indirect ionization: Formation of free radicals through interactions of photons and water which in turn are very chemically reactive and damage DNA or RNA. Indirect ionization is thought to be the main process that produces biological damage as the human body is mostly water.

B. If damage is done to a single DNA strand then repair can occur through the complementary strand. If there is more severe damage and both strands are involved a base deletion, substitution, complete strand break, or chromosomal aberrations, such as translocations may occur as a consequence.

C. Radiosensitivity is the relative sensitivity of cells to ionizing radiation and determined by variety of factors:

Fractionization: If radiation is fractioned over a period of time cells have more time for repair therefore a single high dose has more potential for doing more biological damage.

Oxygen: Free oxygen increases damage by inhibiting recombination of free radicals to form water as well as inhibiting repair of damage.

Cell type: Rapidly dividing cells such as spermatogonia, myeloid cells, endothelial cells, and basal cells of epidermis are more affected by radiation than the slower dividing muscle, bone, or neural cells.

Cell phase: In general, cells are most sensitive during mitosis (M-phase) and RNA synthesis (G2). They are less sensitive during the G1 phase and least sensitive during DNA synthesis (S-phase).

D. The biologic effects of radiation damage can be classified into two categories:

Stochastic effects: Stochastic effects relies on probability; the longer exposed or the higher the X-ray energy the higher probability of damage. This does not have a threshold value and can occur at the low levels of radiography. The prototype example of a radiation-induced stochastic effect is cancer as one harmful event may theoretically induce carcinogenesis at low levels.

Deterministic effects: This effect worsens with dose but does not occur if below a certain threshold. Deterministic effects generally require a much higher dose to make an effect. Examples include sterility, cataracts, and skin erythema. This effect can occur during radiation accidents, radiation therapy, or lengthy fluoroscopic interventional procedures.

E. Biological effects that can occur within the first few days after prolonged endovascular procedure include mild to severe erythema to the skin, temporary sterility, and enteritis depending on the radiation exposure and region of anatomy where the radiation is focused. Effects such as intractable skin ulcers, dry cracked skin and nails, cataracts, and cancer usually take years to develop.

5   Radiation Monitoring Techniques

Personal dosimetry is usually monitored with film badges which are small sealed film packets that absorb X-ray photons. Film badges are worn at the collar level in front of a lead apron. A second badge may also be worn behind a lead apron, especially if a worker is pregnant. Every month the badge exposures are calculated to determine if radiation exposure is at a safe level.

Drawbacks to personal dosimetry include leaving film badges in a radiation field when not working, lost or damaged badges, personnel not wearing or not positioning the badges correctly. All of these problems may increase or decrease the calculation of radiation exposure.

6   Angiography Suites

Angiography suites are specially designed to meet the needs of an interventional radiologist. The angiography system commonly consists of a table as well as a fluoroscopy system or C-arm (an X-ray tube and image intensifier located opposite each other). The table glides from side to side and head to toe to follow an advancing catheter. The C-arm is able to pan around the patient and rotate to obtain oblique projections.

Uniplanar imaging: One fluoroscopic system is used to obtain a two-dimensional image.

Biplanar imaging: Biplane fluoroscopic systems consisting of two X-ray tubes and two image intensifier systems record two angles simultaneously, usually an AP and lateral view. Not only can complex vascular anatomy be imaged but injection of contrast media is reduced as two planes are imaged during injection.

7   Fluoroscopy Adjuncts and Radiation Reduction Methods

Digital subtraction angiography: This is a form of temporal subtraction used to remove the background in angiography. An initial succession of images is taken of the anatomical region of interest then more images are taken of the exact region after iodinated contrast material has been injected into the blood vessels. The images are then digitally subtracted leaving an image of contrast-filled blood vessels.

Image intensifiers: An image intensifier is a vacuum tube that converts X-rays into an image while amplifying the signal in the process. An input layer converts X-rays to electrons. The electrons are then focused and concentrated on an output phosphor. The output phosphor finally converts the electrons into visible light for an image.

Through an amplification of electrons a similar diagnostic image results in a smaller dose to the patient.

Last frame hold: This function allows an angiographer to examine the last image without continually giving radiation. The last frame hold image can be captured but it is of less diagnostic quality than a formal digital photo-spot.

Road mapping: Road mapping employs last frame hold in which an angiographic image obtained is displayed next to a live fluoroscopy monitor in which an angiographer is advancing a catheter. More commonly, the image can be used as a "road map" where it is over-laid onto the live fluoroscopy monitor. This is thought to ultimately help negotiate complex vascular anatomy reducing the overall fluoroscopy time.

Frame averaging: Fluoroscopy images are obtained with relatively lower radiation than typical radiography and produce higher noise. With frame averaging fluoroscopy images are averaged in a series with a resultant reduction in noise. The major drawback is reduced temporal function causing an image lag.

Pulsed fluoroscopy: Instead of continuous fluoroscopy, short X-ray pulses are produced to make an image. Exposure times are shortened and blurring is reduced from motion. This tool can be used with highly pulsatile vessels in which motion is high. Low frame rates can be used to further reduce exposure when high temporal resolution is not needed (such as advancing a catheter through a long vessel).

Collimation: Restriction of the field size keeps the angiographer from irradiating tissue that does not need to be imaged. Magnification modes do decrease the field of view but increase the radiation dose significantly.

Automatic brightness control: This function changes the exposure rate as the attenuation of the tissue changes. A thick area such as the mediastinum would require higher settings compared to imaging over the lung which is done automatically with the automatic brightness control.

Selectable automatic brightness control: Some fluoroscopy systems allow the operator reduce the mA and kV if quality is not essential. This will result in higher noise

8   Radiation Protection

There are three main principles of radiation protection: time, distance, and shielding. In addition, personnel whose presence is necessary should only be allowed in the interventional suite. If there is a pediatric patient, restraining devices (physical or chemical) may be used and aid in reducing the radiation exposure.

A. Time: Simply reducing fluoroscopy time reduces dose to patient as well as to the staff in the room. More experienced physicians are typically able to use less fluoro time for a given procedure. At times work can be performed without continuous fluoroscopy using occasional spot fluoro to verify position.
B. Distance: Increasing the distance form the source reduces X-ray exposure. The principle is governed by the inverse square law, $x_2 = x_1 (d_1/d_2)^2$. This usually applies mostly to accessory staff in the room in avoiding scattered radiation. Dose to the patient can be reduced by increasing the source to object (the patient) distance. The image intensifier is typically close to the patient to reduce geometric blur.
C. Shielding:

   Equipment shielding: Special structural shielding reduces leakage radiation from the X-ray tube. Also, specific organ shielding can be used such as gonadal shielding to protect radiosensitive areas from primary radiation.

   Lead aprons: A lead apron is to be worn by everyone working in a room with fluoroscopy running. The weight may limit mobility but the lead is in the form of rubber and provides some flexibility. Awareness of the apron design is important especially if the back is open as the wearer cannot turn his or her back during fluoroscopy. Wrap around designs are also available are useful when the workers back may be exposed. Skirt and vest combinations distribute weight better on hips while decreasing weight on the shoulders. 0.5 mm lead equivalent thickness is typically used and decreases the transmission to 3.2 % at 100 kV.

   Thyroid shields: Are typically used to reduce radiation to the thyroid, a relatively more radiosensitive organ. Other adjuncts like lead glasses and protective gloves are used less often.

Portable radiation protection barriers: These barriers generally offer more protection than lead aprons and are placed between the X-ray source and personnel needed in room.

Flat panel detectors: X-ray photons are made into a proportional charge by indirect conversion, from a scintillator, or direct conversion to create an image. The technology allows for an improved dynamic range and reduction in artifact. Also, since there is a higher detective quantum efficiency when compared to traditional detectors, the radiation dose is reduced, especially during high dose procedures.

9   Outcomes

Endovascular and other fluoroscopic procedures have become mainstream and are growing in complexity requiring more fluoroscopic time. These two factors have led to more events of radiation-induced damage to the patient and physician. Radiation damage to the skin requiring reparative plastic surgery has been well documented during endovascular procedures. Cataracts have also been reported among those working with ionizing radiation. More importantly, interventionalists may be unaware that these problems may occur with modern equipment and referring physicians may not associate their patient's injury with a recent fluoroscopic procedure.

Ionizing radiation is an essential tool used in the diagnosis and endovascular treatment of a multitude of diseases but is not without risk. Proper education in fluoroscopy, adjuncts to reduce time, and effects of ionizing radiation can reduce radiation exposure to the patient and angiography staff thus reducing injury.

10   Reality

In general, interventional radiologists have a liberal attitude concerning radiation safety. I have seen too many physicians and hospital workers walk into endovascular suites unprotected stating, "I will be here for only a second" or "I have already had my children." We must learn from our predecessors as some early interventionalists have experienced the effects of prolonged exposure including early arthritis of the hands and cataracts. While modern equipment significantly reduces our risks I urge all workers in radiation to strictly adhere to ALARA to reduce radiation risks.

References

1. Brateman L. Radiation safety considerations for diagnostic radiology personnel. Radiographics. 1999;19(4):1037–55.
2. Bushberg JT. The AAPM/RSNA physics tutorial for residents. X-ray interactions. Radiographics. 1998;18(2):457–68.
3. Cousins C, Sharp C. Medical interventional procedures-reducing the radiation risks. Clin Radiol. 2004;59(6):468–73.
4. Miller DL, Balter S, Noonan PT, Georgia JD. Minimizing radiation-induced skin injury in interventional radiology procedures. Radiology. 2002;225(2): 329–36.
5. Koenig TR, Mettler FA, Wagner LK. Skin Injuries from fluoroscopically guided procedures: part 2, review of 73 cases and recommendations for minimizing dose delivered to patient. Am J Roentgenol. 2001;177:13–20.

Chapter 6
Hybrid Cardiovascular Operating Room

S. Rao Vallabhaneni and Amit Kumar

1 Introduction

Most of the departments undertake their endovascular interventions either within an Interventional Radiology suite/Cathlab or within a conventional operating room with mobile imaging system. With the tendency for endovascular interventions becoming increasingly complex and the trend of integrating endovascular techniques with conventional surgery, the limitations of either approach has come into sharp focus. The need to incorporate the features of a Cathlab/Interventional Radiology suite and an operating room into one "hybrid" facility has therefore been recognised.

The term "Hybrid Operating Room" is used to describe an operating room with fixed imaging equipment, specifically designed to carryout both conventional surgery and complex image-guided intervention. Consequently imaging systems that can be used within operating room such as Philips Healthcare Hybrid labs, have become essential equipment.

S.R. Vallabhaneni, M.D., F.R.C.S., E.B.S.Q. (Vasc) (✉)
Royal Liverpool University Hospital, Liverpool, UK
e-mail: fempop@liv.ac.uk

A. Kumar, M.D., F.A.C.S.
Department of Surgery, Columbia Universiy, New York, NY, USA

A. Kumar and K. Ouriel (eds.), *Handbook of Endovascular Interventions*,   69
DOI 10.1007/978-1-4614-5013-9_6,
© Springer Science+Business Media New York 2013

2 "Hybrid Approach" and Its Benefits

When a patient requires both conventional surgery and image-guided intervention, it remains acceptable to stage these on separate occasions in sequence. For example, a patient for infra-inguinal bypass surgery also require angioplasty of the iliac system to ensure adequate inflow. It is acceptable to undertake percutaneous angioplasty of the iliac system in the interventional radiology suite in the first instance and separately undertake femoropopliteal bypass in the conventional operating room. The trend, however, is toward conducting both at the same time within a hybrid operating room. Expeditious completion of treatment, shorter cumulative hospital stay, lower cumulative complication rates, and lower healthcare costs are some of the potential benefits envisaged.

There are some instances where staging is not possible and the very design of the operation is based on a combination of open surgical and endovascular interventions; e.g. carotid to subclavian bypass/ transposition in combination with endovascular repair of thoracic aortic aneurysm with seal zone extending over the left subclavian ostium. Transapical aortic valve replacement is another example requiring a mini thoracotomy to allow an image-guided procedure. Even transfemoral aortic valve replacement is best performed in a fully equipped cardiac operating room so that an occasional serious complication requiring conversion to open surgery could be dealt with safely [1]. Treatment of acute complicated type B aortic dissections is a challenging area and endolumenal and hybrid options have found a rapidly expanded role.

In the treatment of multivessel coronary disease, rather than considering bypass surgery and percutaneous coronary intervention as mutually exclusive choices, treating each lesion by the most appropriate technique for its anatomical features, a hybrid approach, has advantages. Reports of internal mammary bypass to the left anterior descending artery through a minithoracotomy combined with translumenal angioplasty of additional lesions has been reported to decrease morbidity and mortality [2, 3].

The value of image guidance is being recognised in relation to some operations traditionally been performed without imaging, e.g. peripheral arterial embolectomy. Intraoperative imaging and over-the-wire embolectomy ensures that the embolus fragments have been removed completely and that no iatrogenic damage has occurred to the vasculature. This represents a significant improvement over the traditional approach where it is a matter of guesswork or judgement to evaluate the effect of embolectomy. Intraoperative angiography identifies technical issues with bypass grafts and has been shown to reduce early failure rates following coronary revascularisation [4]. This trend is catching on in peripheral bypass surgery.

The current trend of integrating image-guided intervention and conventional surgery to achieve the best results has affected every area of cardiovascular intervention. For most centres, currently the solution is to utilise a mobile c-arm that can be wheeled into the operating room for specific procedures and there are some advantages with this approach. Mobile systems cost only a fraction of that of a fixed system. They can be moved between different operating rooms, supporting the needs of different specialities. Although many endovascular programmes depend upon mobile imaging systems, they have significant limitations, thus creating the need to re-evaluate this working environment.

3 Limitations of Mobile Imaging

The first limitation of mobile systems to note is the obvious inferiority of their images in terms of quality compared to fixed X-ray systems. Despite improvements, mobile imagers are less powerful at usually less than 25 kW compared to fixed systems that operate at 80–100 kW. Imaging an obese patient, particularly in lateral angle, may therefore produce a poor image.

Another drawback of mobile systems is their propensity to overheat during operation. Dissipation of the heat produced at the anode is a significant limiting factor upon the operating power of the X-ray generator. The anode cooling mechanisms of most mobile systems are generally not effective enough to prevent overheating. While conducting long and complex procedures it is often necessary to take steps to slow down the heating process, thereby causing either deliberate slowing down the pace of the procedure or accepting poorer quality imaging or both. Incidents of automatic and unstoppable shutdown from overheating during a procedure are well known. Therefore when complex endovascular procedures are performed using mobile imaging system, availability of backup imaging equipment should be ensured and a lack of this has potential for catastrophic consequences.

Failure of imaging system is only rarely being identified as the primary cause of a serious untoward clinical event, when back-up equipment is available. It is, however, frequently noted as a contributory factor when mobile systems are used. The effects of poor quality imaging or transient failure of imaging on physician fatigue or concentration are poorly understood, but likely to be significant.

Mobile equipment need to be stored or parked at a safe place and kept connected to electrical charge when not in use, creating a logistical problem. Time should be allowed for moving the equipment between the site of parking and operating room, setting up the equipment and network connections.

4   Interventional Radiology Suite

A vast array of consumables such as catheters, sheaths and guidewires are required to conduct complex interventions and in majority of the centres, this inventory is stored within or near the interventional radiology suite. This advantage and the better imaging available, however, are outweighed by many disadvantages. Majority of the problems arise from the fact that rarely consideration has been given at the time of designing the suite, to accommodate complex procedures requiring multidisciplinary input. A number of design considerations to create an ideal environment to carry out such procedures are discussed in the chapter later and it is rare that standard interventional radiology suites satisfy most or even some of them. This realisation has lead pioneering centres to develop Hybrid Operating Rooms.

5   Hybrid Operating Room

The Hybrid Operating Room incorporates as many as possible the best features of both standard operating rooms and standard interventional suites in order to create the best working environment to carry out complex procedures.

6 Design Considerations (Fig. 6.1)

Whether a new hybrid operating room is being designed or an existing operating room/interventional suite is being upgraded, paying attention to detail in designing the facility is crucial for its users to get the best out of it. Rectifying deficiencies later could be difficult, expensive or even impossible.

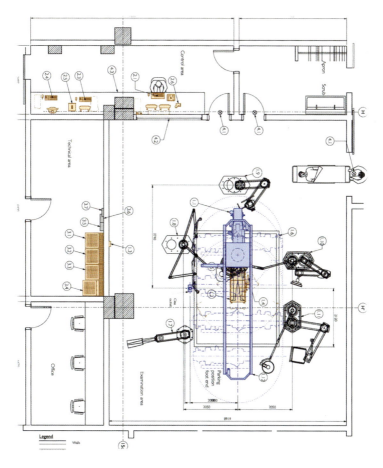

Fig. 6.1 Prototypical design of a hybrid operating room

Deciding the location of hybrid operating room is important. There should be easy access to and from various other departments within the hospital such as emergency rooms, CT/MR scanners, intensive care unit and wards. Support facilities such as blood bank, pharmacy and clinical laboratories should also be accessible without difficulty even out of hours. Despite the need for easy access, operating rooms, including hybrid facilities ought not be located upon corridors with heavy traffic within the hospital for infection control reasons.

Another important consideration that is often difficult to satisfy is the space required to accommodate an ideal hybrid operating room. Space is required for the following purposes (1) Area for induction of anaesthesia/anaesthetic room. (2) Scrub room for personnel to wash hands before and after operations. (3) Prep area for scrub nurses to set up their trolleys of instruments. (4) Control room for locating controls of imaging and archiving system. (5) Storage area, considerable space is necessary to store the vast array of consumables needed to be kept handy for complex interventions (6) Equipment such as cardiopulmonary bypass machines, transoesophageal echocardiography and intraoperative monitoring equipment occupy considerable space. (7) The operating table, imaging equipment and their displays, anaesthetic apparatus, electrodiathermy, intraoperative red cell salvage equipment occupy space too (Figs. 6.2, 6.3, 6.4). (8) Complex and hybrid procedures often require the presence of a greater number of personnel within the operating room compared to standard procedures. Anaesthetists, intensivists, radiologists, cardiologists, surgeons, perfusionists, radiographers, operating department practitioners, surgical assistants, product specialists from companies, observers, proctors and a variety of other personnel are often in attendance.

Different areas of a hybrid operating room are often compartmentalised for convenience and improved working environment. For example, a central large operating room of approximately 60 sq m surrounded by smaller rooms that serve distinct purpose, with the total floor area of the hybrid facility reaching 100 sq m. The minimum recommended space to install a hybrid operating room is 70 sq m, although examples of 45 sq m facilities exist (Fig. 6.2).

Adequate general lighting and operating lighting is clearly imperative (Fig. 6.4). Operating lights are traditionally ceiling mounted and thus compete for space with other components that too require ceiling mounting. Choice of the operating table depends upon the case-mix expected within the hybrid room.

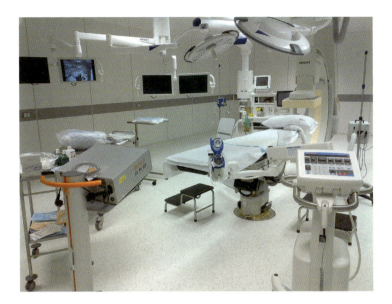

Fig. 6.2 Hybrid OR arrangement

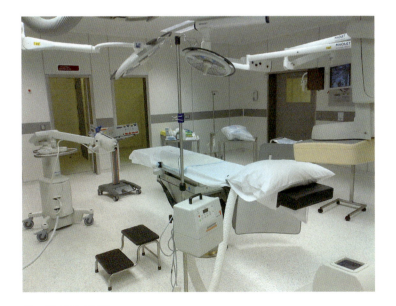

Fig. 6.3 Hybrid OR entrances

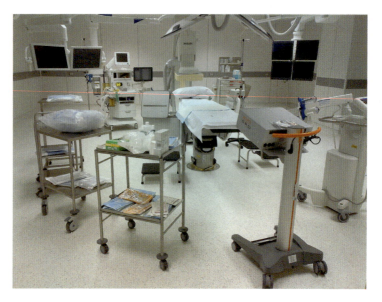

Fig. 6.4 Hybrid OR monitors

Sterility of the operating room is of paramount importance. Ideally, hybrid operating rooms should be served by the traditional double corridor system (Fig. 6.4); a clean corridor for movement of patients, personnel, clean equipment etc. and a separate dirty corridor for the transit of waste and contaminated clinical material. Ventilation should be of positive pressure type with the requisite number of air changes appropriate for the type of operations conducted. Laminar flow systems require special considerations since a c-arm always interferes with laminar flow, whether it is floor or ceiling mounted and whether the airflow is vertical or horizontal.

7   Benefits of a Fixed Imaging System

Complex procedures require more than the basic functions of subtraction angiography. Fixed imaging systems provide better quality images, larger field of view, greater range of magnification and also a range of advanced functions such as post processing, measurement and image referencing functions. Almost all new fixed systems are being equipped with flat panel detectors, which employ completely digital processing. In combination with rotational angiography, this allowed the development of some new and exciting possibilities of generating CT like images, with levels of radiation exposure comparable to that of standard helical multidetector CT. Excellent quality images allow drastic reduction in the dose of radiographic contrast material, thus attenuating their nephrotoxic effects. It is also possible to glean the necessary information through low frame rates, thus reducing exposure to ionising radiation. The combination of reliability and better quality imaging with advanced tools leads to significant reduction of operator fatigue, which is an important factor, particularly in relation to procedures that require concentration over extended periods of time, e.g. side-branched endovascular aneurysm repair.

8 Conclusion

Intraoperative imaging is an essential component of modern cardiovascular therapeutics. The fact that a hybrid operating room is an essential component of the infrastructure of a modern cardiovascular service is being recognised increasingly by clinicians.

References

1. Vahanian A, Alfieri O, Al-Attar N, Antunes M, et al. Transcatheter valve implantation for patients with aortic stenosis: a position statement from the European Association of Cardio-Thoracic Surgery (EACTS) and the European Society of Cardiology (ESC), in collaboration with the European Association of Percutaneous Cardiovascular Interventions (EAPCI). Eur Heart J. 2008;29(11):1463–70.
2. Reicher B, Poston RS, Mehra MR, et al. Simultaneous "hybrid" percutaneous coronary intervention and minimally invasive surgical bypass grafting: feasibility, safety, and clinical outcomes. Am Heart J. 2008;155(4):661–7.
3. Zhao DX, Leacche M, Balaguer JM, et al. Routine intraoperative completion angiography after coronary artery bypass grafting and 1-stop hybrid revascularization results from a fully integrated hybrid catheterization laboratory/ operating room. J Am Coll Cardiol. 2009;53(3):232–41.
4. Mack MJ. Intraoperative coronary graft assessment. Curr Opin Cardiol. 2008;23(6):568–72.

Chapter 7
Vascular Lab: Reading in the Endovascular Era

Renee C. Minjarez and Gregory L. Moneta

1 Noninvasive Testing: Its Continued Need in the Endovascular Era

Accompanying the recent rapid expansion of endovascular therapies is an increased need to utilize the noninvasive vascular laboratory to provide quantitative, diagnostic, and surveillance data for vascular patients treated with endovascular therapies. The general indications for noninvasive vascular laboratory testing remain irrespective of whether an open or an endovascular therapy is being entertained. These indications include the diagnosis or exclusion of peripheral arterial disease, the patterns and extent of disease, and the behavior over time of treated vessels. When considering endovascular techniques, the vascular lab can also help to minimize the use of contrast and radiation by localizing and characterizing discrete lesions prior to a potential or planned intervention. Given the apparent overall

R.C. Minjarez, M.D.
Oregon Health Sciences University, Portland, OR, USA

G.L. Moneta, M.D. (⊠)
Division of Vascular Surgery, Oregon Health Sciences University,
3181 SW Sam Jackson Pk Rd OP-11, Portland, OR 97201, USA
e-mail: monetag@ohsu.edu

A. Kumar and K. Ouriel (eds.), *Handbook of Endovascular Interventions*,   79
DOI 10.1007/978-1-4614-5013-9_7,
© Springer Science+Business Media New York 2013

shorter durability of endovascular peripheral treatments, the vascular lab can also be utilized to identify asymptomatic problems to allow preventative intervention.

While diagnostic standards have been well established for native, untreated arteries, data gained from the noninvasive vascular lab investigating arteries treated with endovascular techniques are in the nascent stages of standardization. A challenge is to better understand the immediate and long-term effects of endovascular treatments on the vascular system. Current follow-up protocols for endovascularly treated vessel are not standardized and in many cases it appears criteria for recurrent stenosis of treated arteries, particularly stented arteries, differ from the well-accepted criteria for native, untreated arteries.

2 What Is the Difference in Duplex Findings of Preintervention Versus Postintervention Vessels?

Some commonalities are now apparent in the adaptation of duplex ultrasound (DUS) to investigate endovascularly treated arteries. Differences between native artery assessment of stenosis and endovascularly treated arteries appear to depend primarily on the presence of stents.

Criteria correlating duplex-derived velocities to angiographic stenoses do not appear applicable to stented arteries, especially for mild to moderate degrees of stenosis. The reason for this is unclear but stents theoretically reduce distensibility and compliance of the artery compared to the immediate upstream and downstream segments from the stent [1]. Physical changes in the treated artery induced by the stent result in alterations in flow characteristics detected by DUS [2]. Peak systolic velocities (PSVs) tend to be higher in stented, adequately treated arteries and in some cases, exceed criteria established for severe stenosis in native arteries. Typically, duplex-derived flow velocities are higher in the stented segment than would normally be expected from color flow images or correlative angiograms. This has been shown to be true for mild to moderate in-stent lesions in the stented carotid artery. This phenomenon, however, is perhaps most dramatic in stented superior mesenteric arteries (SMAs) where widely patent stented SMAs virtually uniformly have flow velocities that would indicate a $\geq70\%$ stenosis in a native SMA [3].

It is notable, however, that DUS is able to accurately identify high grade recurrent stenosis as reflected by an elevated PSV and end diastolic velocity (EDV). These findings have been best demonstrated in the stented carotid artery [4]. In cases where there is severe in-stent restenosis, traditional duplex criteria for native arteries with the exception of the SMA appear to apply also to stented arteries. In other words, very high velocities, whether they be in stented or native vessels, with the exception of the SMA, indicate a high-grade stenosis. Similarly, normal PSVs in stented vessels are reliable indicators of the absence of in-stent restenosis.

Accordingly, there is a need to better standardize DUS criteria for stented arteries to identify recurrent stenoses. In the interim, other factors such as B mode imaging to visually quantify degree of stenosis, PSV and EDV trends, poststenotic turbulence, and other duplex-derived findings should perhaps play a larger role in judging the effect and durability of endovascular treatments.

3 Specific Duplex Ultrasound Criteria

3.1 Carotid Artery Stents

Carotid artery stenting is an alternative treatment to carotid endarterectomy in the treatment of selected symptomatic and asymptomatic carotid artery stenosis. Studies correlating duplex-derived PSVs of stented carotid arteries with in-stent restenosis to angiography have shown velocities in a stented carotid artery are higher than nonstented arteries for similar degrees of angiographic stenosis [4–8]. Therefore, validated DUS criteria established for native artery stenosis overestimate the degree of stenosis in stented arteries and could result in a pessimistic assessment of the durability of stents in selected vascular beds (carotid, SMA, renal) and, in clinical practice, unnecessary angiograms.

Several studies have delineated DUS criteria for carotid artery in-stent restenosis (Table 7.1). Duplex ultrasound evaluations of stented carotid arteries were performed using a 5, 7.5, or 10 MHz transducers and followed standard examination technique. Peak systolic velocities

Table 7.1 Literature review of carotid artery in-stent restenosis (ISR) duplex criteria

	N	Validation test	ISR ≥70% PSV (cm/s)	ISR ≥70% EDV (cm/s)	ISR ≥70% ICA:CCA	ISR ≥50% (cm/s)
Stanziale 2005 [27]	118	Angio	≥350		≥4.75	PSV≥225ICA:PCA≥2.5
Chi 2007 [11]	260	Angio	≥450	NS	≥4.3	PSV≥240ICA:CCA≥2.5
Lal 2008 [6]	189	CTA/Angio	≥340		≥4.15	PSV≥220ICA:CCA≥2.7
AbuRahma 2008 [28]	215	CTA/Angio	≥325	≥119		PSV≥224EDV≥88ICA:CCA≥3.4
Zhou 2008 [10]	22	Angio	≥300	≥90	≥4	
Setacci 2008 [7]	814	Angio	≥300	≥140	≥3.8	PSV≥175EDV≥88ICA:CCA≥3.4
Cumbie 2008 [8]	129	Angio	≥205[a]	NS	≥2.6	

PSV peak systolic velocity, *EDV* end diastolic velocity, *ICA:CCA* internal carotid artery to common carotid artery PSV ratio, *NS* not significant, *CTA* CT angiogram

[a]Indicated ≥80% in-stent restenosis

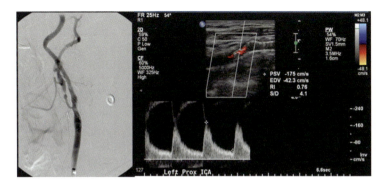

Fig. 7.1 Completion angiography after internal carotid artery (ICA) artery stenting shows <25% residual stenosis. However, postprocedure day 1 baseline duplex ultrasound peak systolic velocity measures 175 cm/s, which would indicate ≥50% stenosis in a native carotid artery. Native artery velocity criteria for internal carotid artery stenosis tend to overestimate actual moderate to mild lesions in stented ICAs

correlating to ≥70% diameter reduction by angiography are typically ≥300 cm/s while EDVs are above 90–150 cm/s (similar to a high-grade stenosis in a native carotid artery). Greater than 50% diameter reduction in stented arteries has been described by PSVs ≥220 cm/s and internal carotid artery (ICA) to common carotid artery (CCA) ratios of 2.4–3.8. These values represent significantly higher numerical values than native artery criteria where a ≥50% internal carotid artery stenosis is defined by a PSV ≥125 cm/s.

Suggested DUS surveillance protocols for the detection of in-stent restenosis for stented carotid arteries are similar to those following carotid endarterectomy. An early, initial postprocedure DUS should be obtained (preferably within 1 month of the procedure) to establish a baseline velocity profile to which follow-up scans can be compared. Additionally, early initial DUS velocities can be correlated to the poststent angiographic images (Fig. 7.1) as well as confirm the technical success of the procedure and extent of contralateral disease. Additional information from both color flow and B-mode imaging can help corroborate velocity data to better define the lumen diameter. Patency and structural deformities of the stented vessel such as poor wall apposition and stent migration may also be detected at the initial and in subsequent duplex examinations.

The interval between duplex surveillance of stented carotid arteries should be dictated by the observed timing of recurrence of stenosis. Armstrong found that time to progression of high-grade stenosis after carotid artery stenting was 14 ± 10 months [9]. Zhou had an average time to reintervention of 11 months (range 1–24 months) [10]. A reasonable schedule for follow-up of the stented carotid artery is 6-month intervals for the initial 2 years then yearly thereafter in patients whose initial DUS indicate a $\leq 50\%$ residual stenosis. If initial DUS indicates $\geq 50\%$ residual stenosis then the interval between DUS can be shortened to every 3–6 months until adequate stabilization or reintervention occurs.

3.2   Renal Artery Stents

Renal artery stenting is used for treatment of renal artery stenosis that may lead to deterioration in renal function and/or severe hypertension. In-stent restenosis caused by intimal hyperplasia can occur in up to 20% of stented renal arteries, typically in the first 3–12 months after placement. Progression of atherosclerotic disease, typically at either end of the stented arterial segment can also occur during the follow-up period and may require treatment. Reintervention is considered to prevent stent occlusion or recurrence of symptoms when there is hemodynamically significant in-stent restenosis or progression of atherosclerotic occlusive disease.

For the diagnosis of native renal artery stenosis, a PSV ≥ 200 cm/s and a renal aortic ratio (RAR) ≥ 3.5 (calculated by dividing the PSV of the renal artery by the PSV of the adjacent aorta) has been shown to correlate with angiographic stenosis of $\geq 60\%$. There are no prospective studies validating the use of DUS velocity measurements to angiographic in-stent restenosis in stented renal arteries. However, large elevations in renal artery stent PSVs are likely to indicate in-stent restenosis (Fig. 7.2).

In one study by Chi et al., patients with renal artery stents underwent angiograms if they had suspicion of in-stent restenosis by native artery DUS criteria standards for renal artery stenosis. Less than half studied with angiography actually had $\geq 50\%$ in-stent restenosis. Based on their analysis of patients studied with both DUS and angiography and who had in-stent restenosis, a PSV ≥ 395 cm/s

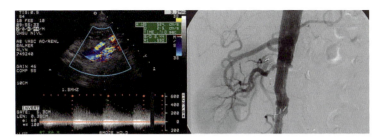

Fig. 7.2 Surveillance duplex ultrasound of renal artery stent demonstrates elevated peak systolic velocity of 524 cm/s and end diastolic velocity of 215 cm/s highly suggestive of a high grade in-stent restenosis. (**b**) Angiogram showing confirmation of the right renal artery in-stent restenosis

would yield a sensitivity of 83%, specificity of 88% with an overall accuracy of 87% to predict a ≥70% renal artery in-stent stenosis. A RAR of ≥5.1 would give an accuracy of 88%, sensitivity of 94%, and specificity of 86% for the detection of ≥70% renal artery in-stent restenosis [11].

Alternatively, findings from the RENAISSANCE renal artery stent trial indicate that native artery criteria (PSV ≥225 cm/s with poststent turbulence and/or an RAR ≥3.5) have a high level of concordance (86.6%) with angiographic stenosis (defined as ≥60%) [12]. Pending a larger prospective trial comparing DUS with angiography to establish in-stent restenosis criteria, the most prudent means of detecting in-stent restenosis seems to be with a combination of clinical status and the PSV and RAR trends. Since restenosis from intimal hyperplasia is most likely to occur in the first year after stent placement, DUS every 3 months in the first year and yearly or every 6 months thereafter is a reasonable approach to DUS surveillance of renal artery stents.

3.3 Superior Mesenteric Artery (SMA) Stents

Superior mesenteric artery stenting is an increasingly utilized treatment of symptomatic chronic mesenteric ischemia (CMI) in patients at high risk for an open surgical revascularization. The celiac artery and SMA are almost always severely stenosed or occluded in clear cases of CMI. Regardless, treatment of the SMA alone, either by

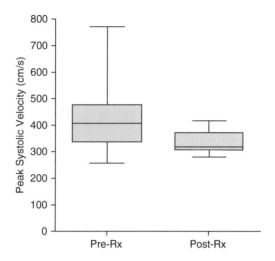

Fig. 7.3 Superior mesenteric artery peak systolic velocities (PSV) before and after SMA stenting in a series of 35 patients. PSV decreased significantly ($p=0.039$) after stent placement but remained above native artery criteria for ≥70% stenosis (275 cm/s) despite a less than ≤30% residual stenosis by completion angiography [3]

surgical revascularization or stenting, appears to be adequate to relieve symptoms in the majority of patients [13]. While associated with lower morbidity and mortality than open surgery, SMA stenting does not appear as durable as surgical reconstruction. Reinterventions on SMA stents for symptom recurrence or restenosis occur in up to a third of patients [14].

There are no established DUS criteria of stented SMAs that have been validated against an angiographic standard. Well-established native artery velocity criteria (SMA PSV of ≥275 cm/s is equivalent to a ≥70% angiographic SMA stenosis) have been applied to stented SMAs to help identify recurrent disease. However, it is unclear if reintervention in stented SMAs with evidence of restenosis based on native SMA DUS criteria for stenosis affects patency rates or recurrence of symptoms [15]. It does appear DUS criteria for native SMA disease likely overestimate the severity of stenosis when applied to stented SMAs. In one study after successful SMA stenting with documented <30% residual angiographic stenosis, SMA PSVs were uniformly found to be ≥275 cm/s on postprocedure DUS examination (Fig. 7.3). Average postprocedure PSVs were 336±45 cm/s after

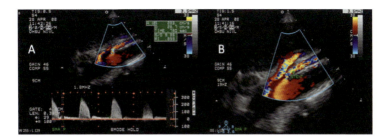

Fig. 7.4 Surveillance duplex ultrasound scan 1 month following angiographically successful (<30% residual stenosis) superior mesenteric artery (SMA) stenting. (**a**) SMA stent peak systolic velocity is elevated at 283 cm/s and waveform analysis shows spectral broadening. (**b**) Color flow image of celiac trunk and SMA origins suggests a widely patent stent consistent with completion angiography

successful stenting, significantly reduced compared to preoperative values, but still in excess of native artery criteria for ≥70% stenosis (Fig. 7.4) [3].

Restenosis can occur at a mean follow-up time of 8.5 ± 1.9 months according to a recent series of 49 patients treated with mesenteric stents. In this group of patients, nearly 30% of treated patients underwent reintervention at a mean of 17 months from the original treatment. Of the patients who underwent reintervention based on ultrasound detected restenosis, there was no significant difference in the PSVs compared to patients that did not undergo reintervention (420 cm/s vs. 403 cm/s). However, EDVs did significantly differ in those undergoing reintervention (169 cm/s) versus those not undergoing reintervention (79 cm/s) [14]. Armstrong had a similar finding of elevated EDV (168 cm/s) in SMA stent patients undergoing reintervention [16]. Given these current figures, a reasonable approach to surveillance seems to be to obtain a DUS soon after placement of an SMA stent to establish baseline PSV and EDV values. Progressive elevation of the PSV and/or EDV may suggest restenosis and can be used to help guide clinical decision making towards repeat angiography and possibly reintervention. B mode imaging and poststenotic turbulence may also play a role to help identify restenosis, but these parameters have not been systematically evaluated. The interval between DUS surveillance scans should be every 3–6 months in light of the observed early mean time to restenosis.

3.4 Superficial Femoral Artery (SFA) Stents

In many centers SFA stenting is now preferred treatment for TASC A and B lesions producing lower extremity symptoms and is frequently used for more extensive lesions as well. The most common mode of failure in the stented SFA is in-stent restenosis which occurs in up to 40% at 1 year. Close surveillance of SFA stents may therefore be important in maintaining patency. Thus far, DUS surveillance of stented SFAs has used criteria extrapolated from those developed for native arteries and vein graft surveillance. Only one study has directly compared DUS with angiography in stented SFAs using DUS as a screening tool to identify recurrent stenoses [17]. Both PSV and velocity ratios were found to accurately predict recurrent stenosis. A greater than 80% stenosis was identified using a PSV of ≥265 cm/s. A velocity ratio between the upstream untreated artery and the treated artery segment of ≥3.5 also had a high sensitivity and specificity for the detection of ≥80% in-stent restenosis. Combining the two does not significantly add to the accuracy of detection of restenosis (Table 7.2). Intimal hyperplasia can at times be seen on color flow imaging during surveillance duplex of SFA stents and may give important clues as to lumen size in the absence of elevated velocities (Fig 7.5).

3.5 Abdominal Aortic Stent Grafts

Endovascular stent graft placement is now preferred treatment of abdominal aortic aneurysm (AAA) in appropriate patients. However, aneurysms treated with endografts are potentially at risk for expansion and possibly rupture due to persistent perfusion of the excluded aneurysm sac by endoleaks. Endoleaks can be caused by inadequate sealing of the graft to the proximal and distal fixation zones (Type 1), collateral flow into the sac, typically from lumbar arteries or the inferior mesenteric artery (Type 2), gaps in the seal zones of the modules of the graft (Type 3), or porosity of the graft material allowing flow into the sac (Type 4). Follow-up protocols to detect or monitor endoleaks have traditionally been based on serial CT scans. However, due to concerns over radiation exposure, contrast-induced nephropathy and cost, the use of serial DUS studies is emerging as a reasonable

Table 7.2 In-stent restenosis (ISR) duplex criteria: renal, SMA, SFA

	N	Validation test	PSV (cm/s)	Additional factors
Renal artery stent				
Chi 2009[11]ISR≥70%	55	Angio	≥395	RAR≥5.1
Rocha-Singh 2008 [12]Stenosis≥70%	100	Angio	≥225	RAR≥3.5
SMA stent				
Armstrong 2007 [16]ISR≥70%	38	Angio	≥300[a] (and EDV≥50)	With recurrence of symptoms, *or* progressive elevation of PSV (>150 cm/s above baseline) without symptoms
SFA stent				
Baril 2009 [17]ISR ≥80%	330	Angio	≥275	velocity ratio≥3.5

PSV peak systolic velocity, *EDV* end diastolic velocity, *RAR* renal aortic ratio, *SMA* superior mesenteric artery, *SFA* superficial femoral artery
[a]PSV ≥300 cm/s frequently observed after angiographically successful SMA stenting

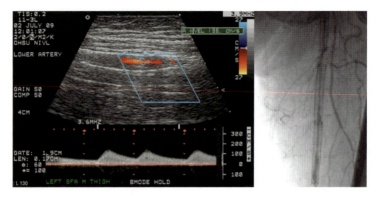

Fig. 7.5 Duplex ultrasound surveillance image of superficial femoral artery stents demonstrates blunted waveforms and spectral broadening consistent with long-segment stenosis. Color flow imaging suggests a narrowed lumen. Angiography confirms diffuse in-stent restenosis in the SFA stents

option for the surveillance of selected patients with aortic stent grafts. Multiple studies have documented potential equivalence of DUS to CT angiogram in the detection of clinically significant endoleaks [18–21]. The efficacy of DUS to detect endoleaks is dependent on operator skill and experience. The patient's body habitus, the presence of bowel gas, and other anatomic limitations may limit ultrasound scanning of aortic stent grafts.

The technologist should be familiar with the type of stent graft implanted. After an overnight fast, the patient is placed supine and scanned with a 2–5 MHz transducer. B-mode imaging is used to scan the aorta in both long axis and cross-sectional views from the proximal to the distal fixation zones of the endograft. Residual aneurysm sac diameter is measured. Color DUS and spectral analysis is used to detect perigraft flow. Special attention should be paid to the proximal and distal fixation zones to assess for Type 1 endoleaks. The anterior lateral area of the sac in the region of the inferior mesenteric artery and the posterior sac where lumbar arteries enter should also be scrutinized for Type 2 endoleaks. Graft module junctions should be assessed for Type 3 endoleaks. Power Doppler may be used to increase sensitivity in the detection of "low flow" endoleaks.

Several small series suggest that contrast-enhanced DUS may be superior to unenhanced color DUS in the detection of endoleaks associated with stent graft repair of AAA. US contrast agents are composed of highly echogenic gas-filled microbubbles that are infused into a peripheral IV either as a bolus or continuous infusion. Contrast-enhanced DUS has been reported to have sensitivity of 90%, specificity of 81%, negative predictive value of 99%, in the detection of endoleaks associated with stent graft repair of AAA requiring intervention [22].

One approach to integrating DUS surveillance of AAA stent grafts is to perform CT angiogram at the initial 1- and 12-month intervals postprocedure. If no endoleak, sac enlargement, or other complication is demonstrated during the first year, then subsequent exams may be performed with ultrasound imaging. If a type 2 endoleak is detected during the first year, then surveillance follows every 6 months with CT until resolution of the endoleak or stabilization of sac size occurs. US surveillance can then be instituted. New endoleaks identified during surveillance with US should prompt a CT scan or an angiogram [20].

4 Role of Vascular Lab in the Operating Room

4.1 Transcranial Doppler (TCD) During Carotid Artery Stenting or Endarterectomy

Carotid artery stenting has been used to treat patients with symptomatic carotid artery stenosis and asymptomatic patients deemed high risk for open repair, either for anatomic or physiologic reasons. Its use may expand following release of the CREST trial data. There are multiple potential technical concerns surrounding carotid artery stenting. These include catheter dislodgment of friable plaque material with embolization to the cerebral circulation, hypoperfusion during balloon inflation, thrombosis with subsequent emboli, and vasospasm leading to reduced flow. Cerebral protection devices such as balloon occluders, flow reversal systems, and filter wires are designed to address these potential complications. However, each device can also cause microemboli or decreased flow despite proper usage.

TCD is an US technique that is used to examine the major cerebral arteries of the Circle of Willis. TCD can be used intraprocedure to track microembolic events as well as low flow with both carotid endarterectomy and carotid stenting. The TCD is used to sample the ipsilateral middle cerebral artery with a low frequency (2.5 MHz) fixed probe. Microembolic signals are then detected according to recommended guidelines [23]. The procedure can be cumbersome intraoperatively and up to 15% of patients cannot be insonated due to a lack of a transtemporal window.

4.2   Carotid Endarterectomy and Intraoperative Assessment with DUS

The success of carotid endarterectomy (CEA) in preventing stroke hinges on the technical success of the operation and minimizing perioperative stroke. Intraoperative assessment of the arterial repair has traditionally been by visual inspection, palpation of pulses, and assessment with a continuous-wave Doppler. Arteriography is also routinely used intraoperatively to assess the repair in some centers. Drawbacks of intraoperative angiography include limited views, access trauma to the repaired artery, and potential for air emboli during injection.

Intraoperative Duplex ultrasound can also be used to verify the technical success of carotid endarterectomy. The procedure is performed with a 7.5 or 10 MHz transducer covered with a sterile sleeve. The transducer is placed directly over the arterial repair and scanning is performed starting proximal to the suture line and continuing to the distal ICA. Special attention is paid to the proximal plaque transection in the common carotid artery and to the plaque transection site at the distal endpoint. Any significant shelves or flow abnormalities are worrisome.

Intraoperative assessment of the CEA with DUS has not been shown to decrease ipsilateral perioperative stroke or perioperative death following CEA but may reduce late recurrent stenosis. It is advocated by some as a useful adjunct in determining what repairs need immediate revision that may impact long-term stenosis-free patency. Mullenix et al. proposed the following duplex findings indicative of an anatomic abnormality that should be immediately revised [24]

- PSV in ICA ≥125 cm/s
- ICA/CCA velocity ratio ≥2
- Spectral broadening throughout systole
- Flap ≥2 mm seen on B mode imaging
- Any major anatomic problem such as kinks or thrombus

4.3 Placement of Inferior Vena Cava (IVC) Filters Using Intravenous Ultrasound (IVUS)

Bedside placement of IVC filters using IVUS is generally safe, economical, and effective and is an alternative to undergoing cavography for the placement of IVC filters [25]. The procedure is particularly applicable to critically ill patients who cannot safely be transported or who may need monitoring or emergency equipment that is not available in the traditional angiography suite. Contraindication to contrast is another indication for ultrasound-guided placement of IVC filters. Venous anomalies identified either by DUS or CT scan should prompt the use of cavography to place IVC filters and are relative contraindications to ultrasound alone guided IVC filter placement.

Several discrete steps are involved in IVUS-guided placement of IVC filters. Bilateral femoral veins are initially assessed for patency with DUS. One side is accessed for filter sheath placement and the other for the IVUS sheath and catheter. Using IVUS the diameter of the IVC is measured and the most inferior renal vein is identified. The filter is positioned and deployed under continuous IVUS monitoring. IVC filter placement and alignment is confirmed with abdominal x-ray.

4.4 Use of IVUS During Endovascular Abdominal Aortic Aneurysm Repair (EVAR)

IVUS can be a useful adjunct during endovascular placement of aortic stent grafts to map aortic anatomy and identify suitable landing zones. The feasibility of "IVUS only" approach has been documented by von Segesser et al. in a series of 80 patients undergoing endovascular aneurysm repair. After a period of using both IVUS and angiography to internally validate the accuracy of IVUS for stent graft placement, the investigators then used IVUS as the sole imaging modality during endograft placement in 47 patients. Complication rates were comparable to those obtained after placement of endografts using angiography. The authors conclude that IVUS is a reliable tool for target site identification, landing zone measurement, neck quality analysis, quality assessment, and troubleshooting [26]. Although a few centers use IVUS as the primary modality of vascular imaging to place endografts, its use is more commonly combined with angiography during EVAR.

5 Venous Treatment: Role of US

Since the advent of endovenous ablation techniques, ultrasound has become an essential tool in the treatment of venous reflux. Ultrasound is important in diagnosis, treatment, and follow-up of venous patients.

5.1 Initial Evaluation and Preoperative Evaluation

In patients with varicose veins a history and physical is performed focusing on any history of previous vein stripping, ablation procedures, or sclerotherapy. This will help guide the identification of abnormal venous segments which may be causing the varicose veins. A history or physical findings suggestive of deep venous thromboses, congenital abnormalities, or arteriovenous malformations are sought in the preoperative evaluation. Using US the deep and superficial veins are interrogated for reflux. Once the refluxing segments are delineated a treatment plan can be formulated. Treatment may be comprised of various techniques including endovenous ablation using laser or radiofrequency, sclerotherapy, microphlebectomy, or perforator ligation and is individually based on the abnormal anatomy identified.

5.2 Endovenous Ablation

Ultrasound is used throughout the performance of endovenous ablation. Ultrasound is used to localize the GSV at the knee or the small saphenous vein near the ankle. Typical probes used are high frequency 10–12 MHz hockey stick or linear array configurations because these offer finer resolution at more superficial depths. The operating surgeon holds the probe in one hand and the micropuncture needle in the other or alternatively, a technician performs the US during the procedure. Accessing the vein can be done in either a transverse or a longitudinal view. Once access is obtained a guidewire is threaded into the vein. Scanning along the vein segment is performed to track the course of the wire to the saphenofemoral junction (SFJ) or the saphenopopliteal junction (SPJ), confirming the wire has not entered a collateral vein and is in the deep system.

After venous access, a sheath is placed into the vein. The tip of the ablation device is placed 2 cm distal to the SFJ/SPJ under direct US guidance. The superficial epigastric vein, circumflex iliac veins may drain into the SFJ and should be preserved to allow flow into the terminal segment of the saphenous vein inhibiting thrombosis and possible extension into the common femoral vein. These tributary veins at the SFJ can usually be easily identified by US.

Once the ablation device is in place, tumescent anesthesia is infiltrated into the fascial sheath surrounding the vein, again using US guidance to direct the needle. Following the ablation, US is once more used to verify that the treated vein is ablated and that the SFJ is patent and that there is no thrombus intruding into the common femoral vein or popliteal vein. Follow-up of these patients includes a subsequent duplex ultrasound 1-week postprocedure to identify any thrombosis at the SFJ or SFP that intrudes into the deep venous system.

6 Conclusion

The noninvasive vascular laboratory will continue to provide clinically important diagnostic and surveillance data for vascular patients treated with endovascular therapies. However, when applied to endovascularly treated arteries, Duplex ultrasound-derived data must be interpreted with the awareness that native artery criteria for stenosis may not apply. In general, DUS native artery criteria for stenosis appear to overestimate the degree of in-stent restenosis. That being said, it appears that very high velocities in endovascularly treated arteries, with the exception of the SMA, indicate a high-grade stenosis. Correspondingly, normal PSVs likely indicate the absence of in-stent restenosis. Of those stented arteries studied, the data has not been consistent enough to allow specific values to be adopted for the duplex characterization of in-stent restenosis. Further research in this area is needed, especially as the number of patients treated with endovascular treatments increases.

DUS is likely to play a larger role in the follow-up of abdominal aortic endografts given the accumulating evidence that it may be as accurate as CT scan in the detection of clinically significant endoleaks. In the operating room, DUS is used to verify the technical success of carotid endarterectomy. Transcranial Doppler has also been used by some as a means of detecting embolic events during carotid artery surgery and stenting. Vascular imaging with IVUS offers an alternative imaging modality to angiography for the placement of IVC filters that might be particularly useful in critically ill patients or those at risk for contrast-induced nephropathy. In the treatment of venous patients, the intraprocedural use of DUS to display venous anatomy makes endovascular venous ablation techniques feasible, safe, and convenient.

References

1. Lal BK, et al. Carotid artery stenting: is there a need to revise ultrasound velocity criteria? J Vasc Surg. 2004;39(1):58–66.
2. Vernhet H, et al. Wall mechanics of the stented extracranial carotid artery. Stroke. 2003;34(11):e222–4.
3. Mitchell EL, et al. Duplex criteria for native superior mesenteric artery stenosis overestimate stenosis in stented superior mesenteric arteries. J Vasc Surg. 2009;50(2):335–40.
4. Chahwan S, et al. Carotid artery velocity characteristics after carotid artery angioplasty and stenting. J Vasc Surg. 2007;45(3):523–6.
5. Peterson BG, et al. Duplex ultrasound remains a reliable test even after carotid stenting. Ann Vasc Surg. 2005;19(6):793–7.
6. Lal BK, et al. Duplex ultrasound velocity criteria for the stented carotid artery. J Vasc Surg. 2008;47(1):63–73.
7. Setacci C, et al. Grading carotid intrastent restenosis: a 6-year follow-up study. Stroke. 2008;39(4):1189–96.
8. Cumbie T, et al. Utility and accuracy of duplex ultrasonography in evaluating in-stent restenosis after carotid stenting. Am J Surg. 2008;196(5):623–8.
9. Armstrong PA, et al. Duplex scan surveillance after carotid angioplasty and stenting: a rational definition of stent stenosis. J Vasc Surg. 2007;46(3):460–5. discussion 465–6.
10. Zhou W, et al. Ultrasound criteria for severe in-stent restenosis following carotid artery stenting. J Vasc Surg. 2008;47(1):74–80.

11. Chi YW, et al. Ultrasound velocity criteria for carotid in-stent restenosis. Catheter Cardiovasc Interv. 2007;69(3):349–54.
12. Rocha-Singh K, Jaff MR, Lynne Kelley E. Renal artery stenting with noninvasive duplex ultrasound follow-up: 3-year results from the RENAISSANCE renal stent trial. Catheter Cardiovasc Interv. 2008;72(6):853–62.
13. Foley MI, et al. Revascularization of the superior mesenteric artery alone for treatment of intestinal ischemia. J Vasc Surg. 2000;32(1):37–47.
14. Peck MA, et al. Intermediate-term outcomes of endovascular treatment for symptomatic chronic mesenteric ischemia. J Vasc Surg. 2010;51(1):140–7. e1-2.
15. Morvay Z, et al. Sonographic follow-up after visceral artery stenting. J Ultrasound Med. 2004;23(8):1057–64.
16. Armstrong PA. Visceral duplex scanning: evaluation before and after artery intervention for chronic mesenteric ischemia. Perspect Vasc Surg Endovasc Ther. 2007;19:386–92.
17. Baril DT, et al. Duplex criteria for determination of in-stent stenosis after angioplasty and stenting of the superficial femoral artery. J Vasc Surg. 2009;49(1):133–8. discussion 139.
18. Collins JT, Boros MJ, Combs K. Ultrasound surveillance of endovascular aneurysm repair: a safe modality versus computed tomography. Ann Vasc Surg. 2007;21(6):671–5.
19. Beeman BR, et al. Duplex ultrasound imaging alone is sufficient for midterm endovascular aneurysm repair surveillance: a cost analysis study and prospective comparison with computed tomography scan. J Vasc Surg. 2009;50(5):1019–24.
20. Schmieder GC, et al. Endoleak after endovascular aneurysm repair: duplex ultrasound imaging is better than computed tomography at determining the need for intervention. J Vasc Surg. 2009;50(5):1012–7. discussion 1017–8.
21. Chaikof EL, et al. The care of patients with an abdominal aortic aneurysm: the society for vascular surgery practice guidelines. J Vasc Surg. 2009;50(4 Suppl):S2–49.
22. Bendick PJ, Bove PG, Long GW, Zelenock GB, Brown WO, Shanley CJ. Efficacy of ultrasound contrast agents in the noninvasive follow-up of aortic stent grafts. J Vasc Surg. 2003;37:381–5.
23. Ringelstein EB, et al. Consensus on microembolus detection by TCD. International Consensus Group on Microembolus Detection. Stroke. 1998;29(3):725–9.
24. Mullenix PS, et al. Intraoperative duplex ultrasonography as an adjunct to technical excellence in 100 consecutive carotid endarterectomies. Am J Surg. 2003;185(5):445–9.
25. Aidinian G, et al. Intravascular ultrasound-guided inferior vena cava filter placement in the military multitrauma patients: a single-center experience. Vasc Endovascular Surg. 2009;43(5):497–501.
26. von Segesser LK, et al. Routine use of intravascular ultrasound for endovascular aneurysm repair: angiography is not necessary. Eur J Vasc Endovasc Surg. 2002;23(6):537–42.

Chapter 8
Fundamental Techniques in Endovascular Treatment

W. Austin Blevins and Peter A. Schneider

1 Endovascular Revolution

Endovascular procedures are an integral part of the practice of vascular surgery. Advances over the last 4 decades, and particularly over the last 20 years, have changed the scope of vascular practice and the treatment of vascular disease. Endovascular techniques were initially only useful in patients with less severe anatomical patterns of disease (e.g., focal stenosis of the iliac or superficial femoral artery). The evolution of techniques, equipment, and attitudes has yielded the current situation in which endovascular intervention is viewed as a reasonable first approach and/or alternative in the treatment of most vascular lesions. Developments in catheters, guidewires, stents, endografts, distal protection devices, and CTO devices and advancing knowledge about how to use them offer promise for further advancements in the next few years.

W.A. Blevins, M.D.
Kaiser Permanente Medical Group, Honolulu, HI, USA

P.A. Schneider, M.D. (✉)
Division of Vascular Therapy, Hawaii Permanente Medical Group,
Kaiser Foundation Hospital, 3288 Moanalua Road, Honolulu, HI 96819, USA
e-mail: Peter.schneider@kp.org; peterschneidermd@aol.com

A. Kumar and K. Ouriel (eds.), *Handbook of Endovascular Interventions*,   99
DOI 10.1007/978-1-4614-5013-9_8,
© Springer Science+Business Media New York 2013

The role of endovascular procedures continues to evolve as new technology is developed and long-term data on procedure outcomes become available. In general, endovascular procedures are less morbid and patients have shorter recovery periods. This early benefit should be weighed against long-term outcomes, as well as the need for additional interventions and more frequent surveillance following endovascular procedures. In many cases endovascular interventions have drastically changed the treatment of specific lesion as is the case with iliac angioplasty and stenting, largely replacing open aortofemoral bypass. The distribution of endovascular and open cases varies from one institution to another. At our facility, arterial revascularizations are comprised of endovascular techniques in 70% of cases and open surgery is used in 30%. Open surgery is used for aneurysm patients with short or otherwise unsuitable necks, carotid stenosis patients who do not qualify for stents, and the majority of patients with branch vessel disease and lower extremity disease, including critical limb ischemia due to tibial occlusive disease.

2   Patient Selection for Endovascular Evaluation

1. Clinical Evaluation—In general, patient selection for endovascular repair is dependent upon specific factors, such as the severity of the clinical problem, the fitness of the patient for surgery, and the anatomic morphology and pattern of the vascular lesions. Much can be learned about these factors at the bedside using history, physical exam, and a handheld Doppler.
2. Duplex Ultrasound—Inexpensive and usually readily available, noninvasive screening tool for identification of luminal narrowing and changes in flow velocity. This modality is operator dependent and vascular labs are required to periodically standardize their results against angiographic studies. When integrated into vascular practice and performed by technologists who understand the treatment options, this tool can significantly streamline the evaluation of patients by indentifying levels and severity of disease prior to treatment.
3. CTA—Improvement in the quality of CT scanners and the ability to create 3D reconstructions of lesions have replaced diagnostic angiography in many practices. This modality provides additional

information about the characteristics of the arterial wall (degree of calcification) as well as anatomic relationships to surrounding structures and can be used with success for case planning. This has been particularly valuable in planning stent-graft treatment of all types of aneurysms.

4. MRA — Similar to CTA, MRA is a noninvasive modality providing excellent soft tissue imaging. MRA is more expensive and its use is limited by the presence of a pacemaker, metal implants, or claustrophobia. Details about lesion morphology can be obtained with newer MRA programs.

5. Angiography — Excellent confirmatory tool of other imaging modalities, though typically redundant from a strictly diagnostic standpoint. Conventional angiography continues to have utility in emergencies such as acute limb ischemia, mesenteric ischemia, and for diagnostic dilemmas. An angiogram is usually performed to plan or to guide vascular repair.

3   Diagnostic Angiography

1. Access — Access site selection should take into consideration the proximity to the site of interest, the possibility of intervention, and the risk of complications. The goal is to utilize the smallest entry method that provides safe and effective access. Large caliber transfemoral percutaneous access (>12Fr) can be obtained now that closure devices are available. Percutaneous brachial access can be obtained up to 7 Fr, but beyond that, consider open arterial exposure. The most commonly utilized sites for diagnostic angiography are the femoral, brachial, and radial arteries (Table 8.1).

2. Femoral — This is the most common and versatile access site. Access can be either retrograde (pointed superiorly toward the aortic bifurcation and against the direction of flow) or antegrade (pointed inferiorly toward the foot and in the direction of flow).

   (a) Landmarks — Identify the inguinal ligament (running between the anterior superior iliac spine and pubic tubercle). Optimal CFA access is 1–2 cm inferior to the inguinal ligament. Caution should be used when using the groin crease as a landmark as this is often displaced distally, especially in obese patients.

Table 8.1 Percutaneous access site selection

Puncture site	Approach	Arteries that can be interrogated	Discussion
Femoral	Retrograde	Aorta and its branches	This is the most common access and can be used to access any arterial bed from the coronary and cerebral to the tibials
Femoral	Antegrade	Ipsilateral infrainguinal	Best approach for a distal tibial or pedal intervention, usually not required for diagnostic angiography. Contraindicated when there is inflow disease or the patient is obese
Brachial/radial	Retrograde	Aorta and its branches including coronary and cerebral arteries	Any vascular bed can be visualized, but it can be a challenge to perform tibial and pedal angiography because of the long distance involved. Brachial puncture has a slightly higher risk

(b) Fluoroscopy—Identify the femoral head. The CFA usually passes over the medial portion of the femoral head inferior to the inguinal ligament and is the area where arterial access should be obtained. Puncturing the artery proximal to the femoral head is too proximal and will likely result in access of the external iliac increasing the risk of retroperitoneal hematoma.

(c) Palpate—Pin the artery between the index and middle fingers of your nondominant hand and use the dominant hand to pass the needle. Ultrasound guidance may be utilized to confirm the relationship to the profunda femoris and inguinal ligament.

(d) Technique—The angle of approach is typically 45° or steeper. Only the anterior wall of the artery is punctured and a guidewire passed once pulsatile return is obtained. Once wire access is obtained, confirm the position with fluoroscopy, remove the access needle, and introduce the access sheath/dilator over the wire. Flush the side port of the sheath after aspirating until return of blood in the syringe to remove air.

3. Brachial—This is an alternate choice of access for patients with unfavorable femoral anatomy or previous femoral bypass procedures. The left arm is preferred because right arm access results in crossing both carotid artery ostia increasing the risk of stroke. Brachial access provides for easier access of down-sloping mesenteric vessels. Treatment of lesions distal to the superficial femoral artery is limited due to the distance traversed and the lengths of available sheaths, catheters, and balloons.

   (a) Landmarks—The brachial artery is usually superficial and easily palpable along the medial arm proximal to the antecubital fossa.
   (b) Technique—A steeper angle of approach is recommended. Wire access and sheath placement are performed similar to femoral access. Following removal of the sheath, meticulous hemostasis is mandatory. Hematoma at a brachial access site can result in median nerve compression.
   (c) Duplex USG—Provides useful visualization to access the brachial artery.

4. Radial—This site is typically reserved for diagnostic angiography of cardiac vessels but may also be used for other types of diagnostic angiography.

4 Venography

1. Venography has largely been replaced by venous duplex in the diagnosis of deep venous thrombosis (DVT). Utility of venography still exists for thrombolytic therapy of acute venous thrombosis as well as to define anatomy for venous bypass or valve reconstruction. Venography is also performed in the evaluation of iliac vein obstruction in preparation for reconstruction and also gonadal vein reflux in pelvic congestion syndrome.
2. Diagnostic venography consists of ascending and descending studies. Ascending venography requires distal access (distal great saphenous or vein of the dorsum of the foot) with infusion of contrast oriented toward the vena cava. The patient should be

placed in 30°–45° reverse Trendelenburg without weight bearing (no footboard). The superficial and deep systems can be visualized. Once images are obtained of the leg, the table is returned to the horizontal position and the leg elevated to obtain pelvic images. More proximal access (the popliteal vein) is usually used for catheter-directed thrombolytic therapy. Descending venography consists of accessing the contralateral femoral vein using and up and over technique to position a flush catheter in the proximal femoral vein. The patient is placed in reverse Trendelenburg and is asked to do a Valsalva maneuver to increase intra-abdominal pressure and decrease return to the vena cava. Contrast boluses are administered to assess valvular competence. Contrast flows distally and through incompetent valves.

5   Contrast Injectors

1. Power Injectors—Power injection is required to opacify large volume arteries such as the aorta. Settings can be adjusted to perform angiography of smaller vessels as well. Caution should be used when there is a risk of damaging the artery. Don't use power injection when the tip of the catheter is within the lesion, when the tip is within an aneurysmal segment with thrombus, when the tip is oriented against the wall of the artery, or if there is redundancy (slack) in the catheter.

   (a) Use of the power injector. The reservoir is loaded with contrast that may be full strength or dilute (e.g., 25% or 50%). The extension tubing is sterile and the line is purged of air when connecting to the angiographic catheter.

   (b) Settings—Pressure, Rate of rise, Volume administered per second, total to be delivered. These settings reflect the vascular bed to be interrogated and the catheter through which it is to be administered. A multi-sidehole flush catheter can be used to high pressure (800–1,000 psi). Evaluation of the aorta requires larger volume: 30 ml for the aortic arch and 20 ml for abdominal aorta. End hole diagnostic catheters are used at lower pressure (250–500 psi) and volume (3–5 ml per second). The rate of rise is used in smaller branch arteries such as carotid or renal to permit the pressure of injection to increase slowly (e.g., over 0.5 s).

2. Hand Injection—Fast and simple. Useful in smaller caliber vessels, when the required volume of contrast is less than 10 ml or in low flow vessels. This approach is usually employed when using an end hole diagnostic catheter.
3. Types of iodinated contrast

   (a) Nonionic versus Ionic—Nonionic contrasts are used today and most are iso-osmolar or slightly hyperosmolar and this significantly reduces discomfort. Incidence of anaphylaxis is similar between the two. A high iodine concentration improves visibility.
   (b) Osmolarity—Iso-osmolar agents are preferred. Better tolerated by the patient and result in less physiologic damage.

6   Basic Equipment for Angiography

1. Needles—No. 18 straight angiography entry needle; the lumen is adequate to pass a 0.035 in. diameter guidewire into the vascular system. Coaxial Micro puncture set (Cook, Inc., Bloomington, Indiana, USA)—21-gauge needle with a 0.018 in. guidewire and a 4 or 5Fr dilator.
2. Access Sheaths—A standard access sheath has a side port for the administration of medications or contrast. Measured based on their ID (inner diameter), 4Fr to 7Fr sheaths are used most commonly for peripheral interventions with larger sheaths required for stent-grafts. Most angiography is performed with 4 or 5Fr catheters and sheaths. A standard access sheath for diagnostic angiography is 12–15 cm in length. Sheaths that support interventions may be obtained up to 110 cm in length.
3. Guidewires—Diameter ranges from 0.014 to 0.038 in. Lengths range from 145 to 300 cm. The length of the wire must be long enough to cover the cumulative distance from the access site to well beyond the lesion as well as the length outside the patient to support the longest catheter that is required for the procedure (65 to 145 cm). Access wires should have a floppy tip and be atraumatic. Multiple characteristics including stiffness (support), coating, tip shape, and steerability need to be kept in mind. General types of guidewires are listed below. Guidewire handling skills are included in Table 8.2.

Table 8.2 Guidewire Handling Skills

1. Wet the guidewire with heparin–saline solution
2. Introduce the tip of the guidewire through the entry needle hub
3. Use fluoroscopic guidance when advancing a guidewire, especially when encountering lesions
4. Maintain hand control of the guidewire until you are certain it is secure in the artery
5. Don't force the guidewire
6. Rapid incremental advancement of the wire increases the chance of kinking the wire or inadvertent passage into a branch
7. Caution when the guidewire tip encounters the lesion
8. Shape the guidewire tip by running a metal clamp over the tip of the wire while holding the wire between the clamp and your thumb
9. Have a torque device available for steerable guidewires
10. Pin the wire during exchanges and when advancing catheters. Remove any slack from the wire without withdrawing the guidewire
11. Use a pin and pull technique to remove catheters to ensure that the tip of the wire does not migrate
12. Wipe the wire with heparin–saline after each exchange
13. Ensure intraluminal position of the wire before passing any endovascular device
14. Handle a hydrophilic coated wire with a pincer grasp (between the thumb and forefinger)
15. Place a towel over the end of the guidewire outside of the patient to prevent the wire from falling off the table. A shodded clamp can also be used for wire identification when using a buddy wire technique (two wires through the same access sheath)
16. Contamination of the wire requires removal of the wire or cutting contaminated end of the wire, provided adequate length remains for exchange
17. Place a catheter over the guidewire when additional stiffness or pushability is needed
18. Exchange a kinked or bent wire
19. Do not give up wire access! Leave the guidewire in place until the procedure is finished
20. The way the guidewire feels as it advanced and the appearance using fluoroscopy give clues to optimal handling of guideiwres and can only be learned on the job

(a) Workhorse/general use: This is typically a medium support guidewire with a soft, somewhat floppy and atraumatic tip.
(b) Exchange: Stiff guidewire that can be used to help straighten anatomy and assist passage of a sheath or a larger endovascular device.

Table 8.3 Catheters in endovascular practice

Catheter type	Catheter	Function	Length
Flush	Pigtail Tennis racket Omni-flush	Aortography	65, 90 cm
Exchange	Straight	Exchange guidewires	70, 100 cm
Selective	Simple curve (bend at tip) or complex curve (complex bend or reverse curve at tip)	Assist cannulation, support guidewire, and are used for crossing the lesion; complex curve catheters are used for cannulation challenging or tortuous carotid arteries	40, 65, 100, 120 cm

  (c) Steerable: A steerable guidewire allows a 1:1 turning ratio between the shaft of the wire and the tip. A common steerable guidewire is the Glidewire which also has a hydrophilic coating. The smaller caliber guidewires can typically be shaped at the tip to adjust the degree of curvature.
  (d) CTO: These are smaller caliber guidewires (0.014 or 0.018 in.) that have a stiff shaft and a relatively stiff tip for use in a chronic total occlusion.

4. Catheters—Measured based on their OD (outer diameter). A 5 Fr OD catheter fits into a 5 Fr ID sheath. A variety of lengths (40–120 cm) and shapes may be obtained. Catheters may have a single hole at the tip for contrast administration or there may be multiple side holes plus an end hole (Table 8.3).

  (a) Flush: Multiple side holes, straight or rounded head shapes, used for administration of contrast into large arteries, like the aorta.
  (b) Selective: Single end hole, multiple head shapes. The shape of the catheter tip may be specialized to a specific task, such as cannulating the carotid or renal arteries. These specially shaped catheters are also integral to supporting cannulation in difficult situations.
  (c) Exchange: Single end hole, straight. These are used to exchange the guidewire, typically to insert a stiffer exchange guidewire in preparation of an endovascular intervention.
  (d) Infusion: Multiple side holes, straight, used for thrombolytic therapy.

References

1. Schneider PA. Endovascular skills. 3rd ed. New York: Informa; 2009. p. 1–471.
2. Hodgson KJ, Hood DB. Endovascular diagnostic. In: Cronenwett JL, Johnston KW, editors. Rutherford's vascular surgery. Philadelphia, PA: Saunders; 2010. p. 1262–76.
3. Singh H, Cardella JF, Cole PEH, et al. Quality improvement guidelines for diagnostic arteriography. Society of Interventional Radiology Standards of Practice Committee. J Vasc Interv Radiol. 2003;14:S283–8.
4. Neequaye SK, Aggarwal R, Van Herzeele I, et al. Endovascular skills training and assessment. J Vasc Surg. 2008;47:1008–11.
5. Dotter CT, Rosch J, Robinson M. Fluoroscopic guidance in femoral artery puncture. Radiology. 1978;127:266–7.

Chapter 9
Carotid Artery Disease

Marius Hornung, Jennifer Franke, and Horst Sievert

1 Anatomy

Familiarity with the extra- and intracranial vessel anatomy is decisive for successful treatment of carotid artery disease. The right common carotid artery originates from the bifurcation of the brachiocephalic trunk, while the left one arises directly from the aortic arch. The common carotid artery does not have any side branches. Usually at the level of the upper edge of the thyroid cartilage, it divides into the internal and external carotid arteries. The internal carotid artery supplies the anterior part of the brain, the eye and its appendages, and sends branches to the forehead and nose. Its size in the adult is equal to that of the external carotid artery, but it can be identified due to the absence of side branches in its extracranial course up to the intracranial branching point. Due to its course, the internal carotid can be divided into four parts:

– *Cervical part*: this portion ascends laterally behind the hypopharynx—where it can be palpated—and in front of the transverse processes of the cervical vertebrae to the carotid canal in the petrous part of the temporal bone.

M. Hornung, M.D. • J. Franke, M.D. • H. Sievert, M.D. (✉)
Cardio Vascular Center Frankfurt, Seckbacher Landstraße 65,
Frankfurt 60389, Germany
e-mail: horstsievertMD@aol.com

A. Kumar and K. Ouriel (eds.), *Handbook of Endovascular Interventions*,   109
DOI 10.1007/978-1-4614-5013-9_9,
© Springer Science+Business Media New York 2013

- *Petrous part*: in its passage through the carotid canal and along the side of the body of the sphenoid bone, it describes a double curvature.
- Cavernous part: This part ascends toward the posterior clinoid process, then passes forward by the side of the body of the sphenoid bone, and again curves upward on the medial side of the anterior clinoid. The ophthalmic artery arises from the internal carotid, just as that vessel is emerging from the cavernous sinus.
- *Cerebral part*: It begins distal to the origin of the ophthalmic artery and continues until the bifurcation into the anterior and middle cerebral artery.

2 Disease Definition

Carotid artery disease describes any alteration of the carotid artery that is clinically indicated to treat. A carotid artery stenosis is a narrowing constriction of the inner surface of the carotid artery, usually caused by atherosclerosis. The carotid bifurcation is a common site for a build up of plaque that can narrow the common or internal carotid artery. Carotid artery dissection is a spontaneous or traumatic separation of the layers of the artery wall. An aneurysm of the carotid artery is a localized, blood-filled, balloon-like bulge of a blood vessel. Aneurysms can be hereditary or caused by disease, both of which lead to the weakening of the blood vessels wall.

3 Disease Distribution

Cerebral ischemic events are the most frequent cause of stroke (80–85%) and currently the third leading cause of death in industrialized countries. It is well accepted that the presence of carotid stenosis is responsible for 20–30% of all strokes. Atherosclerosis causes about 90% of all carotid artery stenoses. Only about 10% are the result from a non-atherosclerotic disease.

Carotid artery dissection is the most common cause of stroke in young adults between 20 and 40 years of age. A total of 70% of all carotid dissections appear in this group.

The most common reason for extracranial aneurysms of the internal carotid artery is atherosclerosis. These aneurysms are mostly seen over the age of 50 and carry a high risk for thromboembolic stroke. The rupture risk is high in mycotic carotid aneurysms, whereas traumatic ones tend to stabilize and show regression.

4   Classification: Degree of Stenosis

Duplex ultrasound has 90–95% sensitivity and specificity in validation of stenoses of the internal carotid artery >50% compared to angiography. Its specificity and sensitivity for differentiating high-grade stenosis from occlusion is more than 90%.

In angiography, the degree of carotid stenosis can be measured using two different methods:

– European Carotid Surgery Trial (ECST) method: Measurement of the minimal lumen diameter in relation to the assumed diameter of the internal carotid artery at the site of maximal stenosis.
– North American Symptomatic Carotid Endarterectomy Trial (NASCET) method: Relation between the minimal lumen diameter and the diameter of the internal carotid artery distal to the stenosis.

Due to the fact that the anatomic relation between the carotid bulb and the distal internal carotid artery is constant, a conversion of these methods is possible:

ECST-stenosis (%)=0.6×NASCET-stenosis (%)+40%

5   Clinical Findings

The clinical symptoms of stenosis of the internal carotid artery are characterized by ischemia in the corresponding region of cerebral flow. Symptomatic stenosis of the internal carotid artery is defined by neurological syndromes of the ipsilateral hemisphere 6 months prior to the intervention:

– Transitory ischemic attack (TIA)=focal neurological deficit for less than 24 h.
– Amaurosis=monocular visual loss
– Stroke=neurological deficit for more than 24 h

With more widespread use of modern imaging techniques for the brain, up to one-third of patients with symptoms lasting less than 24 h have been found to have an infarction. This has led to a new tissue-based definition of TIA: a transient episode of neurological dysfunction caused by a focal ischemia without acute infarction.

6   Diagnosis

Carotid artery disease is usually diagnosed by color duplex ultrasound. In addition to the assessment of the degree of stenosis, this method also makes it possible to identify the plaque morphology (e.g., soft plaque, calcified plaque, or an ulcerated surface). Patients who should undergo duplex evaluation include:

– Symptomatic patients who have suffered a focal neurological deficit or amaurosis fugax.
– In asymptomatic patients, there are no standard diagnostic recommendations to date, except when a bypass operation is planned. In this situation, a duplex ultrasound examination is recommended in patients with history of cerebral ischemia or carotid bruit on auscultation. Besides duplex ultrasound should be performed in patients over 65 years, patients with stenosis of the left main coronary artery or peripheral arterial occlusive disease.

When duplex ultrasound results are unclear, diagnostic accuracy can be increased using supplementary computed-tomography angiography (CTA) or magnetic resonance angiography (MRA).

Cerebral computed tomography (CT) or magnetic resonance imaging (MRI) can also help exclude other causes of neurological symptoms, such as hemorrhage or tumor.

7   Management

7.1   Medical Treatment

Medical treatment is indicated in every patient in order to limit atherosclerotic progression and reduce the risk of a neurological event. This treatment recommendation is independent of the decision on whether to offer interventional or surgical revascularization therapy. Treatments currently available include inhibition of platelets using acetylsalicylic acid, dipyridamole plus aspirin, or clopidogrel. In addition, treatment with statins is advised due to their anti-inflammatory and thus plaque-stabilizing effect on the vascular bed.

Medical treatment alone is recommended in patients with stenosis of the internal carotid artery who either have a low risk of stroke (symptomatic stenoses <50%, asymptomatic stenoses <70%), who carry a high perioperative or peri-interventional risk due to comorbid conditions, or who have a limited life expectancy.

7.2   Endovascular Treatment

The aim of carotid stenting is to prevent stroke due to carotid artery stenosis. Typical candidates are symptomatic patients (TIA or stroke within 6 months) with >50% stenosis of the carotid artery, or asymptomatic patients with >70% stenosis of the carotid artery. Endovascular treatment is the preferred therapy in patients who are at increased risk for carotid surgery. High-risk features include medical comorbidities (severe heart disease, heart failure, severe lung disease, etc.) and anatomic features (radiation therapy of the neck, prior ipsilateral carotid artery surgery, concomitant intra-thoracic or intracranial carotid disease).

7.2.1   Patient Preparation

- Cranial CT or MRI examination
- Duplex ultrasound
- Aspirin 100–300 mg/day and clopidogrel 75 mg/day, starting at least 5 days before a planned intervention, or bolus administration

(aspirin 500 mg, clopidogrel 600 mg) on the day before the procedure.

7.3 Surgical Treatment

There are basically two techniques that can be used for plaque removal and reconstruction of the internal carotid artery or carotid bifurcation:

- Thromboendarterectomy (TEA) with a patch graft
- Eversion endarterectomy (EEA)

The operation can be performed under general or local anesthesia and with or without intraoperative shunting to decrease the risk of cerebral ischemia during the operation.

8 Intervention

8.1 Peri-interventional therapy

- Heparin (70–100 IU/kg) with an activated clotting time (ACT) of 250–300 s
- Electrocardiographic (ECG) monitoring due to potential bradycardia
- Blood pressure monitoring for possible hypotension related to carotid sinus stimulation by balloon inflation
- Intravenous administration of 1 mg atropine 2–3 min before implantation of the carotid stent, to prevent possible bradycardia or asystole (to be used with caution in patients with narrow-angle glaucoma)
- Infusions for hypotension

8.2 Access Route

Establishing a safe vascular access route in order to minimize complications during carotid stent implantation is essential. The access via the femoral artery is the approach most often employed. The common femoral artery is punctured using a Seldinger needle and then a 5–6 F sheath is placed. Afterward, this initial sheath is exchanged during the procedure for a 90 cm long sheath. If a guiding catheter is to be used, a 8–9 F sheath is needed. In patients in whom the iliac arteries are occluded or who have high-grade stenosis in these arteries, or in situations in which the access route via the femoral artery is unavailable for other reasons, access via the brachial or radial artery can be obtained. The right brachial artery is preferable for interventions in both the right internal carotid artery and the left internal carotid artery. If neither access route is possible, direct cervical common carotid access (percutaneous or open surgical) might be considered.

8.3 Engaging the Supra-Aortic Arteries

Angiography of the aortic arch is often performed prior to selective carotid angiography in order to identify possible difficult anatomic conditions that might make it necessary to exchange the typically employed diagnostic catheters (e.g., Berenstein, Judkins Right, Head Hunter, IMS, JB-1) for an alternative one (e.g., Simmons or Vitck catheter). To engage the common carotid artery, the 5 F diagnostic catheter is positioned over a 0.035 in. hydrophillic guidewire in the ascending aorta with the catheter tip pointing downward. This technique reduces the likehood of embolization of aortic plaque or traumatic injury to the intima of the aortic arch and prevents the catheter from becoming caught in a vascular ostium. As soon as the catheter reaches the ascending aorta, it is rotated 180°. This places the tip of the catheter in a vertical, upright position on fluoroscopy. The catheter is then advanced over this wire into the common carotid artery.

To intubate the left common carotid artery, the catheter is slowly withdrawn from the ostium of the brachiocephalic trunk. It should be rotated 20° counterclockwise, so that the catheter tip points slightly anteriorly. When the aortic arch becomes increasingly kinked with advancing age, the ostium of the left common carotid artery is located slightly further posterior. In these cases, it may be necessary to rotate the catheter posteriorly instead.

Once the left common carotid artery has been entered, the catheter should be rotated back 20° clockwise, so that the tip is pointing vertically or slightly posteriorly. The catheter position is checked by administering a small amount of contrast. This can exclude subintimal contrast flow or reduced blood flow. The hydrophilic wire is advanced to the distal common carotid artery, followed by the catheter.

If engagement of the common carotid artery is unsuccessful with the standard catheter, then a switch to a Simmons catheter is usually made. This type of catheter has a large reverse curve, which must be re-shaped in the aorta after wire removal, usually in the ascending aorta. Moving the catheter backward slightly guides the tip into the brachiocephalic trunk, then into the left common carotid artery, and finally into the left subclavian artery. In contrast, Vitek or Mani catheters have smaller pre-formed curves and do not require shaping. Therefore, these catheters are advanced forward, rather than withdrawn from, the distal aortic arch selecting the left subclavian artery first, and so on. Once the desired vessel is engaged, the wire is advanced followed by the catheter. Advancement of the catheter is carried out slowly with assistance from the pulsating blood flow. At the same time, the wire is withdrawn slightly, so that its position is maintained proximal to the carotid bifurcation. Advancement of the catheter and withdrawal of the guidewire are performed several times alternately until the catheter is safely positioned in the targeted vessel (push-and-pull technique).

8.4 Visualizing the Intracranial Vessels

Injections of contrast medium should be carried out manually or with a small amount of automated contrast administration (a maximum of 6 ml per injection). Larger amounts would lead to mixing of the arterial, intermediate, and venous phases, potentially leading to masking of early venous filling or other types of pathology. Some operators conduct four-vessel angiography to show the status of the collateral arteries. However, as this presents an additional procedural risk, the need for it is questionable, particularly in patients in whom MRA has previously been performed. During balloon dilatation, the absence of collaterals may cause short periods of cerebral ischemia due to brief occlusion of the internal carotid artery. However, this reaction is reversible after deflation of the balloon and has no influence on the completion of the procedure. Once the anatomy of the target vessel has been identified, a hydrophillic guidewire is advanced into the external carotid artery so that the diagnostic catheter can be exchanged for a sheath or a guiding sheath. Bony landmarks can be used for guidance instead of road mapping to mark the origin of the external carotid artery during wire placement.

8.5   Vascular Kinking

If the vessel is very tortuous, it can be straightened using a wire. It is also helpful to ask the patient to inhale deeply and hold the breath. An acute vessel angle can be negotiated by careful rotation and advancement of the catheter until it has reached the desired position. If it is still not possible to advance the catheter, a Simmons III catheter should be used to introduce the guidewire into the external carotid artery. The Simmons III catheter can than be exchanged for a 4 F multipurpose catheter. After this, the hydrophillic wire is exchanged for a 0.035 in. Amplatz wire or a softer wire. Finally, the 4 F catheter is exchanged for a 5 F catheter.

8.6   Placing of the Guiding Catheter

An 8 F guiding catheter (e.g., right coronary or hockey-stick guiding catheter) is introduced into the ascending aorta via a hydrophillic 0.035 in. wire. It is advisable to use a 5 F catheter inside of the guiding catheter in order to avoid a step-up from the wire to the guiding catheter. In case of difficult or abnormal anatomy, aortography of the aortic arch can be used to assist in selective exploration. Following angiography of the aortic arch and assessment of the anatomy, the guiding catheter is introduced into the common carotid artery. This should be carried out by careful aspiration and flushing with saline to clear any possible atherosclerotic particles out of the catheter.

8.7   Placement of the Long Sheath

Engagement of the common carotid artery is carried out with a 5 F diagnostic catheter. Access to the external carotid artery is obtained with an angled hydrophilic guidewire and the diagnostic catheter introduced into the external carotid artery as described above.

The wire is then exchanged for a 0.035 in. wire, typically a stiff Amplatz wire. Afterward, the diagnostic catheter is removed and a 6 F 90 cm long sheath is placed using the over-the-wire technique into the common carotid artery below the carotid bifurcation. The sheath should be handled very carefully, as trauma to the common carotid artery ostium or release of atherosclerotic deposits may subsequently lead to neurological disorders. The sheath should be meticulously aspirated and flushed to eliminate possible air or atherosclerotic debris.

When the external carotid artery is occluded, when there is significant stenosis below the bifurcation, or when there is a stenosis at the ostium of the common carotid artery, placing the 6 F 90 cm port in the common carotid artery may represent a considerable challenge. If possible, crossing the stenosis with a stiff wire should be avoided, as this may dislodge plaque material and cause distal embolization. If necessary, the 5 F diagnostic catheter is advanced over a 0.035 or 0.038 in. guidewire for placement further distally, slightly proximal to the stenosis. It can then be exchanged over a 0.035 in. Amplatz wire (extra stiff). If there is an ostial/proximal stenosis of the common carotid artery, it may be necessary to treat this stenosis first in order to obtain access to the distal stenosis. However, if this stenosis is not severe, the bifurcation stenosis should be treated first, then the proximal stenosis on the way back.

8.8 Predilation

Some operators predilate the stenosis using a small angioplasty balloon and a short inflation time of 5–10 s. This provides for better passage and positioning of the stent. The present authors would only recommend predilation if primary stent placement has failed. In our view, primary stent implantation has a protective effect against distal embolization by fixing deposits on the vascular wall.

8.9 Embolic Protection

The possibility of peri-procedural cerebral embolization is an important concern in carotid angioplasty. Balloon dilatation, stent implantation, and manipulation of the vessels by catheters and wires can easily release emboli, which if large enough, can cause severe cerebral damage. For this reason, embolic protection systems are routinely used in most centers. There are currently three different underlying principles on which protection is based: distal occlusion balloons, filter systems, and proximal occlusion balloons.

Distal occlusion balloons were the first embolic protection systems to become available, and were widely used in the initial carotid stent experience. It consists of a 0.014 in. guidewire with an occlusion balloon in the distal section, which is inflated and deflated through a very small channel in the guiding catheter (Guardwire® Temporary Occlusion and Aspiration System, Medtronic Vascular; TriActiv® ProGuard™ Embolic Protection System, Kensey Nash). After the guiding catheter is placed, the occlusion balloon is positioned distal to the stenosis and the balloon inflated until blood flow into the internal carotid artery stops. Stent implantation then follows. After the intervention, an aspiration catheter is introduced up to the occlusion balloon, and the blood in the occluded artery is aspirated. Any particles released during the intervention are thus removed. The advantages of the distal occlusion systems are the low profile, flexibility, and good steerability. Disadvantages include the fact that balloon occlusion is not tolerated in 6–10% of patients, and that the vascular segment distal to the occlusion balloon cannot be imaged during the balloon occlusion procedure.

Most *filter systems* consist of a metal framework that is covered with a polyethylene membrane or a nitinol mesh. The pore size can vary between 80 and 180 μm in diameter depending on the specific device. Filters are usually attached to the distal section of a 0.014 in. guidewire. In their closed state, filters are sheathed by an introducer catheter, and are introduced into the vascular segment distal to the stenosis. Once the stenosis has been crossed, the filter of choice is opened by withdrawing it into a recovery catheter, and then removed from the vessel. A wide range of second- and third-generation filter systems are currently available. The technical characteristics of a good filter consist of:

1. Low profile (less than 3 F)
2. Adequate steerability for maneuvering through highly tortuous vessels
3. When the filter is opened—good wall apposition to allow the best possible protection against emboli.

All distal protection systems, occlusion balloons, and filters have the potential disadvantage that the stenosis has to be crossed before the system can be deployed and protection established. This unavoidable step carries a risk of distal embolization during the initial unprotected phase of the procedure. *Proximal protection systems*, such as the Gore Neuro Protection System (Gore) and the MO.MA System (Invatec), provide protection against cerebral embolism even before crossing the stenosis. This is particularly important in the case of stenoses in which fresh thrombi have been identified. Here, the risk of embolization with a distally placed system may be raised. The use of a proximal occlusion device allows the operator to choose any wire of choice to negotiate difficult stenoses. These systems consist of a long main sheath with a balloon on its distal end that is inflated in the common carotid artery to occlude forward carotid flow. A second balloon, which is inflated in the external carotid artery, prevents retrograde external flow, thus establishing complete arrest of antegrade flow into the internal carotid artery. This principle takes advantage of the cerebral collateral system of the circle of Willis. Following balloon occlusion of the external and common carotid arteries, collateral flow via the circle of Willis produces what is known as back pressure. This prevents antegrade flow into the internal carotid artery. After stent implantation and before deflation of the occlusion balloon, blood in the internal carotid artery, which might contain released particles, is aspirated and removed. One disadvantage of proximal protection systems is that a small percentage of patients are unable to tolerate balloon occlusion due to incomplete intracranial collateralization.

8.10 Stent Implantation

Usually self-expandable stents are implanted in carotid stenting. Balloon-expandable stents are recommended in ostial stenoses of the common carotid artery, stenoses located in the distal internal carotid artery, and sometimes in severely calcified stenoses. The disadvantages of balloon-expandable stents, however, are the repeated balloon dilations that are needed to implant the stent adequately and stent compression that can occur during the long-term follow-up in areas vulnerable to external manipulation.

In vessels which carry the risk to bend or to be manipulated, self-expandable nitinol stents are generally the best choice. They are designed to adapt to the shape of the vessel and therefore have only little tendency to straighten it. Stent-induced straightening of the vessel can give rise to a new stenosis distal to the stent due to kinking or folding of the vessel. Stents with a strong radial force are recommended for treatment of severely calcified stenoses. Closed-cell carotid stents typically have stronger radial force. Their cell structure may also provide better plaque coverage, which may theoretically be advantageous in stenoses with high embolic risk. The clinical value of closed-cell designs versus open-cell designs is currently still unclear. Likewise, the importance of the stent cell size is subject to further research. In case of soft or large plaques and visible thrombus, the combination of a proximal occlusion device and a stent system with small struts is probably favorable to manipulate the plaque as little as possible during the intervention.

The authors recommend a stent diameter 1–2 mm larger than the largest vascular diameter to be stented. Carotid stents with a diameter of 6–8 mm are usually used if the stent is being implanted exclusively in the internal carotid artery, or with a diameter of 8–10 mm if the stent is to cross the bifurcation. Stenting across the external carotid artery does not pose a problem and priority should be given to the stent covering the entire stenosis, which in most cases will mean crossing the bifurcation to cover the distal common carotid artery.

8.11 Post-Dilation

Post-dilation is usually carried out using a balloon with a diameter of 4–5 mm, but not larger than the diameter of the internal carotid artery. A balloon with an unnecessarily large diameter might force particles through the stent cells and cause distal embolization. To prevent dissections, postdilatation should be carried out at nominal pressure, and within the stent borders. A residual stenosis of <30% is acceptable, since an adequate blood flow is established and the potentially emboligenic atherosclerotic deposits are compressed sufficiently to induce neo-intimal formation and eliminate the embolic potential of the lesion. The stent expands further during the following few hours. If contrast-enhancing ulcerations occur outside the stent edges, they do not need to be obliterated and can be left without any untoward effects. Post-dilation of the stent segment in the common carotid artery is not necessary. If significant stenosis or occlusion of the external carotid artery develops subsequently to postdilation, it does not require treatment.

Following post-dilation of the stent, angiography of the carotid arteries and intracranial vessels is carried out. Imaging of the intra-cerebral vessels should always include the venous phase. This allows comparison of conditions before and after stent implantation. For assessment of the intracerebral vessels and in preparation for a possible intracranial emergency intervention in case of cerebral embolism, angiography should be carried out with a lateral and anteroposterior 30° cranial projection.

9 Post-Procedure Management and Follow-up

Following the intervention, blood pressure has to be checked closely for at least 6 h. It should be as low as possible. The post-interventional medication consists of lifelong aspirin treatment (100 mg/day) and clopidogrel (75 mg/day) during the first month after stent placement. Color duplex ultrasound scan should be performed 1 month after the intervention to verify the acute result of the procedure, and thereafter at an interval of 6 months as routine follow-up examination.

10 Acute Complications and Management of Treatment

10.1 Ischemic Events (TIA, Stroke)

Ischemic events are the main complication of carotid stent implantations. Possible predictors of complications and potential sources for thrombotic embolization are:

– Insufficient pre-treatment: aspirin and clopidogrel should be started a week before to avoid fresh thrombus.

- Heavily calcified or ulcerated lesions: In case of large plaque volume or a visible thrombus use a proximal occlusion device and a stent with small struts and a small cell area to manipulate the stenosis as little as possible and to secure the plaque as good as possible.
- Malposition of distal filter devices: Use angiography to verify stabile filter position.
- Malposition of proximal occlusion devices: Contrast dye disappears as soon as the occlusion balloon is not occlusive anymore, concurrently the measured blood pressure rises. Flow arrest has to be re-established as soon as possible because malposition immediately results in zero protection.

Cerebral ischemia can present with a large variety of symptoms. Depending on the occluded vessel, the embolization may bring a sudden change of patient's neurological status. Yet sometimes, the ischemia causes only a subtle change of the neurological status or may even only cause a change in vital signs.

In case of sudden symptom onset due to cerebral ischemia, it is most important to act systematically. The operator should finish the current maneuver, then aspirate and re-establish blood flow (if proximal occlusion is used). After a neurological evaluation of the patient's situation, fluids should be administered and a cerebral angiography has to be performed to compare actual findings with baseline. Depending on the type of occluded artery and the inventory of the cathlab, the operator has different treatment options to restore cerebral blood flow. After advancing a microcatheter to the clot interface, lytic agents and glycoprotein IIb/IIIa inhibitors can be administered distally, proximally and into the clot. If available, intracranial retrieval devices (e.g., Phenox Clot Retriever, Concentric Clot Retriever, Merci Retrieval Device, Penumbra) can be used to try to disrupt and retrieve the thrombus or debris. If clot retrieval fails, placement of an intracranial stent (e.g., Wingspan, Solitaire, Enterprise, Neuroform) may be an option to re-establish cerebral perfusion.

In case of very small vessel occlusions, or asymptomatic postprocedural filling defects that may evolve into significant stroke, the administration of glycoprotein IIb/IIIa inhibitors leads to an increased platelet blockade to prevent further clot formation. However, they also increase the risk of bleeding.

10.2   Stent Thrombosis

Despite combined antiplatelet therapy with aspirin and clopidogrel, as well as peri-interventional use of heparin, in some cases a sudden formation of thrombotic material can be seen after stent-implantation. In these cases the ACT has to be raised again by administration of heparin. The administration of glycoprotein IIb/IIIa inhibitors is effective to prevent further clot-formation which may cause distal embolization and stroke. The application of a bolus of thrombolytics in to the clot, followed by continuous intra-arterial infusion may resolve the thrombus. An additional stent implantation may be indicated to fix the formed clot at its position.

10.3   Spasm

In case of vasospasm during carotid interventions, in most of the cases it is attributed to mechanical irritation of the vessel wall caused by movement of distal filter devices. The most crucial point in preventing spasm is to avoid any unnecessary movement of the filter. If spasm occurs during the intervention, it will be of highest importance that the interventionalist stays calm. In most of the cases vasospasm is self-limiting and does not need any further treatment. In symptomatic spasms, intra-arterial nitroglycerin can be given.

10.4   Bradycardia and Hypotension

Bradycardia and hypotension may occur due to compression of baroreceptors in the carotid bulb during post-dilation. These symptoms may occur either during balloon inflation or after the intervention, or even may reoccur and can last up to 48 h. The administration of Atropine 3–5 min before inflating the balloon is most effective to prevent circulatory disorders. In case of bradycardia and hypotension despite of the application, 0.5–1 mg of Atropine can be administered repeatedly. In rare cases, catecholamines are necessary, occasionally for up to 2 days.

11 Inventory for Carotid Artery Stenting

Basic Inventory
– Sheaths
– Guiding catheters
– Guidewires
– Diagnostic catheters (e.g., Berenstein, Judkins Right, Head Hunter, IMS, JB-1, Simmons, Vittek)
– Embolic protection devices (Table 9.1)
– Carotid artery stent systems (Table 9.2)
– Dilation balloons (different diameters and different lengths)
– Neuro wires (e.g., Taper, Dasher)
– Micro catheters (e.g., Fast Tracker, Prowler)

Extended Inventory
– Covered stents (e.g., Hemobahn)
– Intracranial stents (e.g., Neuroform, Wingspan, Enterprise, Solitaire)
– Clot retrieval devices (e.g., Concentric, Merci, Catch, Phenox)
– Aspiration devices (e.g., Penumbra)
– Coils

Table 9.1 Embolic protection devices

Embolic protection devices			
Type	Product	FDA approval	CE mark
Distal occlusion balloon	PercuSurge (Medtronic)	X	X
	TwinOne (Minvasys)		X
Distal filter	Angioguard (Cordis)	X	X
	Accunet (Guidant)	X	X
	Spider (ev3)	X	X
	FilterWire (Boston)	X	X
	Emboshield (Abbott)	X	X
	Fibernet (Medtronic Invatec)	X	X
Proximal occlusion devices	Gore Flow Reversal Device (GORE)	X	X
	MO.MA (Medtronic Invatec)	X	X

Table 9.2 Carotid artery stent systems

Carotid artery stents			
Stent design	Product	FDA approval	CE mark
Closed cell—woven	Carotid Wallstent (Boston)	X	X
Closed cell	Xact (Abbott)	X	X
	Adapt (Boston)		X
Open cell	Acculink (Guidant/Abbott)	X	X
	Precise (Cordis)	X	X
	Protégé (ev3)	X	X
	ViVEXX (Bard)		X
	Zilver (Cook)		X
	Sinus (Optimed)		X
Hybrid	Cristallo Ideale (Medtronic Invatec)		X

12 Outcomes

In 2003, Wholey et al. published a summary of the results of 12,392 carotid stent implantations in a total of 11,243 patients from 53 centers worldwide. The complications during the first 30 days included: TIA (3.1%), minor stroke (2.1%), major stroke (1.2%), and death (0.6%) [3]. In the same year, Cremonesi et al. published a series of 442 consecutive patients treated with carotid stent implantation with embolic protection. Stroke or death occurred within the first month after the procedure in 1.1% of these patients [4]. The German Association for Angiology and Radiology has developed a prospective registry for carotid stent implantations. The results for the first 48 months, from a total of 38 participating centers, were published in 2004. Carotid stent implantation was carried out in 3,267 patients. The procedure was successful in 98% of the interventions. The peri-interventional mortality was 0.6%, the major stroke rate was 1.2%, and the minor stroke rate was 1.3%. In 2005, Bosiers et al. published the ELOCAS Registry, compiled retrospectively and prospectively from the results of four high-volume centers. A total of 2,172 consecutive patients were treated and 99.7% of the procedures were technically successful. The stroke/death rate was 4.1% after 1 year, 10.1% after 3 years, and 15.5% after 5 years [5]. The CaRESS study was a nonrandomized multicenter study including 143 patients treated with carotid stent implantation and 254 patients who underwent carotid endarterectomy. No significant differences were observed with regard to the stroke/death rates either after 30 days (2.1% stent, 3.6% surgery) or after 1 year (10% stent, 13.6% surgery) (CaRESS 2005). The ARCHeR study was published by Gray et al. in 2006 and consisted of three sequential multicenter studies. In ARCHeR 1, only the use of the Acculink carotid stent was evaluated. In the two subsequent studies (ARCHeR 2 and 3), adjuvant use of the Accunet embolic protection system was also tested. A total of 581 patients with high surgical risk from 48 centers were included between 2000 and 2003. The combined stroke/death/myocardial infarction rate was 8.3% after 30 days. The ipsilateral stroke death rate after the first month and up to 1 year was 1.8%. The repeat stenosis rate was 2.2% within the first year [6]. The CAPTURE Registry/Carotid Acculink/Accunet Post-Approval Trial to Uncover Unanticipated or Rare Events) was published in 2007. A total of 3,500 patients with high surgical risk and a stenosis grade > 50% (symptomatic) or > 80% (asymptomatic) were included. The major stroke/death rate after 30 days was 2.9%. In 2008, Stabile et al. presented the results of the European Registry of Carotid Artery Stenting (ERCAS)—a retrospective analysis of 1,611 consecutive neuro-protected carotid interventions in eight European high-volume centers. All procedures were technically successful and the combined stroke and death rate at 30 days was 1.36%. The results of the EPIC trial (Evaluating the Use of the FiberNet Embolic Protection System in Carotid Artery Stenting) were presented by Myla et al. in 2008. Two hundred thirty-seven patients at high risk for carotid surgery were treated in 26 centers using the FiberNet device for embolic protection. The combined 30-day stroke/death/myocardial infarction rate was 3.0%. In the same year, Hopkins et al. presented the results of the EMPiRE trial (Embolic Protection with Flow Reversal using the GORE Flow Reversal System), which enrolled 245 patients at 28 US sites. The 30-day any stroke or death rate was 2.9% and the primary endpoint including TIA and myocardial infarction was reached in 4.5% of all cases. In 2009, the results of the ARMOUR trial were announced by Hopkins et al. This trial evaluated proximal occlusion with the MO.MA device during carotid stenting in patients at high risk for surgery. The primary endpoint of the study, the rate of major adverse cardiac and cerebrovascular events at 30 days, was 2.7%.

In 2010, *CREST (The Carotid Revascularization Endarterectomy vs. Stenting Trial)*, the largest randomized clinical trial comparing the efficacy of carotid stenting to carotid endarterectomy, could show equivalence between interventional and surgical treatment of carotid stenoses. This trial enrolled 2,522 patients across North America and is the most important data set in a long series of trials that have shown over the last 15 years that carotid stenting has gotten better over time. In CREST, the primary endpoint was composite occurrence of stroke, myocardial infarction, or death from any cause during the 30-day periprocedural period or any postprocedural ipsilateral stroke within 4 years of randomization. The combined primary endpoint demonstrated equivalence between CAS and CEA (7.2% vs. 6.8%; $p=0.51$ for stroke, death, MI, or long-term [4 years] ipsilateral stroke event). The rates of major stroke for CAS and CEA were approximately equal (0.9% vs 0.6%; $p=0.52$), the rate of minor stroke for CAS exceeded that for CEA (total 4.1% vs. total 2.3%; $p=0.01$). CAS was superior to CEA with respect to the incidence of periprocedural MI (1.1% vs 2.3%; $p=0.03$). In addition, cranial nerve palsies were less frequent during the periprocedural period with CAS (0.3% vs 4.7% with CEA; hazard ratio, 0.07; 95% confidence interval, 0.02–0.18). There was no differential treatment effect with regard to the primary endpoint according to symptomatic status.

13   Differential Diagnosis of Atherosclerotic Carotid Disease

Although the following diseases are not frequent, it is important to know which etiological differential diagnosis of atherosclerotic carotid disease exist:

– Fibromuscular dysplasia: The most common non-traumatic, non-atherosclerotic, non-inflammatory lesion of the internal carotid artery is estimated to be 0.02%. The preferred treatment for refractory cases is percutaneous balloon angioplasty. If the arterial wall is damaged or weakened, then stenting of the affected artery may be chosen. Besides high blood pressure control, anti-platelet drugs and blood thinner drugs may be used. Bypass surgery is a considered treatment.

- Vasulitis (e.g., Takayasu's disease): The mainstay of therapy are glucocorticoids. Angioplasty or bypass grafts may be necessary once irreversible arterial stenosis has occurred.
- Thoracic outlet syndrome: Should be treated initially with physical therapy, but may require interventional stent angioplasty or even surgical decompression, including first rib excision and scalenectomy.
- Traumatic injuries: Interventional or surgical treatment is indicated in patients with traumatic carotid artery dissection and hemodynamic significant hemispheric hypoperfusion, or in whom anticoagulant therapy was either contraindicated or failed clinically.
- Vasospastic disorders: Since vasospasms can contribute to the severity of ischemia, percutaneous interventions and stent angioplasty may be indicated.

14   Carotid Artery Aneurysm

Aneurysms of the extracranial carotid arteries are rare. They may cause cerebral embolism. The location of the aneurysm often makes surgical correction difficult and leads to perioperative lower cranial nerve injuries and neurological deficits. Endovascular interventions using uncovered stents are effective in treating dissecting aneurysm with intimal flap or small defects in the arterial wall as the stent mesh impedes flow into the aneurysmal sac, inducing thrombosis, or relocating the intimal flap to occlude the aneurysm. However, flow into wide-necked aneurysms is difficult to exclude with an uncovered stent, so that coil embolization of the sac through the stent is often required. Wide-necked saccular aneurysms or pseudoaneurysms can be more appropriately treated with a covered stent (e.g., Hemobahn), leading to immediate and definitive reconstruction of the arterial wall.

Covered stents have been used in the subclavian and common carotid location for pseudoaneuryms related to trauma with excellent long-term results. A bare stent does not pose a good alternative, as it cannot completely eliminate the risk of embolization since the aneurysm would still communicate with the true lumen through the stent struts. Potential limitations of a covered stent include larger delivery systems compared to bare stents and the need for technical expertise for appropriate delivery.

15 Carotid Artery Dissection

The incidence of spontaneous carotid dissection has been reported to be up to 2.6 per 100,000 and is responsible for up to 20% of strokes in the younger population. Advantages of an endovascular therapy of carotid dissections are that it enables the identification of the true and false lumens by superselective catheterization and angiography, and further allows the recanalization of completely occluded vessels by use of microcatheter techniques, provided the thrombus burden is not prohibitive. Additionally, simultaneous treatment of any coexistent pseudoaneurysmal dilatation by the coil-through-stent technique is possible.

References

1. Bates ER, et al. ACCF/SCAI/SVMB/SIR/ASITN 2007 clinical expert consensus document on carotid stenting: a report of the American College of Cardiology Foundation Task Force on Clinical Expert Consensus Documents (ACCF/SCAI/SVMB/SIR/ASITN Clinical Expert Consensus Document Committee on Carotid Stenting). J Am Coll Cardiol. 2007;49:126–70.
2. Brott TG, Hobson RW, Howard G, Roubin GS, Clark WM, Brooks W, Mackey A, Hill MD, Leimgruber PP, Sheffet AJ, Howard VJ, Moore WS, Voeks JH, Hopkins LN, Cutlip DE, Cohen DJ, Popma JJ, Ferguson RD, Cohen SN, Blackshear JL, Silver FL, Mohr JP, Lal BK, Meschia JF, Investigators CREST. Stenting versus endarterectomy for treatment of carotid-artery stenosis. N Engl J Med. 2010;363(1):11–23.
3. Wholey MH, Al-Mubarek N, et al. Update review of the global carotid artery stent registry. Catheter Cardiovasc Interv. 2003;60(2):259–66.
4. Cremonesi A, Manetti R, Setacci F, Setacci C, Castriota F. Protected carotid stenting: clinical advantages and complications of embolic protection devices in 442 consecutive patients. Stroke. 2003 Aug;34(8):1936–41.
5. Bosiers M, Peeters P, Deloose K, et al. Does carotid artery stenting work on the long run: 5 year-results in high-volume centers (ELOCAS registry). J Cardiovasc Surg (Torino). 2005;46(3):241–47.
6. Gray WA, Hopkins LN, Yadav S, Davis T, Wholey M, Atkinson R, Cremonesi A, Fairman R, Walker G, Verta P, Popma J, Virmani R, Cohen DJ; ARCHeR Trial Collaborators. Protected carotid stenting in high-surgical-risk patients: the ARCHeR results. J Vasc Surg. 2006 Aug;44(2):258–68.

Chapter 10
Endovascular Treatment of Acute Ischemic Stroke

Marc Ribo, Marta Rubiera, and Andrei V. Alexandrov

1 Introduction

Despite heterogeneity of stroke mechanisms, one challenge remains across all reperfusion therapies—the persistence of a proximal arterial occlusion. Thrombus burden in stroke patients is often disproportionately larger than allowed doses of systemic thrombolytic, and many patients do not recover during or shortly after treatment. Moreover, a substantial proportion of patients arrive beyond currently established time frame for systemic thrombolytic, thus necessitating our search for effective and direct ways of dissolving or removing the thrombus from cerebral vessels. This chapter will discuss specifics how endovascular approach can be utilized for stroke treatment.

M. Ribo, M.D. • M. Rubiera, M.D.
Stroke Unit, Neurology Department, Hospital Universitari Vall d'Hebron,
Ps. Vall d'Hebron, 119-129, 08035-Barcelona, Spain
e-mail: marcriboj@hotmail.com; mrubifu@hotmail.com

A.V. Alexandrov, M.D. (✉)
Comprehensive Stroke Center, University of Alabama Hospital,
M226 RWUH, 1813 6th Avenue, Birmingham, AL 35249, USA
e-mail: avalexandrov@att.net

A. Kumar and K. Ouriel (eds.), *Handbook of Endovascular Interventions*, 131
DOI 10.1007/978-1-4614-5013-9_10,
© Springer Science+Business Media New York 2013

2   Anatomy

The arteries commonly obstructed in the main stroke syndromes are the ones which constitute the circle of Willis. These can be divided in to two main groups:

1. *Anterior Circulation*: Including the intracranial internal carotid artery (ICA), this divides in the anterior cerebral artery (ACA) and the middle cerebral artery (MCA) in both sides. Usually there is a communication between both left and right sides by the anterior communicating artery (Acom).
2. *Posterior Circulation*: Including the vertebral arteries (VA) from both sides, which conflux in the basilar artery (BA) on the anterior surface of the brainstem. The BA divides in the two posterior cerebral arteries (PCA).

   There is also a communication between both anterior and posterior circulation by the right and left posterior communicating arteries (Pcom).

   Anatomic variations in the cerebral circulation are very common, and only in about 15 % of cases the cerebral circulation is complete as described previously. Some of the most common anatomic variations are:
3. *Fetal Anterior Circulation*: Both ACAs arise from the same ICA and divide distally by the Acom.
4. *Fetal Posterior Circulation*: The PCA arises from the ICA by the ipsilateral Pcom instead of from the BA.
5. Frequently, some of the communicating arteries (anterior or posterior) from the circle of Willis are hypoplasic or absent. Also, there is very frequently an asymmetry between both VA, being one of them hypoplasic or ending in the cerebellar arteries instead of the BA. In this case, all the posterior circulation may depend on the VA from one side.

3   Diagnosis: Clinical

The ischemic stroke is defined by the occlusion of an intracranial artery. It can be caused by the occlusion of a small penetrating artery, causing the lacunar strokes (about 20 % of ischemic strokes), or the occlusion of one or several arteries from the circle of Willis, causing the devastating large artery stroke syndromes. The large artery strokes usually are caused by an occluding embolus from the extracranial ICA (40 %) or the heart cavities (30 %) or, less frequently, because of the acute complication of an in site atherosclerotic plaque (10 %). These rates may change depending on geographical or ethnical aspects (i.e., high prevalence of intracranial atherosclerosis in Asians and Blacks).

The main objective of the acute stroke treatment is to reperfuse the ischemic brain tissue before the ischemic damage becomes irreversible, allowing an improvement or even a complete resolution of the clinical symptoms of stroke. However, the brain tissue is very sensitive to ischemia, and treatment initiation should be attempted before 4.5 h with systemic thrombolytic (intravenous tissue plasminogen activator (tPA)) or before 6–8 h with endovascular reperfusion procedures (only for the large artery strokes). This timeframe may vary depending on many factors such as the quality of collateral circulation, tissue and perfusion appearance on brain imaging, body temperature, glucose levels, etc.

4 Diagnosis: Imaging

The first step in the diagnosis of a suspected acute stroke is the clinical evaluation aimed to determine occurrence of a neurological deficit, and its disabling nature if it persists. An objective tool such as the National Institute of Health Stroke Scale (NIHSS) is often used to grade and monitor the neurological symptoms of the patient. Then, neuroimaging is required to rule out a hemorrhagic stroke, which during the first 4.5 h from symptoms' onset can rapidly be performed by a *non-contrast* computerized tomography (CT) scan. A CT scan can also detect the presence of early ischemic signs that can further increase suspicion of an acute lesion or a thrombus (i.e., hyperdense MCA sign). These signs, if present within 4.5 h of symptom onset, should not preclude administration of systemic tPA in eligible patients. After 4.5 h, the decision to initiate reperfusion treatments should be considered with more information about the state of the ischemic brain.

Multimodal magnetic resonance imaging (MRI) or CT perfusion/ angio CT allows one to obtain simultaneous information about vessel patency and the degree of ischemia and tissue damage. These multimodal and improved neuroimaging techniques offer the possibility to assess the mismatch area between the irreversibly infarcted tissue and the still salvageable penumbra (tissue at risk until recanalization is achieved).

Transcranial Doppler or Echo-Doppler ultrasound may also help when vascular neuroimaging is not available. This non-invasive technique may detect the presence of an intracranial occlusion and allows continuous monitoring of the vessel state at the patient bed-side. Moreover, continuous insonation of the clot has shown to enhance the thrombolytic effect of tPA achieving complete recanalization earlier.

5 Diagnostic Imaging: Algorithm

6 Management: Medical/Non-Operative/ Non-Intervention

During the first 4.5 h from symptoms' onset, the majority of patients with an acute intracranial occlusion may benefit from the systemic thrombolytic treatment. In about 40 % of cases, iv tPA induces an early recanalization of the occluded vessel, leading to clinical improvement.

Intravenous tPA is therefore a powerful measure that unfortunately has a strict time window and numerous contraindications. Thus, it is currently administered to no more than 10–15 % of all ischemic stroke patients (in some countries this number may fall to as low as 3 % while the range for reported individual hospital utilization rates is 0–33 %). There are other medical measures that are applicable and necessary to keep in mind for all stroke patients: correct management of blood pressure, glycemic and body temperature control.

7 Intervention

In 4.5 to 6–8 h time window (or until 12 h in BA occlusions), or in those patients with contra-indications for systemic thrombolysis (recent surgery, anticoagulant treatment), there is an increasing evidence for primary endovascular reperfusion techniques as being preferred intervention for stroke. Furthermore, those patients treated with iv tPA with lack of recanalization at the end of the tPA perfusion may benefit from an endovascular rescue treatment (bridging IV-IA therapy).

There are two options for the endovascular treatment of acute stroke:

6. Pharmacological: intra-arterial application of tPA, usually associated with mechanical wire disruption of the thrombus (the intra-arterial tPA application usually is administered until 6 h after stroke symptoms' onset)
7. Mechanical endovascular application of devices designed for intracranial thrombectomy (these treatments are available until 8 h from stroke onset). The devices currently accepted for acute stroke are:

   (a) Multi-MERCI® catheter: corkscrew-like apparatus able to be lodged in the clot and withdrawn from the vessel;
   (b) PENUMBRA® catheter: continuous aspiration catheter with a proximal occluding balloon, able to extract the thrombus by aspiration;
   (c) SOLITAIRE® catheter: self-expanding stent able to be fully deployed and then completely retrieved with the embedded clot.

Neuro-interventionalist usually chooses the endovascular reperfusion technique according to personal preferences, and very frequently combines both pharmacological and mechanical treatment, and/or two or more different mechanical devices in the same patient.

The Thrombolysis In Myocardial Infarction (TIMI) scale is used to register the location and degree of occlusion and subsequent recanalization (Table 10.2). The majority of clinical trials consider partial recanalization when TIMI 2a score is achieved, while complete recanalization implies a final TIMI score of 2b or 3.

8 Technique and Pitfalls

8. Usually, conscious sedation should be enough to perform the endovascular procedure and recent studies discourage elective intubation and mechanical ventilation for the endovascular treatment of acute ischemic stroke.

Table 10.1 Qureshi grading scale of severity of occlusion and state of collateral circulation in acute ischemic stroke

Grade	Type of occlusion		
0	No occlusion		
1	MCA occlusion (M3)	ACA occlusion (A2 or distal segments)	1 BA and/or VA branch occlusion
2	MCA occlusion (M2)	ACA occlusion (A1 and A2)	≥2 BA and/or VA branch occlusion
3	MCA occlusion (M1)		
3a	Lenticulostriate arteries spared and/or leptomeningeal collaterals visualized		
3b	No sparing of lenticulostriate arteries and no leptomeningeal collaterals visualized		
4	ICA occlusion (collaterals present)	BA occlusion (partial filling, direct or via collaterals)	
4a	Collaterals fill MCA	Anterograde filling	
4b	Collaterals fill ACA	Retrograde filling	
5	ICA occlusion (no collaterals)	BA occlusion (complete)	

9. The procedure of setting up to do a cerebrovascular intervention is quite similar to doing a carotid intervention, using an 8 French sheath with a similar sized guiding catheter (see Chap. 9).

10. In order to save time, we initially only perform an angiogram of the affected artery, primarily advancing the guiding catheter to the affected carotid or vertebral artery. Then, this guiding catheter will be used to rapidly advance the micro catheter or the selected device up to the arterial occlusion site.

11. It is useful to assess in the initial angiogram the presence of collateral flow using the Qureshi scale (Table 10.1). Good collateral flow has been associated with smaller final infarct and better outcome.

12. During the procedure, the interventionalist should be constantly balancing the possible benefits and harms of pursuing recanalization depending on the elapsed time and the amount of lytics and devices used.

13. Finally, the use of contrast should also be taken into account. Specially when administered through the micro catheter distal to the occlusion, contrast seems to increase the odds of hemorrhagic transformation (HT).

9 Post-Procedure Management and Follow-up Protocol

At the end of the procedure, the patient should be transferred to a Stroke Unit or Neurointensive Care Unit where strict control of blood pressure and glycemia are required. Successive NIHSS examinations may detect neurological deterioration indicating complications of the treatment. We also deploy TCD follow-up assessments of vessel patency to detect hyperemic reperfusion, re-occlusion, or impaired vasomotor reactivity—findings helpful to control blood pressure, decide on the need for an additional intervention, and ventilator management.

At 24 h from symptom onset, or if clinical deterioration occurs anytime, a repeat or new neuroimaging examination should be performed. This will allow determination of the infarct volume and possible complications such as HT or brain edema. Initiation of antithrombotic treatment for secondary prevention should be delayed until this second image is obtained, except in cases where a stent was deployed in which early use of anti-platelets is required to avoid in-stent reocclusion.

10 Intracranial Angioplasty and Stenting

In the last few years, development of intracranial stents is continuously increasing for the treatment of intracranial stenosis as well as acute occlusions. Several clinical trials are evaluating their efficacy in long-term outcome of intracranial atherosclerotic disease and the utility of retrievable stents for acute reperfusion. The indications about when an intracranial stenosis should be stented (i.e., after first event or after recurrence) are still to be defined.

Treatment of acute intracranial occlusions or severe symptomatic intracranial stenosis with angioplasty (with or without stenting) shows promising results. Angioplasty without stenting is probably associated with a high risk of re-stenosis or reocclusion.

11   Complications of Endovascular Treatment

The complications of the endovascular treatment of stroke can be related to the stroke itself or the vascular manipulation.

Stroke Complications

(a) Symptomatic intracranial hemorrhage (sICH): it is probably the most feared complication of reperfusion treatment of acute ischemic stroke. Some hemorrhagic transformations (HTs) are asymptomatic, and may even be related to recanalization. These HTs do not imply a worse clinical evolution and some authors even associate them with a better outcome. On the other hand, sICH is associated with high mortality and worse clinical outcome. If sICH has occurred (confirmed by neuroimaging and clinical evaluation), fresh frozen plasma or coagulation factors can be administered. Poor outcomes are generally expected despite this treatment since sICH often occurs with most severe strokes at baseline. Probably, a very strict control of blood pressure may be the best way of preventing sICH.

(b) Reocclusion: Up to 15–20 % of patients with early recanalization may experience reocclusion, some of them symptomatic. Reocclusion can be found more frequently in partial recanalizations and patients with atherothrombotic tandem extra/intracranial disease. There are some case reports of repeated endovascular reperfusion therapies applied after early reocclusion, but probably the best treatment is to prevent this complication. Some patients with higher risk of reocclusion may benefit from early administration of antithrombotic drugs as glycoprotein IIb-IIIa inhibitors or heparin, or stenting.

(c) Brain edema: In some patients, lack of recanalization or very late recanalization induces high-volume infarcts with brain edema and mass effect. The only treatment that has demonstrated an improvement in mortality and functional outcome is decompressive hemicraniectomy. This may be an option in selected patients with so-called malignant MCA syndrome. Large cerebellar strokes should be evaluated for posterior fossa craniotomy.

Vascular Manipulation

(a) Access site hematoma: is a relatively frequent complication, as the sheath used for stroke treatment is necessarily large

(7–8 French). After extracting the sheath, a good compressive bandage or sealing devices are required.

(b) Arterial vasospasm: advancing a catheter in the intracranial arteries may induce arterial vasospasm. Local administration of vasodilators usually resolves the problem with no further complications. If this is not effective, angioplasty of the narrowed segment may be performed.

(c) Arterial dissection or rupture: this is a feared complication of endovascular treatment. If rupture occurs, arterial exclusion may be performed to stop bleeding, but the prognosis is poor.

12   Outcomes

The evaluation of outcomes in endovascular reperfusion therapies for acute stroke can be focused on recanalization (AOL scale) (Table 10.2), reperfusion (TIMI scale), or clinical outcome. Early clinical evolution (at 24 h and discharge) should be monitored using the NIHSS. Functional long-term outcome is usually determined by the modified Rankin Scale (mRS) score. Good functional outcome usually is defined as mRS < 3 (no symptoms, minimal symptoms, or ability to take care of daily needs despite symptoms).

Table 10.2 Thrombolysis in myocardial infarction (TIMI) reperfusion scale and arterial occlusive lesion (AOL) recanalization scale for endovascular procedures in acute ischemic stroke

TIMI scale		AOL scale	
0	No perfusion	0	No recanalization of the primary occlusive lesion
1	Perfusion past the initial occlusion, but no distal branch filling	1	Incomplete or partial recanalization of the primary occlusive lesion with no distal flow
2	Perfusion with incomplete branch filling:	2	Incomplete or partial recanalization of the primary occlusive lesion with any distal flow
2a	Only partial filling (>2/3 of entire territory visualized)		
2b	Complete filling of all the territory with filling slower than normal		
3	Full perfusion with filling of all distal branches, including M3,4	3	Complete recanalization of the primary occlusion with any distal flow

Clinical trials in endovascular treatment of acute ischemic stroke show recanalization rates of up to 60–80 %, but good functional outcomes of 30–50 % depending of the series. Mortality is up to 25–30 % in most published series. Randomized studies of new devices are lacking.

13   Pharmacy of Management of Acute Stroke

During the first 4.5 h from symptoms' onset, intravenous thrombolysis with tPA (0.9 mg/kg) should be administered to all acute ischemic strokes without contraindication for this treatment.

Intravenous heparin is not recommended for acute stroke treatment; however, it can be used during endovascular procedures to prevent catheter-related thrombosis.

In patients receiving thrombolytic treatment (IV or IA) or mechanical reperfusion procedures, antithrombotic treatments should be delayed until a second neuroimaging test rules out an intracranial hemorrhage. In general, if the etiology of stroke is cardioembolic or a dissection and the final infarct volume is small, early anticoagulation with low molecular weight heparin or unfractionated heparin could be started. In the remaining cases, antithrombotic treatment with aspirin or clopidogrel is indicated.

Early anti-platelet treatment with systemic GP IIb-IIIa inhibitors or a combination of aspirin and clopidogrel could be an option in patients with high risk of reocclusion or intracranial stents.

Antihypertensive drugs, insulin, deep-venous thrombosis-preventive drugs, etc., should not be forgotten in these patients.

Papers to Read

1. Furlan A, Higashida R, Wechsler L, Gent M, Rowley H, Kase C, Pessin M, Ahuja A, Callahan F, Clark WM, Silver F, Rivera F. Intra-arterial prourokinase for acute ischemic stroke. The PROACT II study: A randomized controlled trial. Prolyse in acute cerebral thromboembolism. JAMA. 1999;282: 2003–11.
2. The interventional management of stroke (IMS) II study. Stroke 2007;38: 2127–2135

3. Adams Jr HP, del Zoppo G, Alberts MJ, Bhatt DL, Brass L, Furlan A, Grubb RL, Higashida RT, Jauch EC, Kidwell C, Lyden PD, Morgenstern LB, Qureshi AI, Rosenwasser RH, Scott PA, Wijdicks EF. Guidelines for the early management of adults with ischemic stroke: A guideline from the American Heart Association/American Stroke Association stroke council, clinical cardiology council, cardiovascular radiology and intervention council, and the atherosclerotic peripheral vascular disease and quality of care outcomes in research interdisciplinary working groups: The American Academy of Neurology affirms the value of this guideline as an educational tool for neurologists. Stroke. 2007;38:1655–711.

4. Smith WS, Sung G, Saver J, Budzik R, Duckwiler G, Liebeskind DS, Lutsep HL, Rymer MM, Higashida RT, Starkman S, Gobin YP, Frei D, Grobelny T, Hellinger F, Huddle D, Kidwell C, Koroshetz W, Marks M, Nesbit G, Silverman IE. Mechanical thrombectomy for acute ischemic stroke: final results of the multi MERCI trial. Stroke. 2008;39:1205–12.

5. The Penumbra Pivotal Stroke Trial Investigators. The Penumbra pivotal stroke trial: Safety and effectiveness of a new generation of mechanical devices for clot removal in intracranial large vessel occlusive disease. Stroke. 2009;40:2761–8.

6. Rubiera M, Cava L, Tsivgoulis G, Patterson DE, Zhao L, Zhang Y, Anderson AM, Robinson A, Harrigan M, Horton J, Alexandrov AV. Diagnostic criteria and yield of real time transcranial Doppler (TCD) monitoring of intra-arterial (IA) reperfusion procedures. Stroke. 2010;41:695–9.

7. Qureshi AI, Siddiqi AM, Kim SH, Hanel RA, Xavier AR, Kirmani JF, Fareed M, Suri K, Boulos AS, Hopkins LN. Reocclusion of recanalized arteries during intra-arterial thrombolysis for acute ischemic stroke. Am J Neuroradiol. 2004;25:322–8.

8. Khatri P, Neff J, Broderick JP, Khoury JC, Carrozzella J, Tomsick T for the IMS-1 Investigators. Revascularization end points in stroke interventional trials. Recanalization versus reperfusion in IMS-I. Stroke 2005; 36:2400–2403

9. Saver JL, Jahan R, Levy EI, Jovin TG, Baxter B, Nogueira RG, Clark W, BudzikR, Zaidat OO; for the SWIFT Trialists. Solitaire flow restoration device versusthe Merci Retriever in patients with acute ischaemic stroke (SWIFT): arandomised, parallel-group, non-inferiority trial. Lancet 2012 doi:10.1016/S0140-6736(12)61384-1

10. Nogueira RG, Lutsep HL, Gupta R, Jovin T, Albers GW, Walker GA, Liebeskind DS, Smith WS. Trevo versus Merci retrievers for thrombectomy revascularisation of large vessel occlusions in acute ischaemic stroke (TREVO 2): a randomised trial. Lancet 2012 doi:10.1016/S0140-6736(12)61299-9

Chapter 11
Cerebral Protection Devices

Juan C. Parodi and Claudio Schönholz

1 Introduction

Carotid angioplasty and stenting is an alternative to carotid endart-erectomy in the treatment of carotid artery stenosis. During the stenting process, however, distal embolization usually occurs, and the particles released may cause neurologic problems or death. Thus, the safety of carotid stenting depends partly on the use of a cerebral protection device during the procedure.

In the past decade, several different techniques and devices designed to prevent cerebral damage associated with embolization have been developed (Table 11.1). The principal types of cerebral protection devices are occlusion balloons, distal filters, and flow reversal mechanisms [1]. The following discussion pertains to the use of these different protection devices.

J.C. Parodi, M.D. (✉)
Department of Vascular Surgery, Trinidad Hospital, Don Bosco 3231,
Buenos Aires 1642 4735231, Argentina
e-mail:parodijc@yahoo.com

C. Schönholz, M.D.
Department of Radiology, Medical University of South Carolina,
Charleston, SC, USA

A. Kumar and K. Ouriel (eds.), *Handbook of Endovascular Interventions*,   143
DOI 10.1007/978-1-4614-5013-9_11,
© Springer Science+Business Media New York 2013

Table 11.1 Cerebral protection devices and manufacturer

Distal occlusion balloons
– Theron triple coaxial catheter
– PercuSurge GuardWire
(Medtronic Vascular, Santa Rosa, CA)
Distal filters
– AngioGuard RX/AngioGuard XP
(Cordis Endovascular, Miami Lakes, FL)
– RX Accunet
(Guidant, Indianapolis, IN)
– FilterWire EZ/FilterWire EX
(Boston Scientific, Santa Clara, CA)
– MedNova NeuroShield/MedNova EmboShield
(Abbott Vascular Devices, Abbott Park, IL)
– Spider/SpideRX
(ev3, Plymouth, MA)
– FiberNet Embolic Protection System (EPS)
(Lumen Biomedical Inc., Plymouth, MN)
Proximal occlusion devices with or without reversal of flow
– Flow Reversal System
(W.L. Gore & Associates, Flagstaff, AZ)
– MO.MA
(Invatec, Roncadelle, Italy)

2 PercuSurge GuardWire (Fig. 11.1)

The PercuSurge GuardWire device (Medtronic Vascular, Santa Rosa, CA) provides temporary occlusion of the internal carotid artery (ICA) and aspiration of particles after CAS. The device has three components: an exchange guidewire, a microseal adapter, and a monorail aspiration catheter. The wire is a 0.014- or 0.018-in. angioplasty-style device with a segment that consists of a hollow hypotube made of nitinol. The distal segment of the wire is shapeable, radiopaque, and steerable. Just proximal to the distal segment is an elastomeric latex balloon capable of occluding blood flow when inflated. The proximal end of the hypotube wire incorporates a moveable seal that allows inflation and deflation of the balloon by means of the detachable adapter. After the distal tip is shaped, the guidewire is advanced through the guide catheter under fluoroscopic guidance. The wire is steered through the carotid stenosis and advanced at least 3 cm beyond the target lesion. The predilatation balloon is then

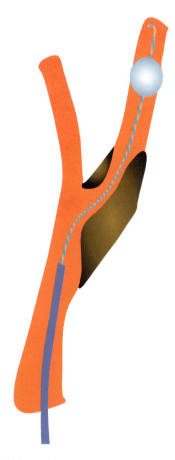

Fig. 11.1 Distal Occlusion Device

passed over the wire into the distal guiding catheter. The microseals'
adapter is attached, and the balloon is inflated to a diameter of
5.5 mm. Contrast is injected to confirm complete occlusion of distal
blood flow [2, 3].

   If flow is observed, an additional 0.5 ml of diluted contrast agent
is added to enlarge the balloon until complete occlusion is achieved.
The microseal is then closed and the adapter removed. The predilatation balloon is passed across the lesion, inflated, deflated, and
removed. The carotid stent is placed over the guidewire and deployed
in the lesion. The stent delivery system is removed, and the post dilatation balloon is passed over the guidewire into the lesion, inflated,

Table 11.2 Distal occlusion balloon

Pros:	• Low Crossing Profile
Cons:	• No protection during initial passage
	• Interruption of flow during protection
	• Inability to perform angiography during procedure
	• Difficulties in crossing tight and/or tortuous lesions
	• Potential to cause spasm and dissection in the distal ICA
	• Potential for particles to embolize to the brain via patent external carotid circulation.
	• Intolerance

deflated, and removed. An Export aspiration catheter with a monorail design (Medtronic Vascular) is inserted up to the level of the distal occlusion balloon. Blood (15–45 mL) is aspirated from the area between the carotid artery bifurcation and the balloon. The aspiration catheter is then removed, and the occlusion balloon is deflated, restoring antegrade flow (Table 11.2).

3   Filters (Fig. 11.2)

Filtering cerebral protection devices are the most commonly used systems to prevent cerebral embolism during carotid stenting procedures [4]. The devices are, in general, sophisticated in construction, but the protection is based on a simple concept of trapping downstream larger particles of debris capable of causing cerebral ischemia. Most of the devices are calibrated to filter particles larger than 100 μm, allowing blood flow to continue during the procedure. At the time of this document being written, there are six FDA-approved filtering devices for carotid stenting in the United States:

1. Angioguard
2. Accunet
3. Filter Wire
4. EmboShield
5. FiberNet
6. SpideRX

The Angioguard, Accunet, FilterWire, and FiberNet have the filters attached to the working wire, while in the other devices the filter is deployed over the wire already in place. The filter devices are

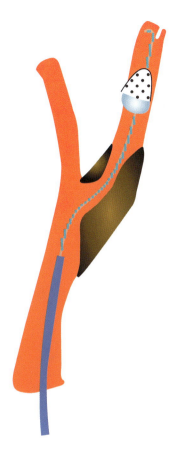

Fig. 11.2 Filters

deployed above the stenosis after passing through the lesion and apposed to the ICA wall. Following the procedure, a recovery sheath recaptures the filters. The carotid flow is maintained throughout the procedure allowing test injections to identify the location of the lesion and proper stent placement. A potential shortcoming of the filter protection technique is the need to cross beyond the stenosis unprotected, and some of the filters have larger crossing profile than the occlusion balloons, potentially increasing the risks. Most of the filters need a longer landing zone above the lesion, which can be problematic in tortuous internal carotids and distal lesions, reducing apposition to the vessel wall, which may lead to embolism around the

Table 11.3 Filters

Pros:	• Preservation of flow
	• Ability to perform angiogram during procedure
Cons:	• No protection during initial passage
	• Possibility of missing small particles
	• Potential for thrombosis of filter
	• Difficulties in crossing tight and/or tortuous lesion
	• Potential for spasm/dissection in distal ICA

device. In addition, concerns for embolism during recapture and retrieval of the filter should be assessed. The filters can promote spasm and/or dissection of the artery or may become occluded by the excessive volume of debris, as they are small devices with limited volumetric capacity. (Table 11.3)

4 Flow Reversal (Fig. 11.3)

The Flow reversal device is a closed system that allows arrest of ICA flow, continuous passive ICA flow reversal, or augmented active ICA flow reversal so that any particles released during CAS will pass retrograde through the catheter and be retrieved in the arteriovenous conduit filter outside the body. The three components of the device were designed specifically to allow retrograde flow in the ICA and minimize margination of particles or collection of material that could subsequently embolize [5].

The first component, the balloon sheath, is a 9.5 Fr, 90-cm-long guide catheter with a funnel-shaped balloon on its tip. This atraumatic balloon allows occlusion of the CCA and flow reversal. It also serves as the access port for the stent delivery system and other therapeutic devices. The second component, Balloon Wire, is a soft atraumatic oval balloon mounted on a 0.019-in. hypotube, which is a low-profile hollow guidewire that allows inflation of the balloon. The distal, shapeable, floppy guidewire facilitates navigation into the ECA. The third component, the external filter, is a conduit that connects the side flow reversal port of the system to a venous sheath.

The external filter has a 180-µm filter that collects particulate debris before the blood reenters the venous system. The first step in obtaining flow reversal is placement of the balloon sheath. This can

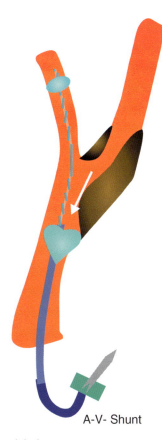

Fig. 11.3 Flow reversal device

be done by using any of the accepted techniques for guide catheter placement in the carotid artery. The balloon wire is then placed through the dedicated proximal port of the device and navigated under fluoroscopic guidance into the ECA as the second step. The third step is purging and attaching the external filter to a 6-F venous sheath. The venous sheath can be placed in the ipsilateral or contralateral femoral vein.

After the device has been positioned, the CCA is occluded with the balloon sheath and the balloon wire is inflated in the ECA. Opening the external filter stopcock initiates continuous flow reversal through the arteriovenous shunt. Patients are observed for evidence of intolerance to flow reversal, which may manifest as cloudiness of conscience, agitation, hemispheric deficit, or seizure. (Table 11.4)

Table 11.4 Flow Reversal

Pros:	• Protection prior to crossing lesion
	• No mechanical device in the distal ICA
	• Micro bubbles trapped in the stent delivery system are aspirated
	• Vulnerable lesions with thrombus may be treated
	• May treat tortuous lesions
Cons:	• Large profile sheath (9 FR)
	• Need for venous sheath placement
	• Intolerance to occlusion
	• Learning curve

4.1 MO.MA (Fig. 11.4)

The MO.MA device has a 100-cm-long catheter with a central lumen large enough for insertion of angioplasty instruments and other devices [6]. The exit port of the working channel is between two independently inflatable balloons that occlude the ECA and CCA. Antegrade flow is blocked before a guidewire crosses the lesion. Any debris resulting from the CAS procedure remains at the carotid bifurcation. The debris can be removed by aspiration with a syringe through the working channel at any time during the intervention (Table 11.5).

4.2 "Seat Belt and Air Bag" Technique (Fig. 11.5)

The seat belt and air bag technique (Fig. 11.5) is a two-device approach to cerebral protection during stenting of the ICA in patients with intolerance using proximal balloon occlusion systems. With use of a 260-cm exchange wire, a Flow reversal system or MO.MA device is placed in the CCA 3 cm below the carotid bifurcation. Flow reversal or occlusion is obtained by inflating balloons in the ECA and CCA. Through an external connector, a filter is delivered to the distal ICA while active suction from a syringe is applied to the guiding catheter. When the filter is beyond the stenosis, antegrade flow is re-established and CAS proceeds under cerebral protection provided by the filter. Theoretically, the simultaneous presence of two protection devices could yield results better than those obtained with either

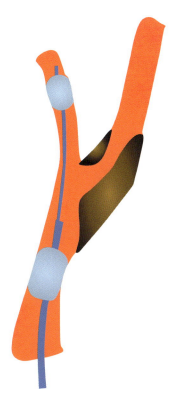

Fig. 11.4 MoMa device

Table 11.5 MO.MA

Pros:	• Lesion crossing protected
	• May treat tortuous lesions
	• May treat lesions with thrombus?
Cons:	• Standing column in the ICA without "active aspiration"
	• Effectively carotid cross-clamping
	• Bulky sheath
	• Cannot be used when there is occlusion of the ECA
	• Cannot be used in lesions of the CCA

device alone. Therefore, the seat belt and air bag approach may be found to represent the ideal means for treating ICA stenosis with a high risk of embolization or patients with a nonfunctioning circle of Willis who are intolerant to balloon occlusion or flow reversal [7].

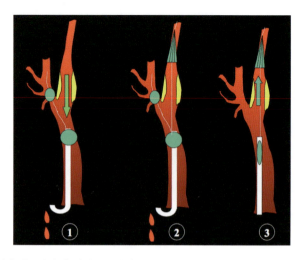

Fig. 11.5 Seat belt & air bag technique

References

1. Schönholz C, Uflacker R, Mendaro E, Parodi JC, Guimarães M, Hannegan C, Selby B. Techniques for carotid artery stenting under cerebral protection. J Cardiovasc Surg. 2005;46:201–17.
2. Whitlow PL, Lylyk P, Londero H, Mendiz O, Mathias K, Jaeger H, Parodi JC, Schönholz C, Milei J. Carotid artery stenting protected with an emboli containment system. Stroke. 2002;33:1308–14.
3. Parodi JC, LaMura R, Ferreira LM, Mendez MV, Cerosimo H, Schönholz C. Initial evaluation of carotid angioplasty and stenting with three different cerebral protection devices. J Vasc Surg. 2000;32(6):1127–36.
4. Uflacker R. How to optimize carotid artery stenting? J Cardiovasc Surg. 2007;48:131–49.
5. Parodi JC, Schönholz C, Parodi FE, Sicard G, Ferreira LM. Initial 200 cases of carotid artery stenting using a reversal-of-flow cerebral protection device. J Cardiovasc Surg (Torino). 2007;48(2):117–24.
6. Diederich K-W, Scheinert D, Schmidt A, Scheinert S, Reimers B, Sievert H, et al. First clinical experiences with an endovascular clamping system for neuroprotection during carotid stenting. Eur J Vasc Endovasc Surg. 2004;28:629–33.
7. Parodi JC, Schönholz C, Ferreira LM, Mendaro E, Ohki T. Seat belt and air bag technique for cerebral protection during carotid stenting. J Endovasc Ther. 2002;9:20–4.

Chapter 12
Vertebral Artery Disease

Jörg Ederle and Stefan Brew

1 Anatomy

The right vertebral artery forms the first branch of the right subclavian artery, which has its origin in the innominate artery. The left vertebral artery arises as the first branch from the left subclavian artery, which arises from the aortic arch.

The vertebral arteries are commonly divided into four parts:

- Prevertebral segment (V1): From the origin in the subclavian artery to the entrance of the transverse foramen at the level of the sixth cervical vertebral body.
- Cervical segment (V2): Passes through the transverse foramina.
- Atlantic segment (V3): Exits from the transverse foramen of C2, curves around the superior articular process of the atlas and enters the vertebral canal.

J. Ederle, Dr. med., Ph.D. (✉)
Stroke Research Group, UCL Institute of Neurology, Queen Square,
London, WC1N 3BG, UK
e-mail: J.Ederle@ion.ucl.ac.uk

S. Brew, M.B.Ch.B., M.Sc., M.H.B.(hons), FRANZCR
Lysholm Department of Neuroradiology, National Hospital for Neurology
and Neurosurgery, Queen Square, London, WC1N 3BG, UK

A. Kumar and K. Ouriel (eds.), *Handbook of Endovascular Interventions*,   153
DOI 10.1007/978-1-4614-5013-9_12,
© Springer Science+Business Media New York 2013

- Intracranial segment (V4): After entering through the foramen magnum, it pierces the dura mater to enter the cranial cavity where it joins with the contralateral vertebral artery to form the basilar artery.

Branches of the vertebral artery given off in the neck supply the spinal cord and the deep muscles of the neck. Intracranial branches include meningeal branches, the posterior and anterior spinal arteries, the posterior inferior cerebellar artery and the medullary arteries.

2 Anatomic Variations

The vertebral arteries are commonly asymmetrical in diameter. In the majority of cases, the left vertebral artery is dominant.

In rare instances, the left vertebral artery originates directly from the aortic arch or the external carotid artery.

The vertebral artery sometimes enters the transverse foramen of C5 or C7.

One vertebral artery may terminate in the posterior inferior cerebellar artery and the basilar artery will subsequently only be supplied by the contralateral vertebral artery.

3 Disease Definition

The causes of occlusive vertebral artery disease are manifold:

(a) Atherosclerosis (most commonly occurring in the V1 segment, but also in V3)
(b) Cervical spine trauma causing artery dissection (affecting the V2 segment)
(c) Degenerative disease of the cervical spine (affecting the intra-foraminal V2 segment)
(d) Head and neck tumours invading the blood vessel

Other extra-luminal causes may mimic occlusive vertebral disease:

(a) Thickened cervical bands (compression of V1)
(b) Subclavian steal syndrome (stenosis of the subclavian artery proximal to the origin of the vertebral artery)

4 Disease Distribution

Atherosclerosis in the vertebral artery is more common than in the carotid artery but only about 20 % of all strokes occur in the vertebro-basilar circulation. The incidence of atherosclerosis increases with age, and men are more commonly affected than women. Cervical artery dissection appears to be occurring predominantly under the age of 50.

The vertebral artery origin is the most common site for vertebral stenosis. However, ulcerated plaque is very rare.

5 Diagnosis

5.1 Clinical

Definitive diagnosis of symptomatic vertebral artery disease is difficult and a neurologist or physician with a special interest in stroke should be consulted prior to any decision for invasive treatment.

Occlusive vertebral artery disease presents with cerebrovascular symptoms (TIA or stroke) originating in the brain regions supplied by the vertebro-basilar system. Often the cranial nerve nuclei are involved and the pattern of bilateral distribution and cerebellar signs may help to distinguish posterior circulation symptoms from anterior circulation symptoms.

Vertebral artery dissection may present with pain in the occipital region, TIA or stroke, or cervical spine syndromes and is commonly associated with a history of trauma.

Disease processes in other vessels (e.g., subclavian steal syndrome) or extra-vascular pathology may mimic occlusive vertebral artery disease in addition to disease-specific presentation.

5.2 Laboratory

No laboratory investigations are specific to vertebral artery disease but may help in distinguishing stroke from metabolic causes and assessing vascular risk factors. They include full blood count, glucose, electrolytes, liver and renal function.

5.3   Imaging

- **Duplex ultrasound** often does not allow for a complete visualisation of the vertebral artery, though it may show the V1 segment and Doppler waveform may be useful.
- **CT** angiography has been shown to have a high sensitivity for detecting vertebral artery stenosis. The anatomy may be reconstructed with post-processing software.
- **Contrast-enhanced MRI** has a slightly higher sensitivity than CTA in detecting moderate to severe vertebral artery stenosis. It is more time consuming and some patients may not be eligible for MRI. CT, MRI and ultrasound have the advantage of visualising the vasculature as well as surrounding tissue. Special sequences may be helpful to investigate possible dissection. MRI of the vertebral artery origin is often prone to artefacts mimicking stenosis.
- **Diagnostic angiography** is the investigation of choice for the confirmation of occlusive vertebral artery disease but carries up to 2 % risk of iatrogenic stroke. It is increasingly limited to confirming suspicions of occlusive disease raised by non-invasive imaging and resolving discrepancies between different non-invasive investigations. A complete investigation encompasses imaging the collateral circulation, including the carotid arteries. Imaging of the contralateral vertebral artery is particularly important to assess the pattern of fusion of the vertebro-basilar junction.

The definite diagnosis of dissection should only be made if intramural haematoma, two lumina or an intimal flap have been demonstrated on imaging. Subclavian steal requires imaging of the proximal subclavian and innominate arteries. Thickened cervical bands may be investigated with dynamic angiography (head rotation and/or arm elevation).

Structural brain imaging is essential to confirm cerebrovascular symptoms. DWI is useful for detecting recent ischaemia.

6   Management

Medical management of atherosclerotic disease in general includes risk factor control (hypertension, hypercholesterolaemia, smoking) and anti-thrombotic treatment and also applies to vertebral artery disease.

There is no consensus on best medical management of patients with vertebral dissection and local guidelines need to be consulted.

Invasive treatment of atherosclerotic vertebral disease depends on underlying pathology and should be considered in symptomatic patients with recurrent symptoms despite maximal medical therapy.

6.1 Intervention: Technique and Pitfalls

6.1.1 Pre Procedure

It is vital that all patients are assessed prior to the procedure by a neurologist or physician with a special interest in stroke medicine to ensure that the stenosis is symptomatic and that medical therapy has been optimised. All patients should be on dual anti-platelet agents, ideally aspirin and clopidogrel. The need for intervention is doubtful if the contralateral vertebral artery is of normal calibre and there is a conventional pattern of fusion at the vertebro-basilar junction, as haemodynamic ischaemia is unlikely in this circumstance and embolic infarction from vertebral artery origin atheroma is rare. Intradural vertebral stenosis presents specific issues; they may cause symptoms if unilateral, despite conventional anatomy, but on the other hand their treatment carries greater risk than extracranial vertebral disease and requires different techniques. These are not addressed here.

6.1.2 Procedure

An anaesthetist, ideally experienced in neuroanaesthesia, should be present. The procedure should be performed without sedation wherever possible, to maximize the chances of identifying neurological deficits that occur intra-procedurally. Arterial pressure should be monitored and rampant hypertension must have been controlled.

- Arterial access should usually be femoral. Use a long 6 Fr. Sheath (Cook Shuttle), partly for the flexibility it subsequently gives in terms of choice of device, and partly because of the matching catheters in various shapes which avoid the need for an exchange technique. In some instances, a conventional arterial sheath and guiding catheter may be preferable.

- Heparin is administered.
- Initial angiography should be performed from the ipsilateral sub-clavian artery, in some instances supplemented by the contralat-eral subclavian and vertebral artery. Views of the intracranial arteries should be included, looking for the pattern of flow at the circle of Willis, and providing a baseline to identify subsequent emboli.
- All equipment should be available and ready for use; the stent should be selected, and appropriate pre- and post-dilatation bal-loons selected.
- The lesion is then crossed with a 0.014 wire, usually without distal protection.
- Systolic blood pressure is then reduced by around 20 % to reduce risk of reperfusion injury.
- Pre-dilatation is performed if required. Very tight and calcified lesions should be pre-dilated, though some operators advise it as routine.
- The stent is positioned across the stenosis and deployed as quickly as possible, as flow is often impeded at this point. Both short, accurately sized balloon-expanded stents positioned flush with the subclavian wall, and Carotid Wallstents draped proximally into the subclavian artery are suitable. The latter approach has the advantage of avoiding the difficulties that may result from recoil of the artery and withdrawal of the stent into the stenosis and also allows for easier access in those instances of re-stenosis.
- Post-dilatation is performed if there is significant residual narrow-ing or failure of apposition of the stent to the vessel wall.
- Final angiography is performed, including the intracranial arteries, to look for emboli.
- Haemostasis is ensured with a closure device.

6.2 Post-Procedure Management and Follow-up Protocol

Patients should be admitted to HDU/ITU overnight, for neurological observation and monitoring of arterial pressure and should remain in hospital for 48 h, under the care of their neurologist. All patients receive a full neurological assessment before discharge. Any new neurological deficit warrants MRI scan, including DWI.

The neurology team should review all patients as outpatients. Dual anti-platelet agents continue for 12 weeks and aspirin should continue for life. A Doppler ultrasound scan carried out over this interval assesses the patency of the stent.

7 Complications and Management

The immediate complications of vertebral artery intervention include cerebral infarction and haemorrhage. Haemorrhage may result from hyperperfusion and is minimised by careful intraprocedural blood pressure monitoring and management. Acute onset of new neurological symptoms should prompt at least CT, and ideally MRI including DWI and neurological assessment. A neurosurgeon should be available for management of intracranial haemorrhage. Intra-arterial and intra-venous thrombolysis for ischaemic complications should be readily available. The support and availability of a neuroanaesthesist and neurointensivist in the intra- and immediate post-procedural period cannot be over emphasised.

The main long-term complication is in-stent restenosis. This should only be treated by angioplasty if the patient is symptomatic.

7.1 Outcomes: Open Versus Endovascular Treatment

Non-randomised case series of endovascular treatment reported a 30-day stroke or death rate of about 3 %. The Carotid and Vertebral Artery Transluminal Angioplasty Study (CAVATAS) compared endovascular treatment to medical therapy alone and reported no 30-day strokes following endovascular treatment. However, transient vertebrobasilar symptoms occurred in two patients within 30 days of treatment. Beyond 30 days, two further vertebrobasilar territory TIAs were recorded in both the endovascular treatment and medical therapy groups. The rate of restenosis following endovascular treatment was high.

Vertebral endarterectomy has been shown to be feasible and may have a favourable outcome. It is often difficult to access the site of stenosis, which makes surgery technically challenging and it is rarely carried out. CAVATAS did not include a surgical arm for vertebral artery disease because centres were not willing to offer surgery to these patients.

8   Role of Endovascular Treatment

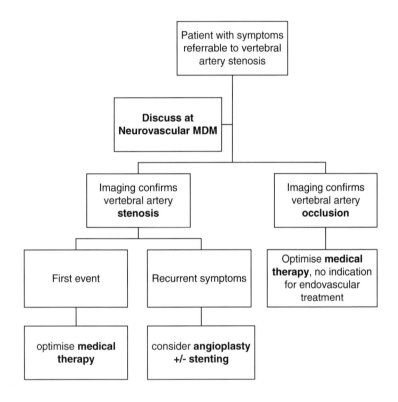

Landmark Papers

1. Blacker DJ, Flemming KD, Wijdicks EF. Risk of ischemic stroke in patients with symptomatic vertebrobasilar stenosis undergoing surgical procedures. Stroke. 2003;34(11):2659–63.
2. Coward LJ, Featherstone RL, Brown MM. Percutaneous transluminal angioplasty and stenting for vertebral artery stenosis. Cochrane Database Syst Rev 2005;(2): CD000516

3. Coward LJ, McCabe DJ, Ederle J, Featherstone RL, Clifton A, Brown MM. Long-term outcome after angioplasty and stenting for symptomatic vertebral artery stenosis compared with medical treatment in the Carotid And Vertebral Artery Transluminal Angioplasty Study (CAVATAS): a randomized trial. Stroke. 2007;38(5):1526–30.
4. Flossmann E, Rothwell PM. Prognosis of vertebrobasilar transient ischaemic attack and minor stroke. Brain. 2003;126(Pt 9):1940–54.
5. Khan S, Rich P, Clifton A, Markus HS. Noninvasive detection of vertebral artery stenosis. A comparison of contrast-enhanced MR angiography, CT angiography, and ultrasound. Stroke. 2009;40:3499–503.

Chapter 13
Below the Elbow Occlusive Disease

Roberto Ferraresi and Altin Palloshi

Critical hand ischemia (CHI) is a disabling disease because of its effects on hand function. It may be caused by above and/or below the elbow (BTE) vessels occlusive disease. Whereas above the elbow vessels treatment is well-known, the data about BTE vessel disease and treatment are poor. Based on our experience in below-the-knee arteries disease treatment with percutaneous transluminal angioplasty (PTA), we applied this technique in patients with CHI due to pure BTE vessels occlusive disease (Table 13.1). In this chapter, we suggest that BTE occlusive disease is a new underrecognized pattern of atherosclerotic disease, similar to below the knee vessel one, and describe our preliminary experience using endovascular treatment.

R. Ferraresi, M.D. (✉)
Department of Cardiology, Instituto Clinico Citta Studi,
Via Ampere 47, Milan 20131, Italy
e-mail: ferraresi.md@gmail.com

A. Palloshi, M.D.
Clinical Cardiology-Heart Failure Unit, Instituto Scientifico-Universita
Vita/Salute San Raffacle, Milan, Italy

A. Kumar and K. Ouriel (eds.), *Handbook of Endovascular Interventions*,   163
DOI 10.1007/978-1-4614-5013-9_13,
© Springer Science+Business Media New York 2013

Table 13.1 Clinical data of patients with pure BTE occlusive disease

	N	%
Patients	24	100
Age (years)	62 ± 11	
Females	3	12,5
Diabetes	19	79
Duration of diabetes (years)	19 ± 7	
ESRD	20	83
Haemodialysis	17	71
Peritoneal dialysis	3	12,5
Duration of dialysis (years)	$4,8 \pm 3,9$	
Diabetes + ESRD	17	71
Connective tissue disorders	2	8
Coronary heart disease	16	66
Cerebrovascular disease	6	25
Inferior limb ischemia	20	83
Previous below the ankle amputation	8	33
Previous above the ankle amputation	11	46

1 Anatomy

BTE vessels include the radial, ulnar, interosseous, and hand arteries (arches, metacarpal, and digital arteries). The most common anatomical variations are the accessory brachial artery and the high origin of radial, ulnar, or interosseous arteries, also known as brachioradial, brachioulnar, or brachioulnoradial arteries. Variations in the distal distribution of the radial and ulnar arteries are common (Fig. 13.1); in normal subjects there is always a significant anastomosis between the radial and the ulnar artery in the hand.

2 Disease Definition and Distribution

Table 13.2 shows the data of our CHI patients (24 patients, 30 hands) with pure BTE vessels disease. In each patient it is essential to clarify the causes of the impaired blood flow to the distal tissues, giving to each one the right weight.

(a) **Ulnar and Radial Arteries Occlusive Disease**: In the majority of the cases both arteries are affected. These arteries and their distal arches have the same size of coronary and tibial arteries

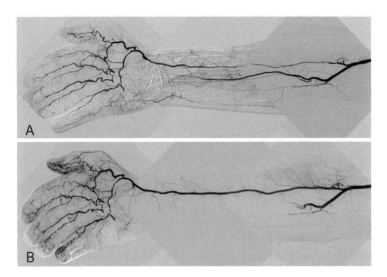

Fig. 13.1 67 years old male type 2 diabetes, ESRD in hemodialysis. Presentation: 4th finger apical gangrene. Retrograde femoral approach. (**a**) Basal ulnar artery occlusion, dominant radial artery giving both palmar arches presenting diffuse disease of the mid and proximal segment. (**b**) Final result

Table 13.2 Vascular data of 30 ischemic hands

	N	%
Finger gangrene or ulcer	30	100
Radial artery disease	28	93
Ulnar artery disease	29	97
Interosseous artery disease	0	0
Ipsilateral closed AVF	7	23
Ipsilateral functioning AVF	2	7

leading to the possibility to treat them with PTA. Interosseous artery was always patent, but its wrist collaterals were insufficient to supply adequate blood flow to the distal bed.

(b) **Small Hand Vessels Occlusive Disease**: The extension of occlusive disease to metacarpal and digital arteries plays a major role in generating CHI. Due to their small diameter (<1.5 mm) these vessels are nowadays not amenable to percutaneous treatment.

(c) **Arteriovenous Fistula (AVF)**: In patients with end stage renal disease (ESRD) in hemodialysis with a functional ipsilateral arteriovenous fistula (AVF) the possibility of a steal syndrome must be considered. A successful PTA of the ***non-AVF related BTE artery*** can relief the ischemia saving the AVF for hemodialysis. In case of PTA failure or persistent CHI despite successful BTE vessels PTA, AVF reduction with banding or by a DRIL procedure or if all else fails with closure is mandatory.

3 Disease Distribution

The true incidence is unknown. However it is seen most frequently in patients with coexisting diabetes and end stage renal disease (Table 13.1)

4 Diagnosis: Clinical and Laboratory

BTE arteries occlusive disease presents with symptoms related to chronic CHI: pain at rest and tissue loss. On palpation of the radial and ulnar pulses, one finds the presence of diminished or absent flow. The laboratory abnormalities are those related to ESRD, diabetes, or connective tissue disorders.

5 Diagnostic Imaging: USG/CT/MRI/Diagnostic Angiography

Ultrasound is the cornerstone of noninvasive evaluation of the BTE arteries. It provides quantitative and qualitative information and locates stenosis and occlusions. All major arteries of the upper extremity are identified, including the digital vessels.

CT scan or MR angiography are generally not as helpful, given the reduced sensitivity of these modalities for small vessel occlusive disease..

Diagnostic angiography is essential in confirmation of the diagnosis and treatment choice. It can be performed either via retrograde femoral or antegrade brachial approach (see below, VIII). We generally perform in one step diagnostic angiography and PTA. Multiple views, subtraction techniques, and magnification should be utilized to provide necessary details.

In the presence of an active AVF, before contrast dye injection, inflate a sphygmomanometer at the arm level at a pressure similar to patient systolic blood pressure.

6 Management

Currently, only symptomatic CHI patients should be treated. Data for asymptomatic cohort is missing.

7 List of the Open Operative Choices

1. Thoracoscopic sympathectomy
2. Autogenous vein bypass grafting
3. Arterialization of the venous system of the hand

8 Intervention: Techniques and Pitfalls

Prior to scheduling these patients, it is worthwhile to start them on ASA and Plavix (75 mg once a day) for 5 days. During the procedure they should receive intravenous heparin so as to maintain an activated clotting time between 250 and 300.

A. **Retrograde femoral approach**
   Initial attempts at pursuing this technique had a high incidence of failure, due to the typical diffuse and calcific nature of the BTE vessels disease, which needs high pushability and device control. Furthermore because of the high vascular comorbidities of these patients it may be challenging to transit through the aortic arch and supra-aortic vessels. Consider this approach only for focal disease (Fig. 13.1) and use a long sheath or guiding catheter positioned in the brachial artery.

B. **Antegrade Brachial Approach**
   This is the best approach for occlusions and diffuse disease of BTE arteries, which are difficult to recanalize; it usually extends from the origin of the radial and ulnar arteries to their hand arches (Figs. 13.2–13.4).

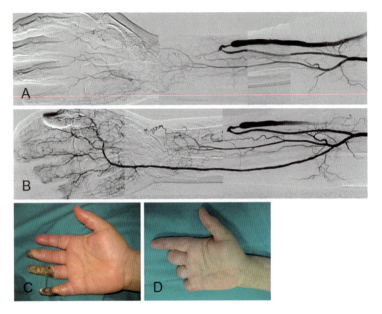

Fig. 13.2 67 years old male type: 2 diabetes, ESRD in hemodialysis. Presentation: 3–4–5th fingers gangrene. Antegrade brachial approach. (**a**) Basal: long ulnar artery occlusion, distal radial artery occlusion: active mid-radial AVF. (**b**) Final Result. Observe vascular exclusion of the necrotic fingers. (**c**) Basal hand. (**d**) Two months later: complete healing of the surgical wounds

1. Access the brachial artery at the antecubital level in an ante-grade direction, using a 4-Fr. micropuncture system and ultra-sound. Insert the sheath for only 3–4 cm in order to better visualize the brachial bifurcation. We strongly recommend not to upgrade the sheath size.
2. Perform angiography with gentle flush of contrast dye (6–8 mL at 2 mL/s).
3. In case of anatomical variations of brachial artery bifurcation try to access the target artery or shift to femoral approach.
4. Direct gently the sheath near the ostium or into the proximal part of the target artery: radial or ulnar one.

C. **Cross the lesion**

1. Try to cross the lesion using a 0.014″ hydrophilic coronary wire (i.e., PT2, Boston Scientific, USA).

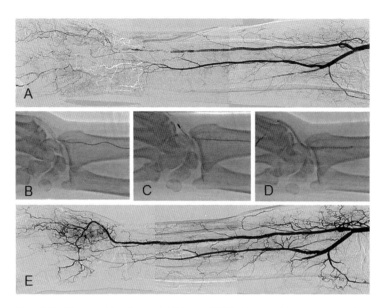

Fig. 13.3 70 years old male, type 2 diabetes, ESRD in hemodialysis. Presentation: 2nd and 3rd finger gangrene with phlegmon. Antegrade brachial approach. (**a**) Basal ulnar and radial artery occlusion, diffuse hand vessel disease. (**b**) 1.5 mm diameter, low profile coronary balloon is unable to cross the lesson. (**c**) A 1.25 mm diameter burr (Rotablator) is advanced through the calcified lesson. (**d**) Final dilatation with a 2.5 mm diameter balloon at 14 atm. (**e**) Final result

   2. Change the wire for a stiff 0.014″ one (i.e. Confianza Pro 9–12 gr, Asahi, Japan) if the first wire fails to cross the lesion. This often requires a-0.014″ microcatheter or coronary balloon support.

   3. In case of failing to cross the lesion antegradely it is possible to puncture with a 21-gauge needle the radial or ulnar arteries at the wrist level and advance retrogradely a 0.014″ wire. Once the lesion is crossed advance the wire into the sheath and switch to antegrade technique.

D. **Pre-dilatation**

   1. Once the lesion has been crossed, advance a 1.5–2.0-mm diameter low-profile balloon. If you encounter resistance in highly calcified lesions, try with a coronary low-profile balloon.

   2. **Rotablator**. In case of failure in crossing or in dilating the balloon through a tight calcified lesion an attempt could be made with Rotablator (Fig. 13.3). Exchange the 0.014″ wire with the dedicated 0.009″ one and advance the 1.25-mm burr through

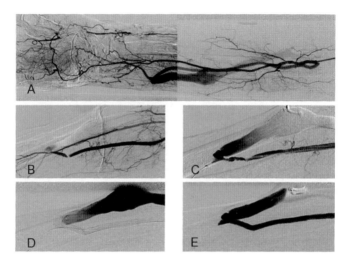

Fig. 13.4 70 years old Female, type 2 diabetes, ESRD in hemodialysis. Presentation: 2nd finger gangrene. (**a**) Basal ulnar artery occlusion, functioning radial AVF. Unsuccessful PTA of ulnar artery. (**b**) 15 min after the procedure the patient declared hand pain and unfilled AVF. A new angiogram showed radial artery dissection obstructing the flow to the hand and to the AVF, (**c**) A 4 mm diameter nitinol self expanding stent was positioned through the dissection covering the AVF anastomosis. (**d**) A second stent was positioned proximally, overlapped with the first stent. (**e**) Final result

the 4-Fr. sheath. Use the Rotablator only for short segments in order to minimize the risk of debris embolization and no reflow phenomenon.

E. **Final treatment**

1. **Local anesthesia**. BTE vessels dilatation can be very painful; before final dilatation inject a single intra-arterial bolus of 50 mg lidocaine through the sheath. This will provide local anesthesia.

2. **Dilatation**. Select an appropriately sized balloon in diameter (2.0–3.0 mm) and length (2.0–22.0 cm). In case of lesion affecting all the radial or ulnar artery long, cone shaped balloons offer the best conformability (i.e., Amphirion Deep, Invatec, Italy). Consider drug eluting balloons to prevent restenosis. No data are available about inflation time: we recommend 2′-4′.

3. **Stenting**. No data concerning stenting in BTE arteries are available. We have deployed only one self-expandable stent (XPert, Abbott, USA) to cover a distal radial obstructive dissection (Fig. 13.4).

F. **Wound treatment**
Antibiotic therapy and optimal wound care (ulcer debridement, amputation of necrotic phalanges) are essential to obtain symptoms relief and hand healing (Fig. 13.2).

9   Complications and Management

When working on BTE arteries any complication has the potential to precipitate an acute deterioration of CHI leading to fingers or even hand amputation. Nonetheless this should not dissuade us from providing the appropriate care.

1. **Dissection**: we had one obstructive dissection of the radial artery, probably due to wire advancement prior to sheath insertion in antegrade brachial approach (Fig. 13.4). The dissection involved the active AVF interrupting its flow. We covered the dissected segment with two self-expandable nitinol stents, one of those positioned across the AVF anastomosis. Fifteen months later the stents and the AVF are patent without restenosis sign.

2. **Subacute thrombosis and rupture**: one patient with scleroderma on the second day after radial PTA with a 2.0 mm diameter balloon had a subacute thrombosis causing acute hand ischemia. After redilatation of the artery with a 2.5-mm diameter balloon at 12 atm we observed a rupture of the distal radial artery at the arch level. Sealing was obtained with 5-min low pressure inflation.

3. **No reflow phenomenon**: In two cases of long chronic total occlusion PTA (one with balloon angioplasty and one with extensive Rotablator use) at the end of the procedure we observed a patent artery with no reflow phenomenon. Months after, both patients had a clinical worsening of the hand ischemia leading to multiple fingers amputation.

4. **Access site complications**: Using a 4-Fr. sheath and manual compression at the end of the procedure we did not observe any access site complication.

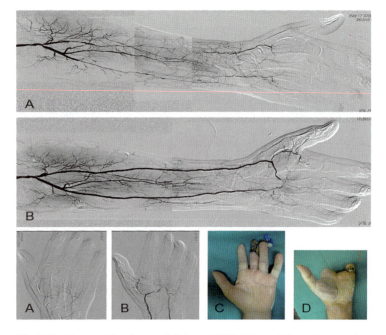

Fig. 13.5 60 years old male, type 1 diabetes, ESRD in hemodialysis. Presentation: 3rd finger gangrene. Antegrade brachial approach. (**a**) Basal diffuse occlusive disease of BTE vessels involving metacarpal and fingers vessels. (**b**) After successful angioplasty of radial and ulnar arteries direct blood flow to one palmar arch without significant improvement of the distal flow to metacarpal and finger vessels. (**c**) Basal hand. (**d**) Eight months later progression of gangrene with multiple fingers ampulations

10 Outcomes

A. Procedural and clinical success

BTE vessels angioplasty was technically successful in overall 77% (23/30) of cases. The flowchart summarizes the procedural success rates matched with the clinical outcome (hand healing). Three groups were identified:

1. **Successful PTA with good hand vessels run off**. 18/30 patients (60%) had successful PTA and good patency of metatarsal and digital arteries: in all these patients hand healing was achieved within few weeks (Figs. 13.1–13.3).

2. **Successful PTA with small hand vessels occlusive disease.**
In 5/30 patients (17%), a successful BTE vessels PTA was clinically insufficient to determine hand healing (Fig. 13.5). In all these patients there was a calcified occlusive **small vessels disease** involving all metacarpal and digital vessels without a significant improvement of the distal flow. This finding is similar to what described in below the knee angioplasty in ESRD patients in whom clinical efficacy of PTA is limited because of the severely diseased pedal arteries.

3. **Unsuccessful PTA.** In 7/30 patients (23%), PTA was unsuccessful due to uncrossable calcified chronic total occlusion (5/30) or no reflow (2/30). No one of these patients achieved hand healing except the patient in Fig. 13.4. This example stresses the importance of a detailed pathophysiological reconstruction of the causes of CHI in every patient. In this case the causes of CHI were (1.) ulnar artery occlusion (2.) steal from the AVF. After failure of the ulnar (non-AVF related artery) PTA the only reasonable solution could be the AVF reduction or closure. Acute closure of radial artery imposed stenting of the dissected segment; we believe that the struts of the stent covering the AVF anastomosis increased resistance to venous flow reducing the steal effect and improving blood flow to the hand through the patent distal radial artery. Due to this new balance between steal and antegrade flow the patient had an improvement of symptoms with complete hand healing at one month; Fourteen months later the patient is still asymptomatic with a functioning AVF and no signs of stent restenosis.

B. **Follow-up/Restenosis**

Because of their heavy comorbidities, our patients underwent a pure clinical follow up, thus the true restenosis rate may be underestimated. At 12 ± 8.6 months follow up 8/23 (35%) patient had a recurrence of symptoms. Ultrasound confirmed restenosis. All these patients underwent a new successful PTA yielding relief of symptoms. Afterward three patients had clinical relapse secondary to restenosis which was successfully treated with re-PTA.

11   Flowchart Summarizing Technical and Clinical Results of BTE Vessels PTA (See Below)

The flowchart—technical and clinical results of BTE vessels PTA

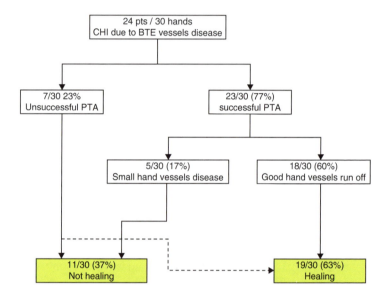

References

1. Ruengsakulrach P, Eizenberg N, Fahrer C, Fahrer M, Buxton BF. Surgical implications of variations in hand collateral circulation: anatomy revisited. J Thorac Cardiovasc Surg. 2001;122:682–6.
2. Chang BB, Roddy SP, Darling 3rd RC, Maharaj D, Paty PS, Kreienberg PB, Ozsvath KJ, Mehta M, Shah DM. Upper extremity bypass grafting for limb salvage in end-stage renal failure. J Vasc Surg. 2003;38:1313–5.
3. Kind GM. Arterialization of the venous system of the hand. Plast Reconstr Surg. 2006;118:421–8.
4. Ferraresi R, Ferlini M, Sozzi F, Pomidossi G, Caravaggi C, Danzi GB. Images in cardiovascular medicine Percutaneous transluminal angioplasty for treatment of critical hand ischemia. Circulation. 2006;114:232–4.
5. Gandini R, Angelopoulos G, Ros VD, Simonetti G. Percutaneous transluminal angioplasty for treatment of critical hand ischemia with a novel endovascular approach: "the radial to ulnar artery loop technique". J Vasc Surg. 2010;51:760–2.

Chapter 14
Aortic Arch-Occlusive Disease

Amit Kumar and Kenneth Ouriel

1   Anatomy

The aortic arch, also referred to as the supra-aortic trunk includes the innominate artery, the subclavian arteries, as well as the common carotid arteries up until their bifurcations. As the aortic arch progresses from an anterior to a posterior position, so do the origins of the great vessels. 20–30 % of patients show anatomic variations with the most common being the bovine arch, in which the innominate artery and the left carotid arise from a common ostium or a common trunk. Other variations seen are:

(a) Separate origin of the vertebral artery, most commonly of the left vertebral, which arises between the left common carotid and the left subclavian artery.

A. Kumar, M.D. (✉)
Department of Surgery, Columbia University, 21 Audubon Ave. Suite 209,
New York, NY 10032, USA
e-mail: endovascularasoa@gmail.com

K. Ouriel, M.D.
Syntactx, New York, NY, USA

A. Kumar and K. Ouriel (eds.), *Handbook of Endovascular Interventions*,
DOI 10.1007/978-1-4614-5013-9_14,
© Springer Science+Business Media New York 2013

(b) Truncus bicarotidus: The two carotid arteries take origin together and the two subclavian arteries take origin together.

(c) Right sided aortic arch—usually have an associated congenital cardiac defect.

2 Disease Definition

Occlusive lesions of the arch are typically due to:

(a) Atherosclerosis (80 %)

(b) Inflammatory diseases—Takayasu's disease or due to therapeutic irradiation.

3 Disease Distribution

Involvement of the arch occurs at an earlier stage than occlusive lesions elsewhere and single vessel involvement presents even earlier. There is an equal distribution amongst the sexes in contrast to occlusive lesions found elsewhere where there is male predominance.

4 Diagnosis: Clinical and Laboratory

Atherosclerotic arch occlusive disease presents with symptoms related to the vessels involved. Unifocal disease is present in about 60 % of cases and multifocal disease in the others.

Multifocal involvement often presents with vertebrobasilar insufficiency related to flow limitation, while unifocal involvement manifests symptoms related to the vessel affected—either as ischemic or embolic events.

Takayasu's arteritis typically involves all three trunks proximally. This is in distinction from Giant Cell Arteritis which affects the more distal vessels as well as a slightly older population compared to Takayasu's which typically affects women in their second and third decades. Takayasu's typically presents with symptoms related to poor flow.

On palpation of the outflow vessel, one finds the presence of diminished or absent flow. Auscultation often demonstrates a bruit over the affected vessel.

The only significant laboratory abnormality noted is in the inflammatory arteritis which will show an elevated ESR.

5   Diagnostic Imaging: USG/CT/MRI/Diagnostic Angiography: Ultrasound

Diagnostic imaging—USG/CT/MRI/Diagnostic angiography: Ultrasound is often used for screening; however, it has the drawback that bony structures impede adequate visualization.

CT scan is quickly replacing invasive angiography for diagnostic purposes in most institutions. It has the advantage of allowing visualization of the pathology from several different angles with new reconstructive software. In addition it has the benefit of providing details of the extent of calcification of the vessels, especially important in open reconstructions vis-à-vis clamp site. CT imaging of the brain should also be done in patients with occlusive disease who have cerebrovascular symptoms.

MR angiography with gadolinium is another modality which allows noninvasive imaging of the arch. It also provides additional benefit of visualizing the stage at which inflammatory occlusive disease is, acute inflammatory phase or the burned-out sclerotic phase, the former being a stage at which intervention should be avoided.

Diagnostic angiography helps in confirmation of the diagnosis, however much of cross-sectional imaging has made this redundant from a diagnostic viewpoint. The steps involved are:

1. Femoral artery access
2. Introduction of starter wire into the ascending aorta just distal to the aortic valve
3. Pigtail flush catheter over the wire in the distal ascending aorta
4. Flush arch aortogram with prolonged run time as the branches fill through collaterals.
5. The aortogram settings are in Table 14.1.

Table 14.1 Arch aortography

Location of arteriorgram	Catheter position	Contrast volume (ml)	Contrast time (s)	Image acquisition[a] (frames/s)
Arch aortogram	Ascending aorta	30 ml	2	4
Innominate arteriogram	Innominate artery	18	3	3
Subclavian angiogram	Subclavian artery	12	3	3
Carotid angiogram	Common carotid artery	10	2	3

[a]No time delay in the injection is needed

6 Management

Indications for treatment:

1. Symptomatic disease

   (a) Cerebrovascular—ocular, hemispheric, or vertebrobasilar symptoms
   (b) Upper extremity ischemia

2. Asymptomatic disease— >75 % stenosis

7 List of the Open Operative Choices

Transthoracic reconstruction

1. Innominate artery disease
2. Multivessel disease

Remote cervical reconstruction

1. With single vessel occlusive disease
2. Patients with prohibitive operative risk factors

8 Intervention: Techniques and Pitfalls

Prior to scheduling these patients, it is worthwhile to start them on ASA and Plavix (75 mg once a day) for 5 days. During the procedure they should receive intravenous heparin so as to maintain an activated clotting time between 250 and 300. The size of the stent is determined by the size of the blood vessel (Table 14.2).

Table 14.2 Vessel Size

Vessel	Size (mm)
Innominate artery	8–11 mm
Subclavian artery	6–8 mm
Axillary artery	5–7 mm
Brachial artery	5–7 mm

8.1 Orificial Lesions

A. Subclavian Artery Lesions

1. Occlusion: These are typically lesions which are difficult to recanalize. They usually extend from the origin of the subclavian artery to just proximal to the origin of the vertebral and the internal mammary arteries. Retrograde recanalization allows for more pushability to recanalize the occlusion

   (a) Access the brachial artery, preferably using a 4-Fr. micropuncture system under ultrasound visualization.
   (b) Femoral artery access is often useful using a 5-Fr. sheath and a pigtail catheter. Perform a flush aortogram to determine the location of the ostium of the artery as a target for the recanalization.
   (c) Exchange the brachial artery sheath to a to a 6-Fr. shuttle sheath (35–55 mm) over a 0.035″ non-hydrophilic wire.
   (d) Using a Kumpe catheter and a hydrophilic glide wire, attempt to recanalize the occluded lesion.
   (e) Change the wire to a stiff 0.014″ wire if the glide wire is unable to recanalize the lesion. This often requires the placement of a 0.014″ microcatheter (Quick Cross catheter, Spectranetics) for support.
   (f) Once the lesion has been recanalized, exchange the catheter for the dilator of the sheath and push the sheath forward across the lesion.
   (g) Introduce a balloon expandable stent (6–8 mm) once the sheath has traversed the lesion and the dilator removed. A balloon expandable stent is more appropriate for ostial lesions as they are more precise and also because they provide more radial force against these tough calcified lesions.
   (h) Position the stent at its appropriate location and pull back the sheath.
   (i) Deploy the stent and confirm position and patency

2. Stenosis: These can typically be treated through a common femoral approach, but difficult arches (Type III) are sometimes easier to treat through the brachial approach.

   (a) Common femoral artery access is obtained.
   (b) A starter wire is placed over which the access needle is exchanged to a 6-Fr. sheath (35 cm).
   (c) Over the wire a pigtail catheter is placed and a flush aortogram is done.
   (d) Once the anatomy has been delineated, the appropriately shaped selective catheter (Kumpe/Simmons 1/Vitek) is preloaded through a guiding catheter (6 Fr.). These are loaded on the wire in exchange for the flush catheter, making sure that the wire has been exchanged to a stiffer variety for support.
   (e) The lesion is accessed.
   (f) If the lesion is very tight, the catheter needs to be exchanged to a balloon (4–6 mm) to predilate the lesion.
   (g) The guiding catheter is then pushed across the lesion as the balloon is being deflated so as to minimize the risk of plaque embolization.
   (h) Once the guiding catheter is across the lesion, the stent system is delivered over the wire and after appropriate positioning the guide catheter is then withdrawn to the orifice of the lesion.
   (i) The balloon expandable stent is deployed and position confirmed.

B. Common carotid artery lesions

These may be approached through a retrograde or antegrade manner.

1. Retrograde approach: Initial attempts at pursuing this technique had a high incidence of neurovascular complications and is not a technique we perform except in cases of tandem lesions of the internal carotid artery and common carotid artery.
2. Antegrade approach: This is commonly used approach and is similar to that used for treatment of stenotic lesions of the subclavian with the exception of the use of embolic protection devices.

(a) Common femoral artery access is obtained.

(b) A starter wire is placed over which the access needle is exchanged to a 6-Fr. sheath (35 cm).

(c) Over the wire a pigtail catheter is placed and a flush aortogram is done.

(d) Once the anatomy has been delineated, the appropriately shaped catheter (Kumpe/Simmons 1/Vitek) is preloaded through a guiding catheter (6 Fr.). These are loaded on the wire in exchange for the flush catheter.

(e) Using a 0.014″ wire the lesion is traversed. If needed one can switch to a 0.035″ hydrophilic wire—with either a straight or a floppy tip.

(f) The guiding sheath is then appropriately positioned just proximal to the lesion. The protection device is deployed in the prepetrous portion of the internal carotid artery similar to its position for internal carotid interventions. This is still important at this stage as the highest risk of embolizing is at the time of balloon inflation or stent deployment.

(g) Over the same wire the stent is introduced and deployed.

(h) The protection device is collapsed and withdrawn after the position of the stent is confirmed angiographically.

C. Innominate Artery Lesions

These lesions require caution as they are at risk of embolization to the anterior cerebral circulation. Another important consideration is that of cerebral protection and the use of an embolic protection device.

(a) For this the right brachial artery access is obtained using a micropuncture system and ultrasound.

(b) This is exchanged over to a 6-Fr., 35-cm sheath.

(c) A 6-Fr. IMA guide is passed through this sheath over a hydrophilic 0.035″ wire and positioned at the origin of the CCA. The 0.035″ wire is exchanged for the filter wire which is then positioned in the usual prepetrous portion of the ICA.

(d) Common femoral artery access is obtained with a short 8-Fr. sheath.

(e) A flush aortogram of the arch is performed and the pigtail is exchanged over a stiff wire to a combination of a guiding catheter mounted on a selective catheter.

(f) The guide catheter should be positioned outside the ostium of the vessel.

(g) Recanalization (if an occlusion is being treated) is then attempted using a 0.014″ or a 0.035″ wire system.

(h) Once the wire traverses the lesion it should be directed into the external carotid artery. The catheter is then progressed across the lesion and the wire changed to a stiff non-hydrophilic one so as to track the guiding catheter on the selective catheter across the lesion as well. This allows one to introduce the stent in a protected manner to the lesion.

(i) Remove the selective catheter and place stent delivery system.

(j) Once positioned, the guiding catheter is pulled back and the stent position confirmed angiographically and then deployed.

(k) A completion angiogram is done.

(l) The protection device is then collapsed and withdrawn from the brachial approach and the wire is removed from the external carotid artery followed by removal of the entire system from the groin.

Distal lesions: These are accessed in the same way as the proximal orificial lesions. However, they differ in the nature of the stent to be deployed. Self-expanding stents are more commonly used in these locations. This is because these parts of the artery take a tortuous route, often in close proximity to overlying bone which puts at increased risk the deformation of the balloon expandable stents. In addition the same degree of accuracy is not needed for these lesions.

9 Complications and Management

When working on this part of the aorta with the cerebrovascular system a part of the circuit of treatment, any complication has the potential to be debilitating. With the ongoing increase in diabetes all over the world, not to mention the high rate of smoking in the majority of the world, this shall only increase the number of procedures that shall be done and thus the number at risk of complications. Nonetheless this should not dissuade us from providing the appropriate care.

9.1   Embolization

This is clearly one of the most important risks in treating arch occlusive disease. In stenting lesions of the subclavian artery origin there
is a risk of embolizing to the vertebral artery or into the arm.
Embolization of the vertebral artery is prevented by placing a protective occluding balloon at the origin of the vertebral artery so as to
prevent embolization. In addition a blood pressure cuff being inflated
at the time of deployment in the ipsilateral arm reduces antegrade
flow volume and provides some protection to the arm as well.
Another method of providing protection to the ipsilateral vertebral
artery is to you a cerebral protection device.

9.2   Dissection

A problem seen when one treats a highly calcified lesion especially
occlusions. However, this can also happen simply from wire access
of the subclavian artery such as in coronary angiography when trying
to access the internal mammary artery. The concern with dissections
is that the side branches will be involved and occlude a disastrous
complication for LIMA grafts or vertebral arteries which might be the
sole source of flow to the posterior part of the brain. The treatment is
to stent the culprit lesion. Tacking of this flap should resolve the distal
dissection.

9.3   Restenosis

There are certain lesions which are more prone to restenosis, such as
long lesions, lesions which have residual stenosis, and lesions which
have been stented. Typically restenosis is seen in the arch vessels
which have been treated, with an incidence of upto 19 %. Lesions
recurring after balloon angioplasty alone can be stented, typically
with a balloon expandable stent, especially if it is a lesion at the
orifice. In stent stenosis can be redilated with a slightly larger balloon
than used previously.

9.4   Pseudoaneurysm

This is treated with placement of a covered stent or open repair.

9.5   Rupture

This is a consequence of overdilation of the stenotic or occluded lesion. Typically seen with the use of balloon expandable stents or with simple overdilation of a lesion with the balloon. In either case the key is in not losing wire access. If this complication is suspected do not remove the balloon which was used for the dilatation too far from the lesion. Inject contrast through the sheath/guide catheter, reintroduce the balloon and inflate to a lower pressure so as to stop the extravasation and place a covered stent across the rupture site. If this does not work, the patient will need an emergent exploration by a vascular or a cardiac surgeon.

9.6   Stent Migration

This can happen in several circumstances.

(a) Migration at the time of delivery/typically happens in the hand mounted balloon expandable stents. The goal in such cases is to either push or pull the undeployed stent using either a snare or a balloon to a position where either the stent can be deployed in the least harmful way or to a position where it is surgically retrievable or better if it can be delivered into the sheath and then the sheath removed with the stent inside.

(b) Migration at site of deployment/When a balloon expandable stent is deployed in a very calcified lesion, it often jumps. This can happen with migration of the stent into the aorta or distally further downstream into the branch vessel. It is usually too risky to move the stent once it has migrated.

Table 14.3 Imaging system position for optimal visualization

Vessels	View
Aortic arch	LAO
Innominate artery bifurcation	RAO
Subclavian artery/vertebral artery/internal mammary artery	Contra-lateral oblique

9.7   Hyperperfusion Syndrome

This is rarely seen in the arch vessels. When seen in the upper extremity it should be treated symptomatically. When seen in the cerebrovascular circulation, it should be treated in the same way that hyperperfusion of the brain is treated with internal carotid artery revascularization/lowering of the blood pressure, with intravenous medications if necessary.

9.8   Misdiagnosis

This is a very important reason for inadequate treatment of patients. More so than in any part of the body, the overlap of the vessels needs to be accounted for and correct orthogonal views to be taken (Table 14.3)

9.9   Access site Complications

Please see Chapter 36.

10   Outcomes

Endovascular treatment of ostial lesions (within 5 mm of the origin of the vessel) has shown technical success of upto 100 %. It is more likely to succeed in stenotic lesions compared to occluded ones. The periprocedural complications range 0–14 % with low to no operative mortality compared with a mortality rate of 0.5–6 %, with open repair (transthoracic and cervical). The stenting of these lesions showed a patency rate comparable to open bypasses, 80–96 % at 3 years, with a higher reintervention rate of 7 % and an overall symptom recurrence rate about 4 %.

11 Flowchart Summarizing the Role of Endovascular Treatment (See below)

The flowchart—endovascular treatment of aortic arch occlusive disease

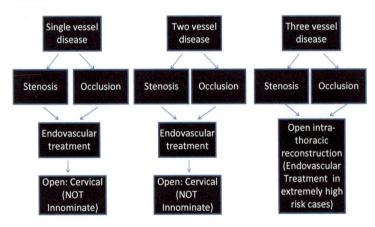

References

1. Bakken A, Palchik E, Saad W, et al. Outcomes of endovascular therapy for ostial disease of the major branches of the aortic arch. Ann Vasc Surg. 2008;22(3):288–394.
2. McNamara TO, Greaser III LE, Fischer JR, et al. Initial and long-term results of treatment of brachiocephalic arterial stenoses and occlusions with balloon angioplasty, thrombolysis, stents. J Invasive Cardiol. 1997;9:372–83.
3. Sullivan TM, Gray BH, Bacharach JM, et al. Angioplasty and primary stenting of the subclavian, innominate, and common carotid arteries in 83 patients. J Vasc Surg. 1998;28:1059–65.
4. Berguer R, Morasch MD, Kline RA, et al. Cervical reconstruction of the supra-aortic trunks: a 16-year experience. J Vasc Surg. 1999;29:239–48.
5. Berguer R, Morasch MD, Kline RA. Transthoracic repair of innominate and common carotid artery disease: immediate and long-term outcome for 100 consecutive surgical reconstructions. J Vasc Surg. 1998;27:34–42.

Chapter 15
Descending Thoracic Aortic Aneurysms

C.I. Ochoa Chaar and Michael S. Makaroun

1 Anatomy

The descending thoracic aorta (DTA) usually starts at the lower border of T4 vertebral body, just distal to the take-off of the left subclavian artery and ends at the aortic hiatus of the diaphragm at the level of T12. The DTA lies in the left chest posteriorly and has a relatively straight configuration until it moves anteriorly and medially at the diaphragmatic hiatus. With aneurysmal degeneration, elongation and tortuosity are to be expected. Distal to the left subclavian artery, the branches of the aorta are predominantly paired intercostal arteries. The artery of Adamkiewicz is a large intercostal artery that deserves special attention because it is a major blood supply to the spine. It arises most commonly on the left side at the level of T9–T12. Thus, aneurysms that are confined to the descending thoracic aorta occur in a straight artery with no major branches making endovascular treatment an attractive option. The proximal extent of the aneurysm and the relation to the left subclavian artery are essential in determining the

C.I.O. Chaar, M.D.
Presbyterian University Hospital, Pittsburgh, PA, USA

M.S. Makaroun, M.D. (✉)
Division of Vascular Surgery, Presbyterian University Hospital,
200 Lothrop, A-1011, Pittsburgh, PA 15213, USA
e-mail: makarounms@upmc.edu

A. Kumar and K. Ouriel (eds.), *Handbook of Endovascular Interventions*,   187
DOI 10.1007/978-1-4614-5013-9_15,
© Springer Science+Business Media New York 2013

suitability of endovascular therapy. Understanding the anatomic variations of the arch is crucial as discussed in another chapter. (Aortic arch occlusive disease—Kumar and Ouriel)

2 Disease Definition

An aneurysm is defined as an enlargement of more than 50 % the normal diameter of the adjacent artery. In the thorax, aneurysmal dilatation of more that twice the normal size is considered significant. Most descending thoracic aneurysms are degenerative and related to atherosclerosis. Familial clustering occurs in up to 20 % of cases. Marfan, Ehlers-Danlos, and Turner syndromes are associated with descending thoracic aneurysms. Aortic dissection and trauma also cause aneuryms of the DTA that typically have a higher rate of growth and warrant close monitoring.

3 Disease Distribution

Descending thoracic aneurysms are uncommon. In the absence of screening studies and since DTA aneurysms have traditionally been reported with aneurysms of the entire thoracic aorta, the exact incidence is difficult to pinpoint but is estimated to be 3–4 per 100,000 and increasing. The incidence of thoracic aneurysms appears to be higher in the Far East than in the USA. Patients are predominantly males in the 7th and 8th decade of life. Women represent 35–40 % of patients, a higher frequency than with abdominal aneurysms.

4 Classification with Regards to Proximal Fixation Site

An anatomic classification system was suggested by Ishimaru to document the proximal landing zone for thoracic endovascular aneurysm repair (TEVAR). The arch is divided to five zones depending on the branches to be covered as follows (Fig. 15.1)

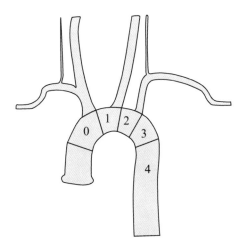

Fig. 15.1 Classification system of the proximal landing zone of TEVAR

(a) Zone 0: The proximal edge of the graft is proximal to the innominate artery. All 3 branches of the arch are covered.
(b) Zone 1: The graft is proximal to the left common carotid artery. The left common carotid and the left subclavian arteries are covered.
(c) Zone 2: The graft is proximal to the left subclavian artery. Only the left subclavian artery is covered.
(d) Zone 3: The graft is located less than 2 cm distal to the left subclavian. All three aortic arch branches are kept patent.
(e) Zone 4: The graft is located more than 2 cm distal to the left subclavian artery.

5   Diagnosis: Clinical

Most thoracic aneurysms are discovered incidentally on imaging studies as they are rarely detectable by physical exam. Patients can present with chest pain, back pain, or flank pain. Uncommonly, the aneurysm can compress adjacent structures and cause hoarseness (recurrent laryngeal nerve), dysphagia (esophagus), dyspnea (bronchus), or superior vena cava syndrome. Rarely, distal embolization from thrombus in the aneurysm sac can cause mesenteric or lower extremity ischemia. Rupture typically causes severe chest pain and shock.

6 Diagnosis: Imaging

CT angiography provides virtually all the required information for diagnosis and operative planning and has become the test of choice for imaging all thoracic aortic pathology. Multi-row detector CT scans with thin-slice axial reconstructions (0.6–2.5 mm) can be obtained with a single breath hold and give accurate measurements of the aneurysm size and its relation to major aortic branches. Three dimensional and multiplanar reconstructions can improve the evaluation of the aneurysm especially with tortuous and angulated anatomy and provide excellent assessment of the proximal and distal landing zones for endografting. MRA is an alternative to CTA in specialized centers. It is inferior to CTA in assessing aortic wall characteristics and calcifications.

7 Management

Since most aneurysms are asymptomatic and discovered incidentally, management decisions are based on their natural history. No prospective studies are available and the risk of rupture is estimated based on size from observational retrospective series. A 1–3 % yearly risk is estimated for an aneurysm 50–60 mm in diameter. It increases to 5–7 % when the size of the aneurysm is larger than 60 mm. The decision to intervene should be individualized taking into consideration the patient's age, comorbidities, and life expectancy. Traditionally, using open repair, the risk benefit ratio in an average patient would suggest a procedure when the aneurysm reaches 60 mm. Patients with Marfan syndrome are treated earlier when the aneurysm reaches 50 mm in size. A rapid growth more than 10 mm per year is another indication for surgery. Saccular aneurysms are presumed to have a higher rupture risk and are treated at a smaller size. Aneurysms that cause symptoms should be treated regardless of size.

8 Open Surgery

Open repair of descending thoracic aneurysm is performed through a left thoracotomy or a left thoracoabdominal incision depending on the extent of the aneurysm, using single lung ventilation. Exposure may require the resection of a rib with extensive disease. Proximal control is obtained distal to the left subclavian artery or between the left subclavian and the left common carotid artery. The aneurysm is replaced with a dacron graft using monofilament sutures. Several techniques are employed to decrease major complications such as ischemia to the viscera and the spinal cord:

(a) A lumbar drain draws CSF out of the spinal canal and can be used to maintain a low intrathecal pressure around 10 mm Hg. This increases the perfusion pressure to the spinal cord and has been shown to reduce the incidence of spinal cord ischemia and paraplegia. Elevating the systemic blood pressure also helps improve spinal cord perfusion. The lumbar drain is usually removed on postoperative day 3 providing some additional protection in the postoperative period in cases of delayed onset of paraplegia.

(b) Left heart bypass using biomedicus pump drives the blood from the left pulmonary vein/left atrium to the left femoral artery. It provides both retrograde perfusion to the visceral organs and "unloads" the pressure from the heart contracting against a cross-clamped aorta.

(c) Reimplantation of the lower thoracic intercostal arteries preserves blood supply to the spinal cord.

9 Intervention: Techniques and Pitfalls

Thoracic endovascular aneurysm repair (TEVAR) can be performed under general, regional, or local anesthesia. There are three endografts currently available commercially in the US for the treatment of descending thoracic aneurysms: Gore TAG, Medtronic Talent, and Cook TX2. There are inherent differences between these devices that are important to understand and are illustrated in Table 15.1.

Table 15.1 Characteristics of the thoracic endografts

	TAG	Talent	TX2
Composition	ePTFE with sutureless nitinol stents	Dacron polyester sewn to nitinol stents	Dacron polyester sewn to stainless steel stents
End configuration	Covered flares with sealing cuff at the base	Bare Spring	Covered stent with barbs proximally, bare stent with reversed barbs distally
Measurements	Inner diameter (ID)	Outer diameter (OD)	Outer diameter (OD)
Neck—Length	≥20 mm	≥ 20 mm	≥25 mm
Neck—Diameter	23–37 mm (ID)	18–42 mm (OD)	24–38 mm (OD)
Graft size (mm)	26, 28, 31, 34, 37, 40	22–46 in 2 mm increments	28–42 with 2 components
Graft length (mm)	100, 150, 200	112–116	108–216
Introducer sheath size	20–24 F, Length=30 cm, flexible	No sheath—Catheter size 22–25 F (OD)	Graft loaded into a 20–22 F (OD) Flexor introducer sheath
Delivery system	Device constrained by a sleeve on delivery catheter	Xcelerant	H&L-B One-shot introduction system
Deployment	Rapid from center to both ends	Controlled – Proximal to distal	Controlled – proximal to distal
Companion balloon	GORE Tri-lobe balloon	Reliant balloon	CODA balloon

9.1 General Guidelines

1. The recommended landing zone length of various endografts is intended for regions with good circumferential apposition. The required length is increased around angulated areas such as the dome of the arch.
2. Measurements and oversizing are different for different grafts.
3. If the proximal landing zone of the endograft is in zone 2, coverage of the left subclavian artery may be tolerated in some cases with good collaterals but the patient should be carefully evaluated first. Prophylactic revascularization of the subclavian artery with a carotid-subclavian bypass or subclavian transposition is mandatory in cases with:

    (a) A dominant left vertebral artery with an atretic right vertebral.
    (b) A left vertebral artery that ends in a PICA
    (c) An existent LIMA graft to a coronary artery usually the LAD.
    (d) Patients who may have compromised spinal perfusion related to a current AAA or prior AAA repair.

4. Lumbar drains for spinal cord protection are recommended for cases with higher risk for paraplegia such as long thoracic coverage, current AAA, or prior AAA repair.
5. Extensive thrombus or calcifications in the landing zones may preclude successful endovascular therapy.

9.2 Technique of TEVAR

1. Although a complete percutaneous approach is feasible, most TEVAR procedures are performed through a cut down on one femoral artery for the device and a small percutaneous sheath access on the contralateral side for an angiography catheter.
2. In 10–15 % of cases, small or severely calcified external iliac arteries especially in women, necessitate that a conduit (10 mm dacron graft) be constructed through a retroperitoneal incision to the common iliac artery.

3. The following steps are usually followed:

   (a) Expose the desired access artery or construct a conduit.
   (b) Place a 5-F sheath on the contralateral side and advance a marker pigtail catheter to the aortic arch.
   (c) Give heparin (100 U/kg)
   (d) Perform an angiogram in an LAO projection (45–60°) to accurately determine the exact position for deployment. If the deployment is strictly in the mid DTA, reference points may have to be different than branches of the aorta. Adjust final therapeutic plans if need be.
   (e) Insert an ipsilateral guidewire and exchange it through a catheter to a 260-cm length stiff guidewire (Amplatz, Lunderquist, or Meier). We prefer the precurved Lunderquist.
   (f) Insert the device under fluoroscopic guidance to the desired target zone and deploy according to the device's instructions after angiographic confirmation. Deploy the graft under fluoroscopic visualization.
   (g) If the distal landing zone is close to the celiac axis, a lateral view may be necessary.
   (h) Insert a balloon as needed and balloon preferably inside the grafts only. Overlap zones should always be ballooned.
   (i) Perform completion angiography looking for endoleaks
   (j) Remove the introducer sheath under fluoroscopic visualization
   (k) Remove all wires and catheters and repair the arteries as appropriate. The arteriotomy can be closed with 5–0 prolene sutures. A closure device may be used for the contralateral groin puncture
   (l) If a conduit is used, the conduit can be divided flush and oversewn or an ilio-femoral bypass can be performed if needed
   (m) Heparin reversal is optional and depends on whether it appears required.

9.3   Deployment Tips and Cautions

1. Overlap zones of multiple segments must be long enough (at least 5 cm) and the inner device preferably oversized to the outside device to avoid type III endoleaks. If multiple segments are planned the smaller devices should be deployed before the larger ones.

2. Severe tortuosity may prevent delivery of the device to the target zones. Possible maneuvers that may help:

   (a) Multiple stiff wires to straighten the aorta
   (b) Brachial femoral wire to guide delivery. If one is used, catheter protection of the branch to aortic junction is mandatory.
   (c) Long Sheaths

3. Placement of a wire access in the celiac artery can help distal deployment accuracy in cases where a very close deployment is desired. Similar wire access to the left subclavian artery or the left carotid artery retrogradely may be beneficial in difficult cases to:

   (a) Mark deployment zones accurately
   (b) Provide access for occlusion of the subclavian artery after deployment to prevent type II endoleak
   (c) Provide access for endovascular salvage of a covered essential vessel if need be.

4. In cases of difficult deployments in Zone 2 where accuracy is essential, certain maneuvers intended to decrease the forward aortic flow may help especially in deploying grafts that are susceptible to a windsock effect such as the Talent device. These include:

   (a) Reducing the systemic pressure to about 80 mmHg systolic
   (b) Rapid heart pacing that essentially stops forward pulsatile flow.
   (c) Transient cardiac arrest with adenosine. This is losing favor recently.

5. Although numerous improvements are planned for all three devices in the near future, the following device specific tips apply at the time of writing.

   (a) TAG: Deployment of the TAG prosthesis is rapid and occurs from the middle towards the ends. Complete stabilization of the device is critical and thus is typically a two person maneuver. Placing it near the greater curvature prior to deployment helps decrease incidence of misplacement. Large cavities in the aneurysm typically on the greater curvature side may result in "sucking" the graft to line up the cavity. The extension required to correct any distal deployment normally deploys very accurately.

(b) TALENT: Deployment of the Talent endograft requires at least some pressure control to avoid pressure on the partially opened graft and avoid misplacement. Distal but not proximal repositioning is feasible after deploying the proximal two stents.

(c) TX2: The proximal stent is somewhat long and stiff and preferably should be in a cylindrical portion for its entire length requiring a slightly longer landing zone than the other two grafts. It can be deployed however accurately with proper planning.

10 Post-Procedure Management and Follow-up Protocol

Patients after TEVAR can be admitted to a surgical floor with telemetry unless they have a spinal drain. Admission to an ICU may be required for some select patients. Most patients can be discharged in 24–48 h. The patients are followed with a CTA and 4 view chest X-rays at 1 month, 6 and 12 months and yearly thereafter. We no longer obtain a 6 months follow-up if the 1 month CT shows no abnormalities.

11 Complications and Management

(a) Endoleak: The incidence of endoleak is 3.9-12.2 % after TEVAR. Type I and III endoleaks should be treated with ballooning or extensions to improve apposition Type II endoleaks are less common with TEVAR but require angiography if the source is unclear. They should be treated if associated with aneurysm expansion. They may resolve spontaneously.

(b) Migration: The incidence of migration (>10 mm) with currently available devices ranges from 0.7 to 3.9 %. Most are not clinically significant and are not associated with aneurysm expansion.

Those associated with endoleaks and loss of seal should be treated.

(c) Spinal cord ischemia: The incidence is 3–8 % after TEVAR with most neurological deficits being reversible. Spinal cord ischemia increases when long segments of the aorta are covered. Concurrent AAA or prior repairs as well as coverage of the left subclavian artery may increase the risk of paraplegia. If spinal ischemia develops after TEVAR, a lumbar drain should be placed and controlled hypertension may reverse the deficit.

(d) Stroke is usually related to manipulation and instrumentation in the arch and occurs as frequently as with open surgery.

(e) Iliac artery injury is one of the most dreaded complications of endovascular therapy. The management of access problem is addressed in a separate chapter of this book.

(f) Miscellaneous: Graft infection, aortoesophageal fistula, and retrograde aortic dissection are rare complications that require conversion to open surgery and explantation.

12   Outcomes

Three multicenter, prospective, nonrandomized trials have evaluated the effectiveness of the devices available for the treatment of descending thoracic aneurysm. In the three trials, TEVAR has significantly decreased the perioperative mortality and morbidity of repair of DTA aneurysms as compared to open surgery. The benefit is sustained as demonstrated by the 5-year follow up results of the TAG device. The aneurysm related mortality at 5 years is 2.7 % for TEVAR and 11.7 % for open repair ($p = 0.008$). Total morbidity was lower with all three devices when compared to open surgery. The incidence of spinal cord ischemia was lower with TEVAR compared to open repair in the TAG trial. That finding was not reproduced in the other two trials. A summary of the outcomes of the three trials is shown in Table 15.2.

Table 15.2 Outcomes of TEVAR

Trial	TAG	Talent	TX3
	Pivotal (191)	Valor (195)	International clinical trial (160)
30 days mortality	1.5 %	2.1 %	1.9 %
30 days morbidity	28 %	30.3 %	9.4 %
30 days—SCI	3 %[a]	8.7 %	5.6 %
LOS	7.6 days	6.4 days	NS
Late mortality	32 % (5 years)	16.1 % (12 months)	8.4 % (12 months)
Aneurysm related mortality	2.8 % (5 years)	3.1 % (12 months)	5.8 % (12 months)
Aneurysm rupture	0 % (5years)	0.5 % (12 months)	0 % (12 months)
Late morbidity	42 % (5 years)	42.7 % (12 months)	NS
Successful delivery	98 %	99.5 %	98.8 %
Endoleak	10.6 % (5 years)	12.2 % (12 months)	3.9 % (12 months)
Reintervention rate	15 % (5 years)	8.7 % (12 months)	4.4 % (12months)

SCI Spinal cord ischemia, *LOS* Hospital length of stay, *NS* Not specified
[a]Statistically significant

References

1. Chaer RA, Makaroun MS. Late failure after endovascular repair of descending thoracic aneurysms. Semin Vasc Surg. 2009;22:81–6.
2. Conrad MF, Cambria RP. Contemporary management of descending thoracic and thoracoabdominal aortic aneurysms: endovascular versus open. Circulation. 2008;117:841–52.
3. Fairman RM, Criado F, Farber M, et al. Pivotal results of the Medtronic vascular talent thoracic stent graft system: the VALOR trial. J Vasc Surg. 2008;48:546–54.
4. Makaroun MS, Dillavou ED, Wheatley GH, et al. Five-year results of endovascular treatment with the Gore TAG device compared with open repair of thoracic aortic aneurysms. J Vasc Surg. 2008;47:912–8.
5. Matsumura JS, Cambria RP, Dake MD, et al. International controlled clinical trail of thoracic endovascular aneurysm repair with the Zenith TX2 endovascular graft: 1-year results. J Vasc Surg. 2008;47:247–57.

Chapter 16
Descending Thoracic Aorta Dissection and Aortic Trauma

Rosella Fattori and Marco Di Eusanio

1 Descending Thoracic Aorta Dissection

1.1 Disease Definition

Aortic dissection is a laceration of the aortic intima and inner layer of the aortic media that allows blood to course through a false lumen in the outer third of the media with simultaneous flow through the true lumen as well. Patients with aortic dissection usually have reentry tears throughout the descending thoracic aorta, which allows decompression of the false channel.

1.2 Predisposing Factors and Pathogenesis

Several risk factors have been identified that can damage the aortic wall and lead to dissection. These include direct mechanical forces on

R. Fattori, M.D. (✉)
Department of Cardiothoracovascular,
University Hospital S. Orsola, Bologna, Italy
e-mail: Rosella.fattori@unibo.it

M. Di Eusanio, M.D.
Department of Cardiac Surgery, University of Bologna, Bologna, Italy

A. Kumar and K. Ouriel (eds.), *Handbook of Endovascular Interventions*,   201
DOI 10.1007/978-1-4614-5013-9_16,
© Springer Science+Business Media New York 2013

Table 16.1 Risk factors for
Type A and B thoracic aortic
dissection

(1)	Hypertension
(2)	Atherosclerosis
(3)	Thoracic aortic aneurysm
(4)	Connective tissue disorders
	Marfan syndrome
	Loeys-Dietz syndrome
	Ehlers-Danlos syndrome
	Turner syndrome
(5)	Bicuspid aortic valve
(6)	Coarctation of the aorta
(7)	Aortitis
(8)	Iatrogenic
(9)	Sheehan syndrome
(10)	Cushing syndrome
(11)	Hypervolemia (pregnancy)
(12)	Polycystic kidney disease
(13)	Pheochromocytoma

the aortic wall and conditions that affect the composition of the aortic wall (Table. 16.1).

Common evolutive scenarios include:

– Frank rupture of the false lumen throughout the adventitial wall
– Impending rupture with peri-aortic hematoma
– False lumen compression of the true lumen and/or origin of aortic branches (arch vessels, splanchnic and limb arteries) with malperfusion syndrome.
– Chronic remodeling and/or dilatation of the dissected aorta

1.3 Classification

Two classification systems are most frequently used in clinical practice: the Stanford and the De Bakey systems (Fig. 16.1).

Stanford type A includes dissections that involve the ascending aorta whereas Stanford type B includes dissections that originate in the descending thoracic and thoracoabdominal aorta.

De Bakey type I involves the ascending aorta, the aortic arch and thoracoabdominal aorta; De Bakey type II only involves the

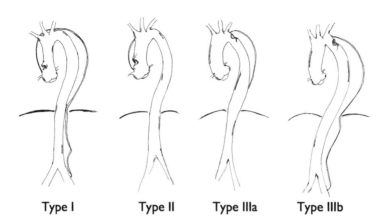

Fig. 16.1 De Bakey classification for acute aortic dissections

ascending aorta; De Bakey type III involves the descending thoracic aorta (subtypes A) or the thoracoabdominal aorta (subtypes B).

A further subclassification is based on the timing of dissection.

1. Acute dissection—presentation within the first 2 weeks.
2. Subacute—presentation between 2 weeks and 2 months
3. Chronic—presenting at greater than 2 months following the initial event.

The present chapter will focus on acute Stanford type B aortic dissection.

1.4 Diagnosis: Clinical

Clinical presentation is variable, from sudden death due to aortic rupture or more typically severe and unrelenting chest/back/abdominal pain. The character of the pain is often described as "ripping" or "tearing," often migratory. Patients may also present with signs or symptoms related to malperfusion affecting the brain, spinal cord, limbs, or visceral organs. These findings may confuse the initial diagnosis. Tachycardia, anxiety, hypertension, or hypotension may accompany the clinical picture. Pulse differential or absence and/or unilateral (left) loss of breath sounds (hemothorax or inflammatory pleural effusion) represent frequent signs of type B aortic dissection.

1.5   Imaging

1.5.1   Chest X-ray

Mediastinal widening is a very sensitive X-ray finding despite its low specificity; the combination of chest pain, pulse differential and *substantial* mediastinal widening is highly (83%) predictive of acute dissection. Therefore, an accurate clinical evaluation may facilitate a prompt diagnosis leading to further imaging evaluation.

1.5.2   CT and MRI

Contrast-enhanced, cardiac-gated multidetector CT with sensitivity and specificity approaching 100% combined with rapidity of execution and wide availability in emergency departments represents the "gold standard" for evaluating acute dissection. MRI, although providing superior anatomical details than CT, is limited by availability and long examination time. High-resolution imaging modalities allow an accurate anatomic selection of candidates for endovascular treatment by delineating the intimal flap and its extension, the femoral access, the involvement of visceral branches, and the distance of the entry tear from arch vessels or the presence/absence of associated intramural hematoma required to identify an adequate proximal neck.

1.5.3   Echocardiography

Although an effective portable diagnostic tool, it does not sufficiently visualize the aortic arch or abdominal aorta or permit 3D reconstructions; nevertheless, its role is essential in guiding endovascular procedures.

1.5.4   Catheter Angiography

Is reserved only for patients in whom other modalities have been unable to identify the required anatomical details (rare) or during endovascular repair.

1.6 Management

– Medical treatment in an intensive care unit is generally recommended for uncomplicated type B aortic dissections. It has been demonstrated that patients may survive their initial hospital stay with aggressive antihypertensive therapy, commonly intravenous labetalol to begin with, and keeping heart rate below 60 bpm significantly decreases secondary adverse events such as aortic expansion, recurrent aortic dissection and aortic rupture. As the aortic dissection is better controlled with anti-hypertensives, the pain shall also resolve.

– Indication for endovascular or open surgical repair is appropriate in patients with acute type B aortic dissection presenting with:

1. Signs of impending aortic rupture at clinical and imaging evaluation and/or
2. Evidence of severely impaired visceral/peripheral perfusion. Results from the IRAD registry demonstrated that, in the setting of acute complicated type B dissection, the endovascular treatment provides lower hospital mortality and morbidity rates than open surgical repair.

   • Key goals for endovascular treatment for type B acute dissection are:

     – Sealing of the proximal tear
     – Depressurization and shrinkage of the false lumen leading to subsequent remodeling and stabilization of the aorta
     – Resolution of dynamic malperfusion without any adjunctive procedure

1.7 Intervention

Endovascular procedures can be performed in the hybrid operating room with a fluoroscopy unit or in the angiographic suite, with the patients receiving general anesthesia and mechanical ventilation.

After injection of 1,250–5,000 U of heparin, a 5.2-French pigtail catheter is introduced into the left or right sub-clavian artery (depending upon the origin of the dissection) for intraprocedural aortography. The femoral artery, with true lumen flow, may be surgically exposed; more recently, the development of vascular closure devices has allowed totally percutaneous endovascular aortic repair to be safely performed. The guidewire is inserted through the femoral access and its position in the true lumen is confirmed by fluoroscopy and transesophageal echocardiography. The sheath with the stent and the pusher are introduced and deployed under induced hypotension (systolic pressure 50–60 mm Hg) to close all thoracic entries up to the celiac artery. Abdominal reentries below the celiac artery allow visceral organs' perfusion and are associated with low-pressure retrograde flow, which usually does not add any risk of aortic proximal dilation.

- In persistent malperfusion after stent-graft, adjunctive endovascular procedures include:

  1. Percutaneous balloon fenestration—Aiming to create a communication between the two aortic lumens homogenizing pressure and flow in both of the lumens and in their branch vessels. A curved, hollow metal needle is employed, introduced into the sheath over a stiff guide wire and advanced above the level to be punctured, under US guidance, usually in the infrarenal aorta or the iliac bifurcation. The metal stylet, with a coaxially mounted 5-F catheter, is inserted to just inside the needle tip. After the puncture the stylet is removed and the 5-F catheter left in position across the flap. With an over-the-wire exchange technique, an appropriate-sized (15–25-mm), low profile balloon is inserted through the sheath and positioned across the flap and inflated. Pressure measurement attesting no gradient between the two lumens assesses the efficacy of fenestration.
  2. Aortic branch stenting—In cases of localized fibrous stenosis in major aortic tributaries or prolapse mechanism of the intimal flap.
  3. Surgical fenestration—Is nowadays rarely performed due to prohibitive mortality rates.

Left subclavian artery(LSA) management:
Entry site in type B dissection is frequently close to the left subclavian artery. Intentional closure of the LSA during an endovascular

procedure is hampered by an increased risk of paraplegia and cerebrovascular accident. Carotid to subclavian by-pass may prevent cerebral ischemia and subclavian steal syndrome; retrograde coil embolization of the LSA is often necessary to avoid retrograde filling of the false lumen and type II endoleak. A vascular plug can be placed at the origin of the LSA through the left brachial artery using 6–8 Fr-guiding catheter.

1.8 Outcome

Two systematic reviews have assessed short- and mid-term results of stent grafts in the management of acute type B dissection. Reported overall outcomes from both reviews were similar with procedural success and 30-day mortality of 95% and 10%, respectively. In a metanalysis study involving 606 patients, Eggebrecht reported 14.5% of major complications intended as life-threatening complications prompting therapeutic consequences. The most critical in-hospital complications were:

– Retrograde extension of the dissection into the ascending aorta ($1.8 \pm 0.9\%$)
– Major neurologic complications (perioperative stroke: $1.1 \pm 0.7\%$) and paraplegia ($0.9 \pm 0.6\%$).

The risk of stroke is increased in patients with:

1. Severely atherosclerotic aortic arch.
2. Left subclavian artery stent-coverage without revascularization.

The risk of paraplegia is proportional to:

1. The length of the aorta covered by the stent-graft (>20 cm).
2. Left subclavian coverage without revascularization
3. Previous abdominal aortic surgery
4. Prolonged hypotension.

The reported 2-years survival was $87.4 \pm 2.1\%$. Interestingly, stent-graft failed to obliterate the false lumen in 25% of patients resulting in a 12% reintervention rate and a $2.3 \pm 0.6\%$ occurrence of aortic rupture during the follow up period. These findings indicate that patients' long-life clinical and imaging surveillance is mandatory.

In the subacute and chronic setting, the INSTEAD trial has recently shown that elective (at least 2 weeks from onset of dissection) endovascular treatment in stable patients with uncomplicated type B acute dissection does not improve 2-years survival and adverse event rates as compared to optimal medical therapy with surveillance, despite a favorable aortic remodeling.

2 Aortic Trauma

Traumatic aortic injury of the descending aorta is a life-threatening condition often involving young persons and leading to immediate death in 75–90% of cases. Vehicle accidents have accounted for more than 75–90% of cases in most series. Other potential causes are fall from height, compression by a heavy object, and a direct blow. In patients with traumatic aortic disruption other traumatic injuries are often present, such as closed head, chest (diaphragm, lung, heart, rib/clavicle fractures), abdominal (spleen, liver, kidney, bowel), and skeletal injuries (extremities, spine, pelvis, maxillofacial).

2.1 Pathology

Three different patterns of traumatic aortic injury have been described.

- Transection. Most commonly, the aorta is transected in a transverse fashion with involvement of all three aortic wall layers with the edges often separated by several centimeters.
- Partial rupture. The aortic lesion is not circumferential and not involving all three aortic layers.
- Intramural hematoma/focal dissection. Limited pathologic pattern, which can result in spontaneous resolution.

Aortic disruption may occur in all aortic segments. The isthmus is the most frequent location for aortic rupture being reported in 80% of the pathological series and in 90–95% of the clinical series. Due to the high immediate mortality of traumatic rupture of the ascending aorta, this location has been reported in the 10–20% of the autopsy series versus 5% of the surgical cases. Other less common locations are distal segments of the descending aorta (12%) or the abdominal infrarenal segment (4.7%).

2.2   Pathogenesis

The most accepted theory poses that differential deceleration and torsion to the different aortic segments may determine appropriate stress and rupture of the aorta at specific sites - the isthmus being the most common due to it being fixed by the ligamentum arteriosum, the left main stem bronchus, and the paired intercostal arteries.

2.3   Diagnosis: Clinical

Aortic injuries are more commonly identified in patients presenting with multi-trauma. Mechanism of trauma involving deceleration forces should be always investigated with appropriate screening leading to further imaging investigations.

2.4   Imaging

(a) Chest X-ray. Despite its high negative predictive value, X-ray findings are not sufficiently sensitive and specific to identify or exclude aortic injury.

(b) CT angiography with multidetector technology and ECG gating, CT has become the gold standard with sensitivity and specificity close to 100%. Direct signs of aortic injury are aortic wall discontinuity and/or filling defects leading to the formation of a pseudoaneurysm; limited intimal flap. Peri-aortic hematoma and mediastinal hemorrhage is often present. Extravasation of contrast medium outside the adventitial layer is a sign of complete rupture. Differential diagnosis should be made between pseudoaneurysm and ductus diverticulum.

(c) MRI. Despite providing excellent assessment of anatomical details, its use has not been widely accepted in this patient population due to the longer times required for data acquisition.

(d) Trans-esophageal echocardiography. TEE reliably images the entire thoracic aorta except the distal ascending aorta and proximal aortic arch. The major disadvantage of TEE is that it requires an experienced operator. The most common feature of aortic injury identified by TEE is a mural flap. Thickening of the vessel wall can represent a contained rupture or a mural thrombus.
(e) Aortography. At present is rarely used for diagnosis.

2.5 Management

Open or endovascular treatment should be immediately performed in patients with traumatic aortic injury and impending rupture as demonstrated on clinical and/or imaging assessment. Operative timing and management of traumatic aortic lesions without signs of impending rupture are matters of debate.

Despite advances in surgical and perioperative care, surgical interventions for acute aortic rupture are still associated with relevant mortality (20%) and paraplegia (7–15%) rates.

Thus, since the 1990s, considering that the risk of aortic rupture is not very high in the first 4–6 h if initial conservative medical treatment with antihypertensive therapy is initiated in intensive care unit, delayed surgical repair has been advocated in patients with traumatic aortic injuries with hemodynamic stability and without imaging of impending rupture.

Over the last few years, endovascular stent graft treatment has become the standard treatment. Advantages of endovascular approach are:

– Less invasive: Avoiding thoracotomy and the use of heparin. Endovascular repair may be applied in the acute patients without the risk of destabilizing pulmonary, head, or abdominal traumatic lesions
– Very low (close to 0) risk of spinal cord injury

Disadvantages with endovascular grafting for traumatic aortic injury are:

– To cover the left subclavian with or without previous revascularization.

– The sharp angle of the aortic arch, which can interfere with stent graft complete expansion. The small size of the aorta and sharp angle of the distal arch may result in insufficient sealing and/or collapse of the stent-graft
– The absence of long term outcome data (<10 years) of stent graft materials, considering the young age of these patients

2.6   Endovascular Technique

Endovascular procedures can be performed in the hybrid operating room with a fluoroscopy unit or in the angiographic suite, with the patients receiving general anesthesia and mechanical ventilation and invasive blood pressure monitoring. The common femoral artery is used for access after surgical exposure or through a totally percutaneous procedure using vascular closure devices. In patients with active bleeding into the pleural space, mediastinal space, or both, no systemic heparin is administered. Angiographic analysis is performed to identify the lesion, its landing zones, and its relation to the side branches. Stent grafts are loaded on an extra-stiff guidewire and delivered under fluoroscopic and trans-esophageal echocardiography with induced hypotension (systolic pressure, <60 mm Hg) to prevent inadvertent downstream displacement of the stent graft during delivery. Compliant aortic occlusion balloons may be used to improve wall adhesion and complete expansion of the stent grafts. Postprocedural angiographic analysis and TEE control are performed to reveal the final result. On the basis of CT/MRI measurement, an oversizing of 10–20% is applied in the choice of stent graft diameter. It is important to consider that in patients with hypovolemic shock and vasoconstriction, aortic dimensions can be underestimated.

2.7   Outcome

In a series of 31 patients receiving endovascular treatment in the acute phase between 1998 and 2007, we recently reported a technical success of 100% with no intraoperative or perioperative deaths. Cerebellar stroke was detected in 1 patient after the intentional closure of the left subclavian artery. At a Follow-up of 32.7±27.5 months, no late deaths, endoleaks, or complications were observed. A recent meta-analysis assessing mortality and occurrence of paraplegia after stent-graft repair and conventional open surgical repair in patients with blunt traumatic thoracic aortic injury indicated that endograft repair represents a first-line therapy for this pathology that may reduce mortality and paraplegia rates by half compared with open surgery.

References

1. Svensson LG, Kouchoukos NT, Miller DC, Bavaria JE, Coselli JS, Curi MA, Eggebrecht H, Elefteriades JA, Erbel R, Gleason TG, Lytle BW, Mitchell RS, Nienaber CA, Roselli EE, Safi HJ, Shemin RJ, Sicard GA, Sundt TM, Szeto WY, Wheatley GH. Society of Thoracic Surgeons Endovascular Surgery Task Force. Expert consensus document on the treatment of descending thoracic aortic disease using endovascular stent-grafts. Ann Thorac Surg. 2008;85:S1–41.
2. Fattori R, Tsai TT, Myrmel T, Evangelista A, Cooper JV, Trimarchi S, Li J, Lovato L, Kische S, Eagle KA, Isselbacher EM, Nienaber CA. Complicated acute type B dissection: is surgery still the best option?: a report from the International Registry of Acute Aortic Dissection. JACC Cardiovasc Interv. 2008;1:395–402.
3. Cambria RP, Brewster DC, Gertler J, Moncure AC, Gusberg R, Tilson MD, Darling RC, Hammond G, Mergerman J, Abbott WM. Vascular complications associated with spontaneous aortic dissection. J Vasc Surg. 1988;7:199–209.
4. Eggebrecht H, Nienaber CA, Neuhäuser M, Baumgart D, Kische S, Schmermund A, Herold U, Rehders TC, Jakob HG, Erbel R. Endovascular stent-graft placement in aortic dissection: a meta-analysis. Eur Heart J. 2006;27:489–98.
5. Nienaber CA, Rousseau H, Eggebrecht H, Kische S, Fattori R, Rehders TC, Kundt G, Scheinert D, Czerny M, Kleinfeldt T, Zipfel B, Labrousse L, Ince H. INSTEAD Trial, Randomized comparison of strategies for type B aortic dissection: the INvestigation of STEnt Grafts in Aortic Dissection (INSTEAD) trial. Circulation. 2009;120:2519–28.
6. Hoffer EK, Forauer AR, Silas AM, Gemery JM. Endovascular stent-graft or open surgical repair for blunt thoracic aortic trauma: systematic review. J Vasc Interv Radiol. 2008;19:1153–64.

Chapter 17
Endovascular Treatment of Symptomatic Abdominal Aortic Aneurysms*

Frank J. Veith and Neal S. Cayne

1 Anatomy

The anatomy of a ruptured aortic aneurysm is no different than conventional aortic aneurysms. However, what is key to treating them is the urgency in delineating the anatomy so as to evaluate the suitability for endovascular repair.

2 Disease Definition

Symptomatic abdominal aortic aneurysms (AAAs) fall into two categories: ruptured AAAs and unruptured but symptomatic AAAs. This differentiation is based on whether or not there is blood outside

---

*From the Divisions of Vascular Surgery, Cleveland Clinic and New York University Medical Center.

F.J. Veith, M.D. (✉)
New York University Medical Center, 4455 Douglas Avenue, Suite 11E, Bronx, NY 10471, USA
e-mail: fjvmd@msn.com

N.S. Cayne, M.D.
New York University, 530 First Avenue, New York, NY 10016, USA

A. Kumar and K. Ouriel (eds.), *Handbook of Endovascular Interventions*,   213
DOI 10.1007/978-1-4614-5013-9_17,
© Springer Science+Business Media New York 2013

the aneurysm wall. That determination can only be made by an urgent high-quality computerized tomographic (CT) scan and to a certain extent on symptoms.

<u>Symptomatic unruptured</u> AAA represents a disease process which may be associated with impending rupture and it carries higher treatment mortality. Symptomatic unruptured AAAs with pain and tenderness require urgent treatment, and this urgency is increased if the patient has severe pain and/or associated hypotension. Symptomatic AAAs should be urgently or emergently treated, either by endovascular aneurysm repair (EVAR) if they have suitable anatomy or by open repair (OR) if they do not.

<u>Symptomatic ruptured</u> abdominal aortic aneurysms (RAAAs) invariably lead to the patient's death. Even when treated by standard open surgical methods, RAAAs have high mortality (35–55%) and morbidity rates. These high perioperative mortality and morbidity rates have not been substantially reduced despite the introduction of many improvements in open surgical techniques and perioperative care.

3 Disease Distribution and Screening

There is an increasing emphasis on screening for abdominal aortic aneurysms given that abdominal aortic aneurysms account for an estimated 2.1% of all deaths in men aged 65 and over each year. However, the true incidence is likely to be underestimated as many of those with ruptured abdominal aortic aneurysms fail to reach the hospital alive. Although dated, in 1992 in England and Wales 4,515 deaths in men and 1,770 in women were certified as being from ruptured abdominal aortic aneurysms.

With a view to reducing the aneurysm related deaths, the Screening Abdominal Aortic Aneurysms Very Efficiently (SAAVE) act was passed in 2007 in the US. <u>This allows a one-time ultrasound scan screening of men aged 65–75 who ever smoked in their lifetime or men and women who have a family history of AAA.</u>

4 Diagnosis: Clinical and Imaging

This is made with the classic triad of known history of abdominal aortic aneurysm combined with abdominal pain and hypotension. Often the history of having an abdominal aortic aneurysm in not known and the patient with hypotension with complaints of abdominal back pain. These patients need to be evaluated for suitability for endovascular repair. This is best done with a CT angiogram. A study by Lloyd et.al. found that in patients with ruptured AAA who did not undergo treatment, 88% of patients with the diagnosis of ruptured AAA died more than two hours after admission. This would suggest that there is adequate time to do a CT. This timing of course depends upon the early clinical suspicion of the problem.

Ultrasound (USG) is useful as a screening tool, however, not adequate for delineating suitability for endovascular repair.

MRI is unsuitable for evaluating for a ruptured AAA given its lengthy time requirements.

Digital subtraction angiography (DSA) is often used as a simultaneous diagnostic and therapeutic modality in symptomatic patients with a known history of an aortic aneurysm.

5 Management

All patients with a presumed diagnosis of a RAAA are taken immediately to the operating room. For preprocedural resuscitation strict restriction of fluid and blood is mandatory. If the blood pressure is in the 50–70 mm Hg range, that is acceptable. If the patient is moving and talking, no fluids should be given. Patients with RAAAs frequently deteriorate with induction of anesthesia. If that occurs and the blood pressure falls below 50 mm Hg or is unobtainable, administration of fluid and blood become necessary.

In the operating room, the patient is prepared for fluoroscopy as if for an open operation, from the neck to the knees.

5.1   Equipment

The set up is standard for an EVAR with the open equipment being present but not opened in case of conversion.

5.2   Anesthesia and Access

Given that there is a possibility of open conversion, it is more suitable to start with general anesthesia and then proceed with open femoral cut-downs. This typically does not affect the duration of the case significantly.

Percutaneous access is used in patients who are hemodynamically unstable, but conscious. While a closure device may be placed prior, this however prolongs the procedure in an unstable patient. We prefer to proceed with the percutaneous option, without a closure device

6   Intervention

Anticoagulation: Administration of heparin is dependent upon the patient's coagulation profile. Patients with auto-anticoagulation from their state of shock can do without further anticoagulation.

Once arterial access has been obtained in both groins, an appropriately sized sheath (18Fr–22Fr) is placed as needed.

6.1   Proximal Balloon Control

The knowledge of this technique is critical for the success of EVAR for r AAA. The balloon can be inserted either in the brachial artery or through the femoral artery. If brachial arterial access is needed this will require an open cutdown. The currently available aortic occlusion balloons require at least a 12-Fr sheath

The currently available compliant aortic occlusion balloons are listed in Table 17.1. The balloon is preferably delivered from the side opposite to the side of the main body. To allow stabilization of the balloon catheter during inflation at the suprarenal or supraceliac level, the supporting sheath should be delivered till the aortic neck so

Table 17.1 Compliant aortic occlusion balloons

Balloon	Company	Sheath size (Fr.)	Maximum balloon diameter (mm)	Catheter shaft length (cm)
Q-50	W.L.Gore	12	10–50	65
Coda	Cook, Inc. (Bloomington, IN, USA)	14	32, 40	100, 120
Reliant	Medtronic	12	46	100
Equalizer	Boston Scientific	65, 110	20, 27, 33, 40	65, 110

as to prevent prolapsed of the balloon into the aneurysm. Often times forward thrust onto the balloon and the sheath is required to prevent prolapsed of the balloon. These balloons usually have low burst pressures, < 5 atm.

EVAR: If constant balloon inflation is required to maintain an adequate blood pressure then the contralateral limb is used to deliver the main body. The balloon is deflated and withdrawn immediately prior to stent graft deployment. Once the graft is deployed, if the blood pressure is such that it still requires balloon positioning, then it is delivered through the side of the main body and reinflated at the infrarenal aortic neck within the stent graft main body. The remaining EVAR is completed as per standard procedure (Chap. 22 — Endovascular treatment of infra-renal aortic aneurysm).

An alternative to using the standard EVAR is the use of an aortouni iliac (AUI) device in circumstances such as inability to access the contra-lateral iliac artery (disease/tortuosity)

Assistive Procedures: These are required in cases where the anatomy might be less than ideal for EVAR. This includes but is not limited to:

1. Hypogastric embolization for extension into the external iliac artery
2. Use of chimney technique:
3. Placement of a Palmaz stent proximally: Any sheath size larger than 16 Fr is adequate for delivering the stent. The Palmaz stent is centered on a 20–25-mm noncompliant Maxi LD balloon (Cordis, NJ, USA) and hand crimped. Holding the stent compressed the balloon is inflated so that the ends prevent "watermelon seed" displacement of the stent during deployment. The stent is delivered protected in the sheath upto the level of deployment, partly in the stent graft main body and partly in the native aortic neck. The sheath is then pulled back and the stent deployed. The deployment

balloon is then exchanged for a compliant balloon so as to mold the Palmaz stent thus anchoring the stent graft to the aortic wall.

If the infrarenal neck is too short, too flared, or too angulated for an endovascular repair, open aortic repair is performed with the balloon being deflated only after proximal control has been established.

7 Benefits of Endovascular Repair (Fig. 17.1a–e)

There are several advantages of endovascular repair of ruptured aneurysms.

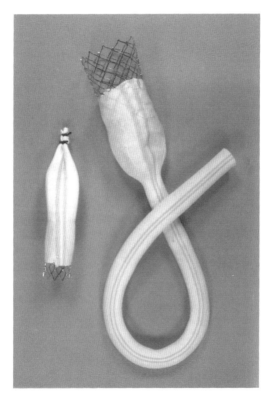

Fig. 17.1 Vascular Innovation (VI) graft. A large Palmaz stent is attached to the PTFE graft. A surgeon-made occluder device is shown on the left. However, there are many other commercially made occluders available, and any of these can be used to block the opposite common iliac artery

7.1   Proximal Control Without General Anesthesia

Patients with ruptured AAAs may be severely hypotensive. However, many patients may have their blood pressure stabilized at a nonlethal level. This is dueto sympathetically mediated vasoconstriction in response to hypotension. It is not uncommon for this vasoconstriction to be released during the induction of general anesthesia, which results in a sudden drop in blood pressure. Therefore, a relatively stable patient may become severely hypotensive, mandating urgent application of proximal aortic control. However, a guidewire can be inserted in the upper abdominal or lower thoracic aorta through a percutaneous puncture under local anesthesia, while maintaining the vasoconstriction. Allowing proximal control to be applied rapidly and relatively safely by placement of a large sheath and an occlusion balloon using the previously inserted guidewire.

7.2   Deployment of Graft from a Remote Access Site

Endovascular grafts can be inserted and deployed through a remote access site, thereby obviating the need for laparotomy and, more importantly, eliminating the technical difficulties that are encountered when performing a standard repair in the ruptured AAA setting. With the associated bleeding, the anatomy of the retroperitoneal structures is often distorted and obscured by a large hematoma, which may lead to technical difficulties as well as inadvertent injury of the inferior vena cava, the left renal vein or its genital branches, the duodenum, or other surrounding structures. These iatrogenic injuries have been the cause of significant operative morbidity and mortality following standard surgery for RAAAs.

7.3   Reduced Blood Loss

Endovascular repair for RAAAs has been accomplished with less blood loss compared with that which occurs during open RAAA repair. This advantage is more important in patients with RAAAs because these patients have already lost a significant amount of blood following rupture, and coagulopathy or disseminated intravascular coagulation secondary to further blood loss can be serious and lead to lethal complications. There are several reasons why blood loss was limited by EVAR, including the maintenance of the tamponade effect within the retroperitoneum. In addition, back-bleeding from the iliac and lumbar arteries and bleeding from the anastomotic suture lines and from iatrogenic venous injuries are eliminated.

7.4   Minimizing Hypothermia

Hypothermia secondary to poor perfusion and laparotomy can exacerbate coagulopathy, which is one of the causes of mortality following open surgical repair. Endovascular graft repair can minimize the extent of hypothermia by avoiding laparotomy.

8   Follow-up Protocol

Typically these patients will have a CT angiogram done prior to discharge and then at 1 month, 6 months, 1 year, and yearly thereafter.

9   Complications and Management

These are the same as that for EVAR (Chap. 22—Endovascular treatment of infrarenal aortic aneurysm). There is however one complication which is unique to a RAAA.

Abdominal compartment syndrome: There are several reasons as to why these patients develop abdominal compartment syndrome, such as presence of a retroperitoneal hematoma, backbleeding from vessels draining into the open aneurysm sac such as lumbars and the inferior mesenteric artery, shock state of the patient with associated changes in microvascular permeability associated with the aggressive blood and fluid resuscitation these patients receive. Coagulopathy also influences development of abdominal compartment syndrome. This is influenced by, amongst other things, use of a proximal aortic occlusion balloon.

Diagnosis is made by measuring urinary bladder pressures (>30 cm H_2O) or by having a more modest increase in bladder pressure accompanied by end organ dysfunction such as reduced urine output or increasing ventilator requirement

The treatment for this is immediate decompression laparotomy.

10   Outcomes

Over the last 9 years, a collaborative group, the EVAR for Ruptured Aneurysm Investigators, have been pooling their results with the use of endovascular graft repair of RAAAs. The results of this study will be published as a multiauthored report in November 2009 (19). Many of the details of this experience cannot be described here. However, the highlights can be summarized. Data was collected from 49 centers on 1037 RAAA patients who were treated by EVAR. The overall 30-day mortality in these patients was 21% although that figure may be biased by the fact that in many centers worse risk unstable patients were usually treated by open surgery while EVAR was used on more stable patients. However, 13 centers were identified in which EVAR was employed to treat all anatomically suitable RAAA patients. In these 13 centers, 680 RAAA patients treated by EVAR had a 30-day mortality of 19.7%, while 763 RAAA patients treated by open repair had a 30-day mortality of 36,3%. Although the two patient groups may have not been perfectly comparable, this mortality difference is highly statistically significant ($p < 0.0001$). In addition, many of the EVAR treated patients were prohibitive risks for a standard open repair (Fig. 17.2). The low mortality for endograft repair coupled with the inclusion in the EVAR treated group of many high risk RAAA patients strongly suggests that endovascular graft repair, when feasible, will improve treatment outcomes for RAAAs.

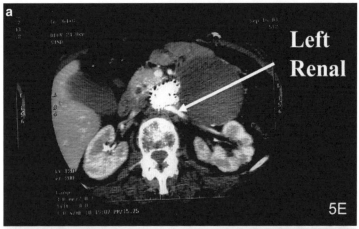

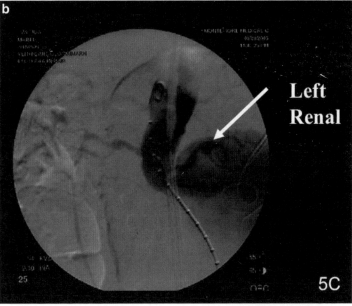

Fig. 17.2 Eighty-six year old Jehovah's Witness with a 10 cm RAAA. (**a**) Contrast CT showing RAAA. (**b**) Contrast CT showing an unfavorable short angulated neck. Open repair was advised but patient refused blood transfusion. The hematocrit fell to 17% and the systolic arterial blood pressure to 60 mm HG. Open repair was thought to carry a prohibitive risk. (**c**)Endovascular repair was performed despite the angulated short neck. Note left renal artery appearing to arise from the aneurysm. The endograft is in place but not yet deployed. (**d**) Contrast CT scan 6 weeks after the procedure. The aneurysm sac is excluded from the circulation. (**e**) Contrast CT scan 6 weeks after the procedure. The aneurysm is excluded. The left renal artery is perfused. The patient remains well over 5 years later

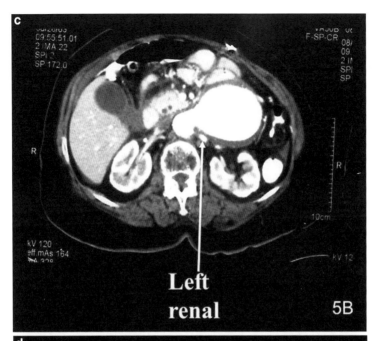

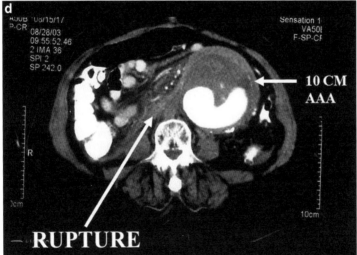

Fig. 17.2 (continued)

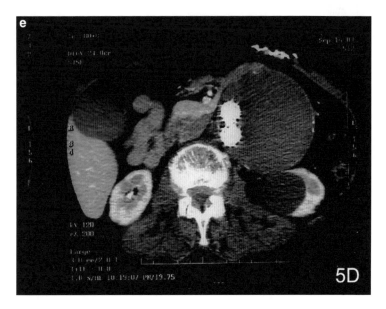

Fig. 17.2 (continued)

References

1. Noel AA, Gloviczki P, Cherry Jr KJ, Bower TC, Panneton JM, Mozes GI, Harmsen WS, Jenkins JD, Hallet Jr JW. Ruptured abdominal aortic aneurysms: the excessive mortality rate of conventional repair. J Vasc Surg. 2001;34:41–6.
2. Yusuf SW, Whitaker SC, Chuter TA, Wenham PW, Hopkinson BR. Emergency endovascular repair of leaking aortic aneurysms. Lancet. 1994;344:1645.
3. Parodi JC, Palmaz JC, Barone HD. Transfemoral intraluminal graft implantation for abdominal aortic aneurysms. Ann Vasc Surg. 1991;5:491–9.
4. Veith FJ, Ohki T. Endovascular approaches to ruptured infrarenal aorto-iliac aneurysms. J Cardiovasc Surg. 2002;43:369–78.
5. Veith FJ, Lachat M, Mayer D, et al. Collected World and single center experience with endovascular treatment of ruptured abdominal aortic aneurysms. Ann Surg. 2009;250:818–24.
6. Hughes LCCW. Use of an intra-aortic balloon catheter tamponade for controlling intraabdominal hemorrhage in man. Surgery. 1954;36:65–8.

Chapter 18
Fenestrated Aortic Endografts: Juxtarenal and Pararenal Aortic Aneurysms

Brian J. Manning and Krassi Ivancev

1 Anatomy

Anatomical variation in the visceral aortic segment is considerable. The celiac trunk follows the classical configuration in only 50 % of cases. The SMA, typically arising approximately 1 cm distal to the celiac artery, may also originate as a celiac-mesenteric trunk, or together with the splenic artery. The renal arteries typically arise at approximately the same level as each other, and usually but not always, distal to the level of the SMA. Each kidney is supplied by a single hilar artery in as few as 55 % of cases, with accessory arteries, double hilar arteries and single arteries with precocious bifurcation being the most common variations. To take account of such individual disparity, often accentuated by aortic tortuosity and aneurysmal distortion, fenestrated stent grafts which allow for preservation of aortic side branches are by necessity custom-made on an individual patient basis.

B.J. Manning, M.D., F.R.C.S.I.
Multidisciplinary Endovascular Team, University College London and
University College London Hospital, 235 Euston Road, London NW1 2BU, UK

K. Ivancev, M.D., F.R.C.S. (✉)
Department of Radiology, Malmo University Hospital, Malmo, Sweden
e-mail: krassi.ivancev@gmail.com

A. Kumar and K. Ouriel (eds.), *Handbook of Endovascular Interventions*,   225
DOI 10.1007/978-1-4614-5013-9_18,
© Springer Science+Business Media New York 2013

2 Disease Definition

Aneurysms with short infrarenal necks are by definition infrarenal, whereas juxtarenal aneurysms arise at the level of the lowest renal artery (Fig. 18.1), with no normal infrarenal aortic neck. According to most recent guidelines, no distinction is made between the terms juxtarenal and pararenal, whilst suprarenal refers to aneurysms present at the level of the renal arteries or at the level of both renal and splanchnic arteries. Such terminology has led to confusion in the literature. Aneurysms which some would term supra-renal are by others

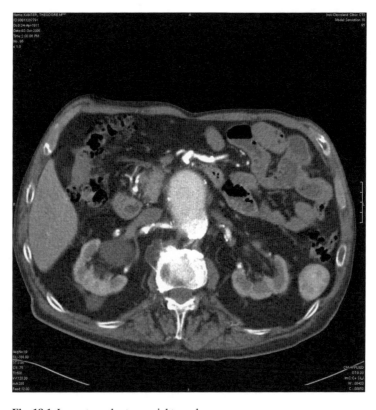

Fig. 18.1 Lowest renal artery—right renal

classified by others as thoracoabdominal type IV, whilst infrarenal aortic aneurysms with short infrarenal necks are often incorrectly called juxtarenal. Although FSGs can be used to exclude juxtarenal and suprarenal aneurysms, initial application of these devices was for infrarenal aneurysms with short infrarenal necks and the largest experience has been in this group of patients.

These aneurysms are most commonly due to degenerative atherosclerotic disease.

Abdominal aortic aneurysms with short or absent infrarenal necks (less than 10–15 mm) are not suitable for treatment with standard "off-the-shelf" endoluminal devices, and prior to the advent of fenestrated stent grafts (FSG), open surgical repair has been the only treatment option. FSGs are so named because they incorporate holes or fenestrations in the graft fabric to allow for continued aortic branch perfusion (usually through stents), whilst achieving a haemostatic seal at the same aortic level.

3   Disease Prevalence

Juxtarenal aortic aneurysms account for approximately 15 % of abdominal aortic aneurysms. Unfavourable anatomy of the proximal aortic neck of an infrarenal abdominal aortic aneurysm is the cause in up to 40 % of the patients who are precluded from an endovascular option.

4   Diagnosis

4.1   Clinical

The diagnosis is usually made incidentally on imaging of the abdomen for other causes. If patients are symptomatic, they will present with abdominal pain or back pain with or without associated symptoms of shock.

4.2 Imaging

4.2.1 Ultrasound

Most abdominal aortic aneurysms are detected by ultrasound, an increasingly so as population screening becomes more widespread.

4.2.2 CT angiography

Assessing suitability for endovascular repair requires CT aortography. In cases where consideration is given to the use of a fenestrated device, thin slice (<3 mm, preferably <1 mm) CT is essential. Both the thoracic and abdominal aorta should be included as well as the iliac and common femoral arteries. Precise measurement of the distance between each visceral aortic branch and the radial position of these branches is required and 3-dimensional CT reconstruction software is essential for this purpose. This allows for a straightened view of the aorta (Fig. 18.2) orthogonal to the line that the proposed stent graft will be expected to take, which enables clear visualisation of the position of each target vessel relative to the proposed device. With currently available multi-detector row CT scanning machines and reconstruction software, further diagnostic imaging is rarely required for planning of treatment.

4.2.3 MR angiography

While adequate imaging is possible with MR angiography, but it is more time consuming.

4.2.4 Digital Subtraction Angiography (DSA)

This has largely been abandoned in favour of CT angiography. However it is occasionally used to supplement the information of the CTA.

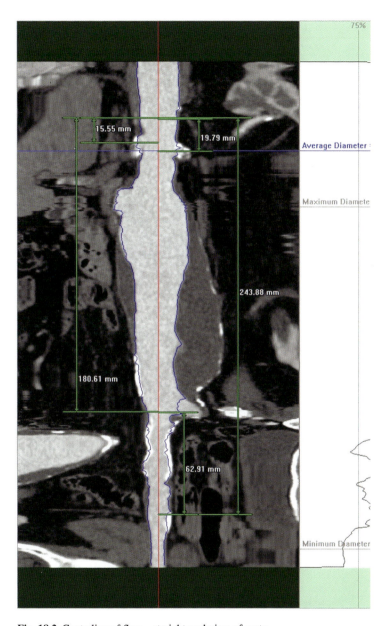

Fig. 18.2 Centerline of flow—straightened view of aorta

5 Management

Open surgical repair must be considered for all patients who present with juxtarenal aneurysms, as this remains the gold standard for good risk patients. This will usually require a period of suprarenal clamping and may or may not require re-implantation of one or both renal arteries. Endovascular repair was initially offered to those deemed unfit for open surgery, but as acceptable early results have been reported, it is increasingly seen as an option for all patients.

Suitability for a fenestrated stent graft is determined largely by the anatomy of the aortic neck, and for the purpose of this discussion we assume acceptable access vessels and a standard anatomy of visceral arteries. The aortic level at which a haemostatic seal between the stent graft and healthy aorta can be achieved will determine the complexity of the endovascular repair required.

1. Adequate infrarenal aneurysm neck: Standard EVAR
2. Short (inadequate) infrarenal neck and healthy neck at the level of the renal arteries: A fenestrated stent graft with two small fenestrations for the renal arteries and a scallop for the SMA
3. Absent infrarenal neck and healthy aorta at the renal arteries: Fenestrated SG as in 2, provided that there is sufficient distance between the renal arteries and the SMA to allow for an adequate haemostatic seal. In most cases where the aorta is aneurysmal at the level of the renal arteries it will be necessary to "climb higher" to achieve a seal zone by means of two small fenestrations for the renal arteries, a larger (strut free) fenestration for the SMA and a scallop for the coeliac trunk.
4. Where the potential for a haemostatic seal zone only occurs at the level of the SMA or coeliac arteries, consideration is given to "triple" (as in 3 above) or even "quadruple" fenestrated stent grafts. The complexity of these procedures is considerable compared with the more standard "double fenestrated" cases (unpublished observations) and other options, particularly the use of thoracoabdominal branched devices (Chap. 19: Branched aortic endografts—thoracoabdominal aortic aneurysms), or of open surgical repair, must be considered.

6   Planning and Sizing

The only commercially available fenestrated stent graft is manufactured by Cook Medical (Perth, Australia) and so the steps for planning are in accordance with the specifications of this device.

1. Inner aortic diameter at the level of the fenestrations will determine the diameter of the sealing stent (or stents, there is an option for 1 or 2 sealing stents in the fenestrated device).
2. The reference point by which the fenestration positions are planned is the edge of the stent graft. This is the position of the most proximal part of the fabric covered sealing stent. A standard scallop is 10 mm wide and 6–12 mm deep. For a typical 12 mm deep scallop then, the graft edge will lie 12 mm cranially from the most caudal or lowest point of the SMA (or usually just distal to this point). The position for each renal artery fenestration is then measured from this point to the centre of the ostium of the artery, giving a "distance from graft edge" measurement for each renal artery, which must measure at least 15 mm. Should the highest renal artery be too close to the SMA to allow for this, then a stent graft with three fenestrations (and a scallop for the coeliac artery) will be required.
3. Fenestrations can be made in various sizes depending on the size of the target vessels. Small fenestrations are 6 mm wide and either 6 mm or 8 mm high, and are usually of a size suitable for the renal arteries. They are always "strut free" and so suitable for stenting. Larger fenestrations range from 8 to 12 mm in diameter. These may be strut free, depending on the position and sizes of other fenestrations in the same device. Such fenestrations are required for more complex devices which involve sealing at the level of the SMA or coeliac arteries.
4. For each target vessel, the radial position of the proposed corresponding scallop or fenestration is planned by assigning the vessel in a clock position, based on a cross-sectional view of the origin of the vessel from the aorta, orthogonal to the line of the SG. By convention, the most ventral point of the aorta in the midline is taken as 12'o clock. If the SMA happens to come off at this point then the clock position of the SMA will be 12'o clock. When this is the case the left renal artery will typically come off in the 3'o clock region (and 86 % of the time will be between 1:45 and 3:45), and the right renal artery at 9'o clock [88 % of the time between 8:45 and 10:45, (unpublished observations)]. The device manufacturers

then use these measurements combined with the requested diameter of the stent graft, to calculate the absolute circumferential distance between fenestrations. All clock position measurements are made in the plane orthogonal to the projected line that the stent graft will take.

5. The fenestrated component must be of a length which lies no closer than 3 cm to the aortic bifurcation, so as to allow the second bifurcated component sufficient room to open and be catheterisation from the side contralateral to the side of delivery.

7   Intervention

1. Access to both common femoral arteries is achieved percutaneously or by means of cut down. A lengthy period of lower limb ischaemia must be anticipated, particularly in planned triple or quadruple fenestration cases. Patients with hypogastric occlusion or peripheral vascular disease may benefit from perioperative extra-anatomic bypass to the lower limbs in such cases. The device is delivered through the side chosen (on the basis of lesser tortuosity or calcification) at the planning stage. Time is taken to correctly orientate fenestrated components and to align the fenestrations with the target vessels. Although the total volume of iodinated contrast material is minimised in so far as is possible, good quality angiography, with visualisation of the fenestrations from multiple view points is essential at this critical point of the procedure. The device is unsheathed fully, maintaining the proximal barestent within the top cap, and keeping both proximal and distal trigger wires in place. A further control handle secures a series of "diameter-reducing-ties" along the stent graft. The purpose of these ties is to prevent full expansion of the graft until such time as target vessels have been cannulated, allowing more space in which to achieve this, and allowing for fine adjustment in the radial orientation of the system.

2. The unsheathed fenestrated component is catheterised from the contralateral groin and a large sheath (20Fr) is delivered into its lumen, whilst firmly holding the position of the fenestrated device. Through this sheath the fenestrations and the target renal arteries are successively catheterised, and long 6 Fr or 7Fr sheaths are positioned extending usually 2 cm into the target vessels (Fig. 18.3).

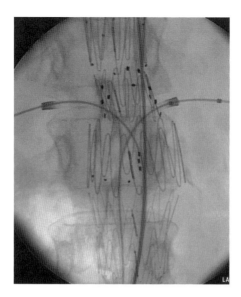

Fig. 18.3 Catheterization of renal arteries through fenestrations

Technically this step is often the most challenging. A curved Rosen wire (Cook Medical, Bloomington, IN, USA) usually provides sufficient stability to allow tracking of the sheaths into the renal arteries, bearing in mind the risk of renal perforation at this stage. If the sheath cannot be delivered we have found it useful to substitute its introducer with a 6×40 mm PTA balloon which is gradually deflated as the sheath is advanced. Once the 6-Fr sheath is in position appropriately sized (usually 6×22 mm) covered balloon mounted stents such as Avanta V12, (Atrium Europe B.V. Manchester, UK) or Jostent, (Abbott Laboratories, IL, USA) are positioned within the sheath, one-third within the aortic lumen and two thirds within the target vessel.

3. Full deployment of the fenestrated component requires release of three wires controlled by locking mechanisms at the hub of the device. Firstly the diameter reducing ties. Secondly the proximal trigger wire which locks the top cap to the bare stent. Once this is released the top cap is advanced deploying the bare stent. The third trigger wire is withdrawn to unlock the distal part of the SG from the delivery system, after which the inner cannula is advanced into the top cap allowing for its safe withdrawal through the stent graft

after which the entire delivery system can be removed, leaving only the deployed stent graft and the 20-Fr sheath behind.

4. Prior to deployment of the covered stents across the fenestrations, a moulding balloon can be applied to the sealing stents, with the fenestration stents protected within their sheaths. The sheaths are then withdrawn to expose the balloon mounted stents which are then sequentially deployed. These balloons are then replaced with larger balloons (e.g. 9 mm for 6 mm stents or 12 mm for 7 mm stents) to flare that part of the fenestration stent producing into the lumen of the fenestrated stent graft, effectively "riveting" the covered stent flush with the fabric of the main device.

5. The remainder of the procedure is similar to a standard infrarenal stent graft deployment, with extra care being taken to avoid dislodgement of the fenestration stents when passing wires and delivery systems through the stent graft (Chap. 22—Endovascular treatment of infrarenal aortic aneurysm).

8   Stent Graft Design Modifications

The fenestrated stent graft differs from the standard infrarenal device in several ways. It is a tapered tubular structure which is not bifurcated, and it usually contains a scallop and up to three fenestrations, (rarely 4). Positioning of the scallops and fenestrations are related and within the constraints implicit in having the fenestrations strut-free, or entirely within the interstices of adjacent stents. For cases requiring large fenestrations, it is therefore not always possible to have these strut-free, unless they can be accommodated between the stents, and to do this may require adjustment of the position and depth of the scallop. Scallops are usually not strut-free and so are not stented, whereas for fenestrations stenting, and in particular the use of covered stents, is routine. The presence of diameter reducing ties is a feature also unique to the fenestrated device as discussed above.

9   Complications and Management

These are discussed in detail in the ensuring chapters, Chap. 19—Branched aortic endografts—thoracoabdominal aortic aneurysms and Chap. 22—Endovascular treatment of infrarenal aortic aneurysm.

10 Follow-up

Follow-up entails surveillance for endoleak, stent graft migrations and sac expansions as is routine for all EVARs. Patients treated with fenestrated devices are best followed with CT, with or without ultrasonography since seal and the level of the fenestrations and the integrity of the stented fenestrations are less reliably assessed by the latter modality in isolation. The particular protocol varies from interventionalist to interventionalist, but can be at 1 month, at 6 months and then at 1 year followed by annual evaluation.

11 Outcomes

Both early and intermediate-term results for fenestrated stent grafts, published to date, have been encouraging. 30-day mortality ranges from 0 to 3.4 %, with target vessels preservation rates of 94–98 %. In the largest single centre experience to date ($n = 119$), there was a single death within 30 days. The 30-day endoleak rate was 10 %, all type 2 endoleaks. Mean follow-up was 19 months and in that time there were no ruptures or conversions, with sac size decreasing in 77 % of cases at 24 months.

References

1. Chaikof EL, Blankensteijn JD, Harris PL, et al. Reporting standards for endovascular aortic aneurysm repair. J Vasc Surg. 2002;35(5):1048–60.
2. Bicknell CD, Cheshire NJ, Riga CV, et al. Treatment of complex aneurysmal disease with fenestrated and branched stent grafts. Eur J Vasc Endovasc Surg. 2009;37(2):175–81.
3. Kristmundsson T, Sonesson B, Malina M, et al. Fenestrated endovascular repair for juxtarenal aortic pathology. J Vasc Surg. 2009;49(3):568–74. discussion 574–5.
4. Muhs BE, Verhoeven EL, Zeebregts CJ, et al. Mid-term results of endovascular aneurysm repair with branched and fenestrated endografts. J Vasc Surg. 2006;44(1):9–15.
5. Semmens JB, Lawrence-Brown MM, Hartley DE, et al. Outcomes of fenestrated endografts in the treatment of abdominal aortic aneurysm in Western Australia (1997–2004). J Endovasc Ther. 2006;13(3):320–9.

6. Greenberg RK, Sternbergh 3rd WC, Makaroun M, et al. Intermediate results of a United States multicenter trial of fenestrated endograft repair for juxtarenal abdominal aortic aneurysms. J Vasc Surg. 2009;50(4):730–737 e1.

7. O'Neill S, Greenberg RK, Haddad F, et al. A prospective analysis of fenestrated endovascular grafting: intermediate-term outcomes. Eur J Vasc Endovasc Surg. 2006;32(2):115–23.

Chapter 19
Branched Aortic Endograft: Thoracoabdominal Aortic Aneurysms

Thorarinn Kristmundsson and Timothy A. Resch

1 Anatomy

The paravisceral aorta includes the take-off of the celiac trunk, superior mesenteric artery, and the renal arteries. Aneurysms including this aortic segment range from suprarenal aortic aneurysm, involving the renal arteries only, to thoracoabdominal aneurysms.

Type I
Type II
Type III
Type IV

It is common for these aneurysms to extend into the common iliac arteries distally (20–30 %). To achieve a seal with an aortic endograft for these disorders, the endograft must incorporate the branching vessels and seal in healthy aorta proximal and distal to the diseased aortic segment and so the aortic wall evaluation extends further proximally and distally. Multiple anatomic variations of the branching visceral arteries exist, the most common being multiple renal arteries. Other common anatomic variations include (a) separate take-off of

T. Kristmundsson, M.D. • T.A. Resch, M.D., Ph.D (✉)
Vascular Center Malmo-Luud, Malmo University Hospital,
Universitetssjukhuset MAS, Malmo, SE 20502, Sweden
e-mail: timothyresch@gmail.com

A. Kumar and K. Ouriel (eds.), *Handbook of Endovascular Interventions*,   237
DOI 10.1007/978-1-4614-5013-9_19,
© Springer Science+Business Media New York 2013

the common hepatic artery and splenic artery from the aorta; (b) replaced right hepatic artery originating from the superior mesenteric artery instead of the common hepatic artery.

2 Disease Definition

Aneurysms of the paravisceral aorta are commonly due to:

1. Degenerative atherosclerotic disease (90 %)
2. Dissection
3. Infection (*Staphylococcus aureus*, *Salmonella*)
4. Trauma.

3 Disease Prevalence

Abdominal aortic aneurysms occur in 5–8 % of the population above 60 years of age. Approximately 5 % of these lesions include the paravisceral aortic pathology. Men are affected more frequently than women. Risk factors include smoking, hypertension, hyperlipidemia, COPD, and peripheral vascular disease.

4 Diagnosis: Clinical

75 % of patients are asymptomatic at the time of diagnosis. These are found incidentally or during clinical exam and confirmed with imaging. Symptomatic disease often presents as abdominal and/or back pain and tenderness over the aorta on physical exam.

5 Diagnosis: Imaging

- **Duplex ultrasound** is often used for screening and follow-up in patients with smaller aneurysms; however, imaging of this segment is hindered by visceral gas.

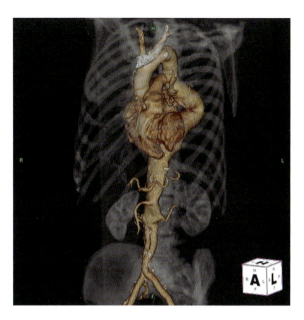

Fig. 19.1 TAAA preoperative image

- **CT angiography** is used for diagnosis as well as pre-procedure planning with axial and multiplanar reconstructions. Post processing is preferably performed on a dedicated 3D workstation allowing detailed reconstructions and center-line-of-flow measurements to define the circumferential as well as longitudinal relationship of visceral vessels as well as appropriate proximal and distal landing zones. Multiplanar and maximal intensity projection reconstructions are used when necessary, particularly in the presence of aortic angulation. CT scanning should be performed from the neck down to the femoral arteries to evaluate the full extent of the disease. In addition this allows evaluation of conduit vessels for delivery of the stent graft system (Fig. 19.1).
- **MR angiography** with contrast enhancement can be used for aneurysm diagnostics, procedural planning as well as follow-up, but it is often more cumbersome and time consuming to achieve a satisfactory result.
- **Diagnostic angiography** has mostly been replaced by CT scans in this patient category since angiography is invasive and places an extra contrast burden on the patient. In selected cases, angiography is used as an additional imaging tool, often in conjunction with

embolization of branching vessels which might be performed prior to the aortic reconstruction

6 Management

Indications for Treatment

1. **Symptomatic disease**

   (a) Abdominal pain and tenderness with confirmation by imaging.
   (b) Ruptured aneurysm (open repair).

2. **Asymptomatic disease**

   (a) Rapidly expanding aneurysm (≥ 5 mm/year).
   (b) Maximal aneurysm diameter >55–60 mm.

6.1 Open Treatment

Open repair is commonly the choice in symptomatic or ruptured aneurysms or in trauma patients due to the need for extensive customization of the graft when performing an endovascular repair.

1. Transabdominal repair: Suprarenal aneurysm requiring a supraceliac or supra SMA crossclamp.
2. Thoracoabdominal repair: For Crawford type 1–4 extent disease. Often performed with left heart bypass, visceral perfusion, and sequential crossclamping of the aorta.
3. Hybrid repair: In high-risk patients not suitable for endografting due to anatomical restrictions. Extraanatomic visceral artery bypass (from iliacs or aorta) combined with endovascular stent-grafting of the aorta.

6.2 Endovascular Treatment

6.2.1 Stent Graft Design (Fig. 19.2)

The implanted devices are constructed using the AAA Zenith endograft platform by Cook (Cook Medical, Bloomington, IN, USA)

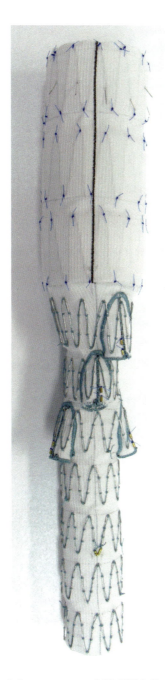

Fig. 19.2 TAAA graft. Image courtesy of COOK Medical Inc

comprising stainless steel Z stents and woven polyester fabric. The key difference between standard infrarenal EVAR and branched stent grafts is the presence of a reducing stent and side branches. The reducing stent, which is located distal to the sealing zone, converts the main body into a 16, 18, or 22-mm cuff bearing segment. This diameter is planned based on the aortic lumen so that it can accommodate both the main body and the bridging covered stents between the graft side branches and the visceral vessels. Aortic sidebranches, as opposed to fenestrations, are used when there is not expected to be any contact between the main body of the endograft and the aorta at the level of the visceral arteries. The diameter of the distal segment is adjusted to be sealed either to the diameter of a previous graft, in those patients who have already undergone open or endovascular infrarenal aneurysm repair or return to a diameter of 22 mm, which will serve as a standard diameter for the overlap of a distal 24-mm bifurcated endograft that is placed simultaneuously. Depending on the proximal extent of the aneurysm, additional endografts may be used proximally. The proximal sealing zone of the graft consists of one or two sealing stents with or without an uncovered proximal stent. Proximal barbs are added to the first sealing stent or to the uncovered stent for fixation to the aortic wall.

6.2.2   Sizing Method (Fig. 19.3)

As stated, the main endograft is modular in design so that the component traversing the visceral segment contains sidebranches (cuffs) to incorporate the target visceral vessels. This endograft segment is then joined proximally and distally with endograft components securing the fixation in the proximal and distal landing zones. The landing zone should be located within normal aorta in an area free of thrombus, angulation, or ectasia and preferably at least 2 cm in length. The branches of the visceral component of the endograft are mated with the target arteries by use of bridging covered stents. The planning of these branches follows two basic coordinates, namely, the distance from the proximal graft edge and their respective clock position in the aorta at the point of emergence. The bridging between the graft side branches and each of the targeted visceral arteries is accomplished with covered stents with diameters preoperatively planned by CT angiography to match both the visceral vessel and the side branch

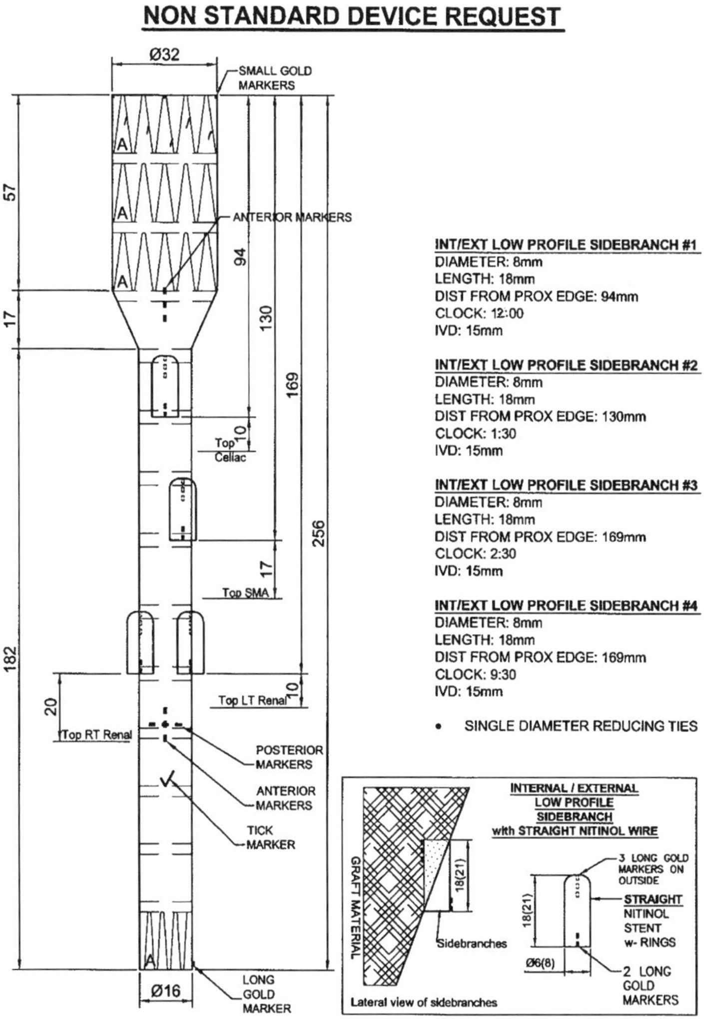

Fig. 19.3 TAAA graft design. Image courtesy of COOK Medical Inc

NON STANDARD DEVICE REQUEST

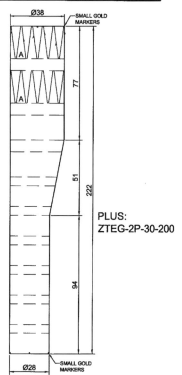

Fig. 19.3 (continued)

diameter. The side branches have 10, 18, or 21 mm in overlap length and are 6 or 8 mm in diameter. In contrast to fenestrations, the use of aortic sidebranches is more forgiving, in a sense that the planned distance to the target vessel (both longitudinally and circumferentially) allows for a greater flexibility when target vessels are catheterized.

6.2.3   Intervention: Techniques and Pitfalls (Fig. 19.4)

Bilateral femoral as well as unilateral brachial/axillary/subclavian access is required in most cases. Visceral branches of the aorta are usually directed caudally and are therefore preferably catheterized from a brachial approach. In select cases, the anatomic features of a

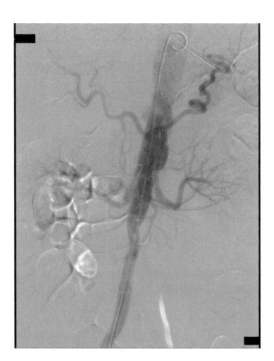

Fig. 19.4 TAAA final angiogram

sidebranch are such that an approach from below is preferred. Either femoral artery is used for introduction of the main stent graft depending on femoral and iliac artery diameter, tortuosity and calcification. The branched graft is positioned and deployed proximally with the side branches 1–2 cm above the target visceral vessels under fluoroscopic imaging with the markers on the graft demonstrating the correct orientation and alignment of the branches with the visceral vessels. From a brachial, axillary or subclavian approach, the aortic endograft is catheterized from above and a 12 F sheath is placed into the endograft lumen. Inside this, a longer 10-F sheath is placed. This large sheath placement is critical to overcome tortuosity in the aortic arch and descending aorta which prohibits accurate catherterization of the endograft cuffs and subsequently the visceral sidebranches. In a first step, the aortic cuffs are cathertized with a combination of a catheter (e.g., Headhunter or Judkins right coronary) and a long hydrophilic guidewire. Once acceess to the cuff is achieved, the target vessel is catheterized. Position is confirmed with angiography and the branch/

ostial interfaces are bridged with extra stiff wires e.g., Jindo (Cordis, Bridgewater, NJ, USA) allowing guide catheters to be placed into the vessels. This allows easy passage of covered stents into the vessels. Through the guide catheters, covered stents are placed, which are deployed to secure the main body aortic side wall to the visceral ostium and bridge the aneurysm sac. After all the target vessels have been stented, the distal section of this composite device are finally placed and deployed. Caution must be taken when completing the repair distally as the delivery system of the distal components crosses the visceral segment endograft and can dislocate the bridgning stents. A common problem of branched stent grafts is the fact that the space between the aortic stent graft and the aneurysmal wall is relatively small. An external side branch may be compressed or kinked by the aneurysmal wall making further catheterization impossible. In such situations internal branches might be preferable. The latter, however, reduce the lumen inside the main graft and might therefore not always be appropriate, especially in the setting of multiple branches. The choice of what type of covered stent should be used to extend the stent graft will depend on whether flexibility or radial strength is preferred. Self-expanding stents are flexible but offer a weak radial force. Balloon expanded stents are stronger but also more rigid which is why they may kink and remain deformed if they get accidentally compressed.

6.2.4   Follow-up Protocol

CT angiography with appropriate recontructions is performed at discharge, 1 month yearly thereafter.

7   Complications and Management of Endovascular Treatment

(a) Failure to catheterizise target vessels—Even though this is a rare event, failure to catheterize the target vessels leads to incomplete aneurysm exclusion as the aortic sidebranch remains open into the aorta. If all endovascular attempts fail one can choose to occlude the sidebranch and revascularize the target vessel by open repair.

(b) Visceral artery dissection and occlusion—Stiff guidewires must be placed into the visceral vessels during the procedure for stability with concurrent risk of damage to the vessels. Selective angiography to ensure correct position is crucial. In case of dissection, adjunctive stenting may be of value.

(c) Embolization—Guide wire and catheter manipulation within the aorta and side branches may result in embolization to the visceral organs and lower extremities. It is vital that the patient is well heparinized during the procedure and that this is monitored by measuring ACT which should be kept at 250–300 s.

(d) Paraplegia/paraparesis—Covering the aortic segment between T8 and L2 increases the risk of paraplegia/paraparesis due to reduced flow in the anterior spinal artery. The rate of paraplegia/paraparesis varies between 1 and 10 % depending on the extent of repair and the underlying disease process (higher in degenerative aneurysm than in dissection). Insertion of a spinal catheter preoperatively with drainage of spinal fluid during and after the procedure for up to 72 h may diminish the risk for spinal ischemia. Optimizing blood pressure (MAP 80–90mmHg) to avoid hypotension is key. Preservation of collateral flow to the spinal medulla through the left subclavian artery as well as internal iliac arteries is crucial and may require adjunctive endovascular or open procedures depending on the disease extent. Drain placement is especially important in patients with previous aortic repair of if the subclavian artery is going to be occluded.

(e) Lower extremity compartment syndrome—If the procedure is long, critical blood supply to the lower limbs is obstructed by the indwelling endograft delivery system. This might result in reperfusion and development of compartment syndrome requiring fasciotomy. Temporary closure of the femoral access site during the process of aortic sidebranch catheterization from above reduces the ischemic time and diminishes the risk for this complication.

(f) Dislocation of stent graft components—Repetitive pulsatile forces are exerted on the endograft during follow up and can result in component separation both in the main components as well as in the cuff to targetvessel junction. It is vital to ensure adequate overlap between components intraoperatively to reduce this risk. Close follow up is mandatory so that any component separation can be detected and treated, primarily with overlapping stents or stentgrafts.

8   Outcomes

Branched endografting of the paravisceral aorta is still in its infancy. The immediate technical success is reported to be in excess of 95 % at centers of excellence. 30day mortality is 6 % and at 1year 16 %. Paraplegia/paraparesis rates are 1–19 % depending on disease extent and etiology. Component separation is rare and target vessel patency at 1 year is over 95 %. Longterm outcomes after 1year are largely unknown.

References

1. Chuter T, et al. Endovascular treatment of thoracoabdominal aortic aneurysm. JVS. 2008;47:6–16.
2. Greenberg R, et al. Contemporary analysis of descending thoracic and thoracoabdominal aneurysm repair: a comparison of endovascular and open techniques. Circulation. 2008;118(8):808–17.
3. Eagleton MJ, Greenberg RK. Late complications after endovascular thoracoabdominal aneurysm repair. Semin Vasc Surg. 2009;22(2):87–92.

Chapter 20
Renal Artery Disease: Stenosis, Dissections and Aneurysms

Christopher S.M. Hay, Joanna R. Powell, and Jon G. Moss

1 Anatomy

Each kidney is supplied by a single renal artery in the majority of cases. These renal arteries generally arise from the aorta at L1–L2 inter space.

Extra renal arteries are present in about 30% of the population. The common variations being:

(a) Extra renal arteries entering at the renal hilum arising directly from the aorta.
(b) Polar branches directly to upper or lower pole from the aorta.
(c) More rarely an extra renal artery may arise from an iliac artery.
(d) Proximal bifurcation of the one or other of the main renal arteries is another common finding to be aware of.

C.S.M. Hay, F.R.C.R.
Royal Infirmary of Edinburgh, Little France, Old Dalkeith Road, EH16 4SA, Edinburgh, UK

J.R. Powell, M.R.C.P., F.R.C.R
Department of radiology, Glasgow Royal Infirmary, Glasgow, Scotland, UK

J.G. Moss, M.R.C.P., F.R.C.R. (✉)
Department of Interventional Radiology, North Glasgow University Hospitals, 1053 Great Western Rd, Glasgow, G12 OYN, UK
e-mail: Jon.moss@ggc.scot.nhs.uk

A. Kumar and K. Ouriel (eds.), *Handbook of Endovascular Interventions*, 249
DOI 10.1007/978-1-4614-5013-9_20,
© Springer Science+Business Media New York 2013

2 Disease Definition

Flow limiting renal artery stenosis (RAS), so as to cause secondary hypertension or renal failure is thought to occur when the renal arteries demonstrate a >50–75% reduction in luminal diameter.

3 Classification of Renal Artery Stenosis

1. Atherosclerotic renovascular disease (ARVD) (90%)
2. Fibromuscular dysplasia (FMD) 10% — A rare non-inflammatory condition that usually affects younger female patients.
3. Other rare causes e.g. Takayasu's disease — more common in India and China.

Atherosclerotic disease and FMD are two very different disease processes and respond differently to intervention. They should therefore be considered as two separate entities.

4 Diagnosis: Clinical and Laboratory

Renal artery stenosis is almost always asymptomatic; however, it should be suspected in certain patients:

1. Uncontrollable hypertension
2. Hypertension and asymmetric renal length on ultrasound
3. 20% or more reduction in eGFR or a 15% rise in serum creatinine at the time of starting an ACE inhibitor or angiotensin 11 receptor blocker
4. Flash pulmonary oedema
5. Kidney damage in the presence of known vascular disease elsewhere (especially if the legs are involved)
6. Malignant or abrupt onset hypertension
7. Hypertension onset when patient is <30 yrs old — consider FMD

Unfortunately there are no specific diagnostic laboratory investigations for renal artery stenosis, and the presence of a reduced eGFR or hypertension is not present in all cases. The diagnosis is usually made following appropriate imaging of the renal vasculature in patients where there is high clinical suspicion.

5   Diagnostic Imaging

5.1   Ultrasound

Assessment of kidney size is accurate and easily achieved, as is cortical thickness (kidneys <8 cm long are unlikely to benefit from revascularization in the treatment of ARVD). Colour flow duplex of the renal arteries is possible but the acoustic window is often limited by adverse body habitus and is also operator dependant. Other non-invasive modalities such as CT and MRI are more useful in diagnosis and planning treatment.

5.2   CT Scan

Multi-detector Computerized Tomographic Angiography (MDCTA) provides fast accurate interrogation of the renal arteries. Multi planar reformatting and 3D rendering allow for intuitive assessment and planning if intervention is required. In severely calcified ARVD, imaging may be degraded by artefact and confident assessment of the degree of stenosis difficult. Attention should also be made to any concurrent renal dysfunction, a GFR of <60 ml/min should prompt concern about possible iodinated contrast related nephrotoxicity and pre-hydration may be necessary.

5.3   Magnetic Resonance Angiography

Evaluation with gadolinium-enhanced magnetic resonance angiography (MRA) is the predominant modality in the assessment of renovascular disease due to its excellent sensitivity and specificity. Renal impairment (GFR < 60 ml/min) prompts careful consideration, as the administration of gadolinium contrast agents carry a risk of nephrogenic systemic fibrosis (NSF) which can result in significant morbidity and mortality. In these cases CTA may be preferable, as iodinated-related nephrotoxicity is usually mild and reversible and can be minimised by pre-hydration.

5.4   Diagnostic Angiography

This remains the gold standard in the assessment of renal artery disease although the above non-invasive modalities have largely replaced it. In severe renal failure, CO_2 can be used instead of iodinated contrast as a contrast agent thus removing any risk of contrast nephropathy.

Steps involved in diagnostic angiography include:

1. Femoral artery access
2. Pigtail flush catheter placed into upper abdominal aorta at the level of L1 vertebrae.
3. Power injection of 20 ml of iodinated contrast at a rate 10 ml/s.
4. Oblique views may be required to accurately interrogate the renal artery origins. For example, the right renal artery often arises from the anterolateral aspect of the aorta requiring a 25 degree left anterior oblique projection. The key to alignment being that the image intensifier be perpendicular to the origin of the renal artery.
5. In cases of non-atheromatous disease selective renal images are usually required. The renal arteries can be easily selected using either a femoro-visceral (Cobra) or a reverse curve (Shepherd's crook) type shape. The reverse curve catheters need to be reformed in the aortic arch or over the iliac bifurcation but are very useful in caudally angulated vessels and very stable once in the renal artery. Hand injection of 10 ml of iodinated contrast is often sufficient for diagnostic needs.

6   Management

Management of patients with atherosclerotic renal artery stenosis remains controversial amongst radiologists and physicians. Individual reports and observational studies report successes from stenting, in terms of blood pressure control and stabilisation of renal function. However two recent randomised control trials, (ASTRAL and STAR) have failed to show any benefit of stenting over best medical treatment alone for a variety of outcomes including blood pressure, renal function and mortality. Therefore debate continues, especially in terms of the optimal time for intervention, the optimal patient on which to intervene and the precise benefits (if any) from stenting. There is however general agreement that stenting may be offered in cases of intractable hypertension, "flash" pulmonary oedema, rapidly deteriorating renal function and those who present with acute renal failure and occluded renal arteries.

Protection devices (filters) and platelet glycoprotein IIa/IIIb receptor inhibitors have been used either together or separately to try and improve the results of stenting by reducing the incidence of cholesterol embolization. There is some very weak anecdotal evidence in their favour which requires further investigation in larger trials.

In summary, careful consideration of the risk to benefit ratio is needed on a case by case basis for renal artery stenting in atheromatous disease.

The results of angioplasty in fibromuscular dysplasia are far more encouraging than with atheromatous disease. Following angioplasty, 10 year cumulative patency rates are as high as 87%. In addition blood pressure cure can be achieved in up to 50% and in the remainder improved blood pressure control with a reduction in the drug burden. Stents are only rarely required in non-atheromatous lesions.

6.1 List of Open Operative Choices

The minimally invasive nature of endovascular renal revascularisation has largely replaced conventional surgical reconstruction particularly, in elderly subjects with multiple co-morbidities. However there is still a need for open procedures particularly in cases of failed or complicated endovascular intervention. The principle options include:

(a) Bypass (aortorenal, spleno/hepatorenal, iliorenal, aortic graft and renal bypass). Extra-anatomical bypass has the advantage of avoiding a heavily diseased aorta
(b) Endarterectomy—seldom practised
(c) Renal auto-transplantation to pelvis—occasionally used for complex FMD with bench surgery
(d) Nephrectomy—occasionally useful with a shrunken kidney causing renin driven hypertension

7 Intervention: Techniques and Pitfalls

A. Ostial Atheromatous Stenosis

Primary stenting is advocated in the treatment of ostial ARVD. These lesions are due to aortic cushions of plaque and simply recoil and restenose if angioplastied alone.

All patients should have non-invasive imaging prior, to establish a diagnosis and plan the stenting. The numbers of renal arteries and the angle at which they arise from the aorta are both vital information. Non-invasive imaging will also dictate optimal C-arm positioning to allow for accurate stent placement ensuring the whole lesion is covered out into the aorta, for 2–3 mm.

Patients will normally be taking an antiplatelet agent (aspirin 75 mg daily or clopidogrel 75 mg daily) which should be continued for life. Pre-hydration with intravenous fluids for 12 h will help minimise the risk of contrast nephropathy. Some advocate the use of *N*-Acetyl cystine (to protect against contrast nephropathy) although the evidence for this is weak.

The small platform stent and angioplasty kits have largely replaced conventional 0.035 systems which will not be discussed further.

(a) Femoral access although in approx 10% of cases the anatomy will dictate an arm approach. Flush aortogram (Fig. 20.1) via 4-French pigtail catheter to confirm anatomy.

(b) Place 7-Fr renal double curved introducer guide catheter leaving the tip adjacent to the renal artery ostium (Fig. 20.2).

(c) Administer 3,000–5,000 units of heparin.

(d) Cross the stenosis with a 0.014 or 0.018 guide wire alternatively if a protection device is going to be used the lesion is crossed with the filter at this stage (Fig. 20.3).

(e) Pre-dilate the lesion with a 3 mm small platform balloon.

(f) Introduce the balloon mounted stent (usually 6 × 18 mm). Position checked by gentle contrast injection via the guide catheter.

(g) Deploy stent allowing for 2–3 mm to project into the aorta (Fig. 20.4).

(h) Check position with gentle contrast injection via the guide catheter (Fig. 20.5).

(i) Remove guide wire. Close and remove protection filter if used.

(j) Manual compression to groin or closure device.

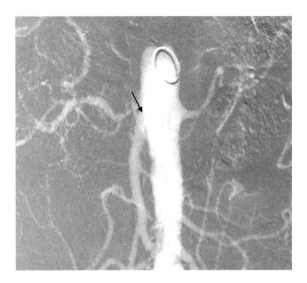

Fig. 20.1 Flush aortogram via 4Fr pigtail catheter. A significant stenosis of the right renal artery is confirmed (*arrow*)

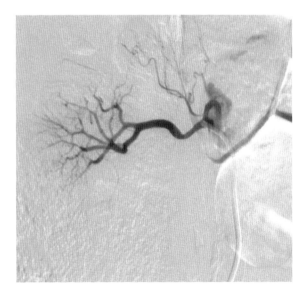

Fig. 20.2 A 7Fr double curved guide catheter is placed at the ostium of the right renal artery

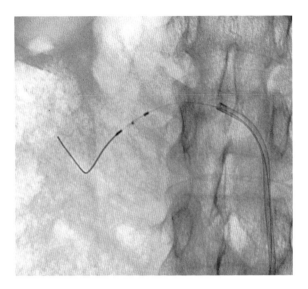

Fig. 20.3 Renal protection device is advanced past the lesion (a 0.018 or 0.014 guide wire alone is an acceptable alternative)

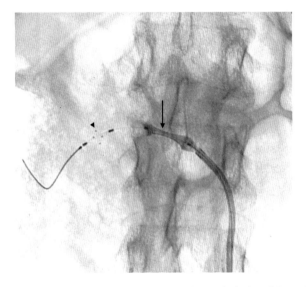

Fig. 20.4 After pre-dilation the balloon mounted stent is deployed (*arrow*) note the open configuration of the renal protection device (*arrowhead*)

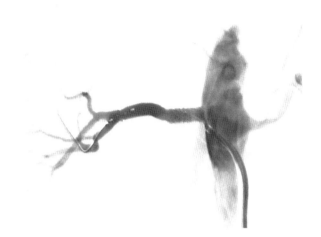

Fig. 20.5 Check angiogram via the guide catheter. Guide wire or protection device must remain in the distal vessel so as to allow access to distal vessel if dissection or rupture occurs

B. Non Ostial Atheromatous Lesions

These rare lesions may respond well to simple angioplasty and stents should be reserved for primary failures (e.g. recoil). Predilation is not required and normally a 6 mm balloon is used.

C. Fibromuscular Dysplasia

Work up should include selective renal angiography as disease affecting the second or third order vessels may be missed by non-invasive methods. Technique is the same as above except that branch lesions may require more complex techniques using "kissing" balloons. Anti-platelets agents are not required.

8   Post-procedure Management

8.1   Acute Management

Immediately post-procedure patients should be monitored for bleeding/ haematoma around the arterial puncture site. The patient is required to lie flat in bed for a 2–6 h post-procedure (depending on local practice). During this time the nursing staff perform routine observations e.g. pulse and blood pressure.

A large diuresis can occur after revascularisation with a drop in blood pressure and careful attention to fluid replacement and anti-hypertensive treatment is required.

8.2 Follow-up Protocol

There is no consensus regarding follow up. Blood pressure and renal function should be monitored. Routine renal artery imaging is not required but may be indicated if there is a clinical deterioration. Re-stenosis is often asymptomatic but when associated with recurrent symptoms e.g. worsening renal function then re-intervention should be considered (angioplasty, stenting or surgery).

9   Complications and Management

1. *Puncture Site Haematoma.* Careful pressure on the puncture site and the use of closure devices in selected patients will minimise this complication. Bleeding times are often prolonged in patients with impaired renal function.
2. *Renal Artery Dissection.* Usually inconsequential if a stent is to be placed.
3. *Renal artery Rupture.* A feared complication usually resulting in a nephrectomy in the past. Most can now be managed with either simple balloon tamponade or a covered stent.
4. *Acute Renal Failure.* In the first few days this is usually contrast related and recovers with supportive management. A more insidious loss of renal function over several weeks often indicates cholesterol embolization for which the prognosis is more guarded.

10   Outcomes-Endovascular Versus Open Surgery

When considering the management of ARVD it is worth considering that

• Maximal medical management may well be as effective as revascularization.

- Both endovascular and, open surgical revascularisation carry risks although these are often perceived to be more serious with surgery.
- Surgical series have published good results but these are from centres of excellence, in highly selected patients.
- For many elderly patients with multiple co-morbidities surgery is simply not an option.

It is our opinion that carefully selected patients may benefit from stenting and angioplasty. Surgery may have a place in complex disease or where stenting has failed, again careful patient selection on a case by case basis is recommended.

Primary angioplasty in FMD demonstrates good medium and long term patency rates and effective treatment of hypertension and renal failure. We would recommend this treatment over and above open surgery as primary treatment.

11   Renal Artery Dissections

The most common cause of renal artery dissection is secondary to endovascular treatment. Primary angioplasty of non ostial lesions and FMD may result in intimal dissection. This requires emergent treatment as the kidney will perish rapidly (60–90 min warm ischemic time).

Another scenario in which renal artery dissections are seen is as a part of aortic dissections. These are more complicated, but are treated in the same way, with the exception that the descending aortic dissection may need to be treated simultaneously.

As previously mentioned the guidewire should remain past the treated lesion until a satisfactory check angiogram has been performed. This wire will allow for access to the distal luminal vessel.

Management

1. A repeat balloon angioplasty over the existing wire with a prolonged inflation time may "stick" the intima back into position restoring flow.
2. If flow can be restored then stenting is recommended unless the angioplasty has resulted in a near-perfect angiogram. A suitable sized (6–8 mm diameter) balloon expandable stent will often provided the support necessary.
3. A second stent projecting into the aortic lumen as for the treatment of ostial stenosis may be required.

12 Renal Artery Aneurysms

Renal artery aneurysms are rare and may be idiopathic (degenerative) or occur secondary to FMD. These are typically extra-parenchymal and usually occur at the first and second order bifurcations. More peripheral aneurysm formation can be seen in some of the vasculitides (e.g. PAN and Behcet's disease), infection and trauma (including iatrogenic e.g. renal biopsy).

12.1 Diagnosis

MRA or MDCTA is usually sensitive enough to detect most aneurysms allowing for planning management and surveillance.

12.2 Management

Renal artery aneurysms are often asymptomatic. Extra parenchymal aneurysms >2 cm are at increased risk of rupture. These may be treated by either open surgical or more recently endovascular techniques. Options include coil embolization with and without stent scaffolding and stent grafting.

Flow chart summarising endovascular treatment for renal artery stenosis.

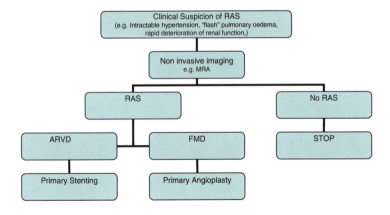

References

1. The ASTRAL Investigators. Revascularization versus medical therapy for renal-artery stenosis. N Engl J Med. 2009;361(20):1953–62.
2. Bax L, Woittiez AJ, Kouwenberg HJ, et al. Stent placement in patients with atherosclerotic renal artery stenosis and impaired renal function: a randomized trial. Ann Intern Med. 2009;150(12):840–8.
3. de Fraissinette B, Garcier JM, Dieu V, et al. Percutaneous transluminal angioplasty of dysplastic stenoses of the renal artery: results on 70 adults. Cardiovasc Intervent Radiol. 2003;26(1):46–51.
4. Hirsch AT, Haskal ZJ, Hertzer NR, et al. ACC/AHA 2005 Practice Guidelines for the management of patients with peripheral arterial disease (lower extremity, renal, mesenteric, and abdominal aortic): a collaborative report from the American Association for Vascular Surgery/Society for Vascular Surgery, Society for Cardiovascular Angiography and Interventions, Society for Vascular Medicine and Biology, Society of Interventional Radiology, and the ACC/AHA Task Force on Practice Guidelines. (Writing Committee to Develop Guidelines for the Management of Patients With Peripheral Arterial Disease): endorsed by the American Association of Cardiovascular and Pulmonary Rehabilitation; National Heart, Lung, and Blood Institute; Society for Vascular Nursing; TransAtlantic Inter-Society Consensus; and Vascular Disease Foundation. Circulation. 2006;113(11):e463–654.

Chapter 21
Mesenteric Vessels

Bram Fioole and Jean-Paul P.M. de Vries

1 Anatomy

1. The three major arteries of the mesenteric circulation arise from the ventral surface of the aorta.

   (a) The origin of the celiac artery (CA) is at the level of the 12th thoracic vertebra and behind the median arcuate ligament. Following a short anterior course, the CA commonly divides into three main branches: the common hepatic artery, the left gastric artery, and the splenic artery. These arteries supply the foregut.

   (b) The superior mesenteric artery (SMA) originates at the level of the first lumbar vertebra. It lies anterior to the left renal vein and posterior to the body of the pancreas. The SMA supplies the mid-gut (small intestine from the second part of the duodenum to the midtransverse colon), and sections of the pancreas.

   (c) The inferior mesenteric artery (IMA) arises from the aorta approximately 5 cm above the aortic bifurcation (level of the

B. Fioole, M.D., Ph.D • J.-P.P.M. de Vries, M.D., Ph.D (✉)
Department of Vascular Surgery, St. Antonius Hospital,
Koekoekslaan 1, Nieuwegein, 3435, The Netherlands
e-mail: volo61wv@kpnmail.nl

A. Kumar and K. Ouriel (eds.), *Handbook of Endovascular Interventions*,   263
DOI 10.1007/978-1-4614-5013-9_21,
© Springer Science+Business Media New York 2013

third lumbar vertebra) and supplies the left hemicolon and the proximal part of the rectum.

2. Numerous arterial interconnections exist between the three mesenteric main branches and form an abundant collateral circulation. The gastroduodenal and pancreaticoduodenal arteries form a collateral network between the CA and the SMA. The middle colic artery also links the SMA to the IMA via the left colic artery. The arterial complex of Drummond (the marginal artery in the vasa recta of the colon and the central anastomotic artery or loop of Riolan) and the arc of Riolan are interconnections between the superior and inferior mesenteric circulation.

2   Disease Definition

Mesenteric ischemia: significant stenosis or occlusions of at least two mesenteric arteries or single-vessel obstruction without sufficient collateral circulation leading to symptoms like food fear, loss of weight, and postprandial pain.

3   Disease Distribution

Unselected autopsy studies have estimated the prevalence of mesenteric atherosclerosis in at least one mesenteric artery to be up to 6–10%. The exact incidence of chronic mesenteric ischemia (CMI) has been estimated to be 1 in 100,000 of the general population per year. CMI accounts for 0.1% of all hospital admissions and 1% of the admissions in patients with acute abdominal pain. The average age of patients with CMI diagnosed is 60 years, whereas acute mesenteric ischemia (AMI) is often determined in older patients.

4   Diagnosis: Clinical and Laboratory

CMI is an uncommon disease. The symptoms may be nonspecific and vary from the classical triad: postprandial abdominal pain leading to food fear, weight loss, and upper abdominal bruit to nonspecific abdominal pain and intermittent diarrhea. Laboratory findings will not be anomalous in patients with CMI.

5   Diagnostic Imaging

A critical point in treating patients with chronic CMI—both open and with endovascular means—is adequate diagnostic imaging. Imaging studies to identify the presence of mesenteric artery obstructive disease include Duplex ultrasound (DUS), magnetic resonance angiography (MRA), or computed tomography angiography (CTA). CMI is suspected in patients with clinical suspicion of mesenteric ischemia and at least two mesenteric arteries demonstrating a hemodynamically significant stenosis or occlusion. Single-vessel visceral obstruction without sufficient collateral circulation may also lead to symptomatic CMI although this is uncommon.

1. DUS is a good noninvasive modality for obstructive disease of the CA and SMA. Sensitivity, specificity, and predictive values are all >80%. A normal duplex examination excludes the diagnosis of CMI in most of the patients. Drawbacks of DUS are the fact that the IMA may be difficult to visualize and the fact that the side branches and collaterals cannot be determined.
2. MRA combines excellent sensitivity, specificity, and predictive values with limited contrast load. It allows the determination of obstructive disease in all main visceral arteries and major collaterals. However, high-resolution MRA is not universally available, technician dependent, and some patients are excluded (metal artifacts, cardiac prosthetic valves, claustrophobia).
3. Multidetector CTA has replaced diagnostic catheter-based contrast arteriography as the imaging study of choice during last years. Besides its accuracy of detecting visceral artery obstruction (including side branches and collaterals) it will exclude other potential intra-abdominal processes in patients with abdominal complaints. CTA is sufficient to plan open visceral reconstructive surgery and useful as follow-up modality of endovascular and open revascularization procedures.
4. Diagnostic catheter based digital subtraction angiography (DSA) has been replaced by noninvasive CTA and/or DUS. In most of the patients with indication for DSA, diagnostic imaging will be combined with direct endovascular treatment in the same setting.

6   Management Paradigm and Indications (Table 21.1)

Patients presenting with longstanding symptoms suggestive of CMI and proven visceral obstructive disease on vascular imaging must be discussed in a multidisciplinary workgroup consisting of interventional

Table 21.1 Table which summarizes the role of endovascular treatment

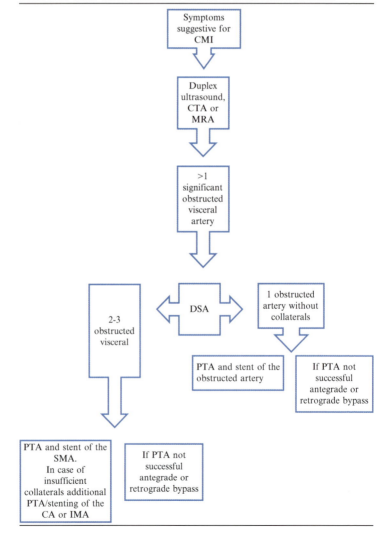

radiologists, gastroenterologists, and vascular surgeons. Other diagnoses have to be excluded by abdominal CT and (on indication) gastroscopy or colonoscopy, or both. Gastric and jejunal exercise tonometry can be used as a functional test (similar to the treadmill test in patients with peripheral arterial disease) and is used by the authors on indication. In patients with high suspicion for CMI the diagnosis can be obtained by digital subtraction angiography (DSA); endovascular treatment is performed in the same session.

7 List of the Open Operative Choices

Open surgical treatment with bypass or endarterectomy has been the standard for many years. Although the long-term outcome after open revascularization is both anatomically and functionally adequate, it is associated with substantial perioperative morbidity and mortality. Open surgery includes antegrade bypasses (bifurcation or tube grafts) from the aorta to one or more of the visceral arteries. An alternative approach is a retrograde bypass form one of the common iliac arteries to one of the visceral arteries. The SMA is the preferred target revascularization artery, both in antegrade and retrograde bypass surgery. Local thrombus in one of the visceral arteries can be treated with local thromboembolectomy. This is mainly performed in patients suffering form AMI instead of CMI. During last decade, endovascular treatment of CMI has replaced open surgery as the preferred treatment modality by nature of it being less invasive, as well as the lower morbidity and mortality rates.

8 Endovascular Intervention: Technique and Pitfalls

1. Heparin 5000 IU
2. Arterial access via a common femoral artery or brachial artery approach, or combined approach.
3. Introduction of a 6F sheath.
4. Diagnostic catheter over a 0.035-glidewire.
5. Anteroposterior and lateral abdominal aortography.

6. Selective cannulation of all three mesenteric arteries with a reversed curved or angled catheter. Evaluation of the outflow bed and collateral circulation.

7. A stenosis of >70% on DSA or a mean pressure gradient of at least 10 mm Hg across the lesion is considered hemodynamically significant.

8. Sufficient collateral circulation is identified when rapid filling occurs of the diseased visceral artery by the gastroduodenal or pancreaticoduodenal arteries, the marginal artery of Drummond or the arc of Riolan. In case of small collaterals without rapid filling of the diseased visceral artery collateral circulation must be considered insufficient.

9. At this point the diagnosis CMI is assessed or rejected.

10. Endovascular treatment will be focused on the SMA. In case of successful treatment of the obstructed SMA combined with sufficient collaterals to the CA and IMA, the procedure can be stopped. Only in case of persistent complaints of CMI during follow-up a second visceral artery obstruction (in the CA or IMA) must be treated. Recanalization of long-segment occlusions can be very challenging, especially via a common femoral artery approach. In patients with a long-segment SMA occlusion and a significant celiac artery (CA) or inferior mesenteric artery (IMA) stenosis both latter arteries can be treated and collateral circulation to the SMA must be assessed. In patients with single-vessel disease without sufficient collateral circulation, this mono-artery obstruction must be treated.

11. After crossing the stenosis or occlusion with a 0.035-inch wire, PTA and stent placement (PTAS) will be performed. Primary placement of a short balloon expandable stent (diameter 4–7 mm) is preferred, since recoil in visceral arteries is observed frequently. All stents should be slightly oversized (max. 10% compared to the measured diameter of the visceral artery). The stenosis can be predilated if necessary, to lower the risk of dislodgement of plaque material/ debris during advancement of the stent. The use of embolic protection devices is not indicated.

12. Technical success is defined as proper placement of the stents and a residual diameter reduction <30% after PTAS or a pressure gradient <5 mm Hg across the lesion.

9 Post-procedure Management and Follow-up Protocol

1. Clinical success is defined as technical success in at least one visceral artery, proven sufficient collateral circulation to the other visceral arteries, and the resolution of symptoms and weight gain at least 3 months after the procedure, or both.
2. All patients are prescribed aspirin (100 mg daily) after (and preferably also prior to) the procedure. In addition to aspirin, clopidogrel (75 mg daily) is prescribed for 3 months in patients who underwent stent placement. After re-endothelialization of the stent, clopidogrel might be stopped.
3. If the endovascular treatment fails, a visceral bypass must be considered.
4. Regular follow-up consists of a history and physical examination 3 months post-intervention and yearly thereafter. If the patient has complete symptom relief, one might omit additional imaging. An asymptomatic single-vessel restenosis has not been associated with death or adverse cardiologic events. Only asymptomatic patients with hemodynamically significant three-vessel visceral obstructions should be considered for prophylactic mesenteric arterial revascularization, because of the increased risk for acute thromboemboli or occlusions during follow-up. This has to be done on a case to case to basis.

10 Complications and Management

1. **Dissection** Dissections might lead to flow obstructive lesions. In most patients this complication can immediately be treated by additional stent placement. In rare cases this complication results in conversion to open repair, and local arteriotomy with tacking of the intimal core or short bypass grafts are the solutions.
2. **Distal Embolization** is a rare complication. As mentioned before, the use of embolic protection devices is not indicated. Thrombosuction or thrombolyses are endovascular solutions. In order to prevent irreversible intestinal ischemia conversion to open embolectomy or visceral bypass might be indicated in case of complete occlusion without collateral circulation.

3. **Rupture** of a target artery is also a very rare complication. Most ruptures can be treated endovascularly by means of a covered stent.
4. **Access site complications** consist of:
   (a) Dissection or obstruction, for which endarterectomy and patch plasty of the brachial or femoral artery is indicated.
   (b) Hematoma, for which surgical intervention is rarely indicated.
5. **Restenosis** is observed frequently. Primary 2-years patency after endovascular treatment for CMI is only 60%, but in-stent stenoses can often be treated successfully with repeated endovascular techniques. Moreover, over 60% of visceral artery restenoses are asymptomatic. A minority of patients with symptomatic restenoses will eventually need open visceral bypass revascularization.

11   Outcomes: Endovascular Versus Open

Open revascularization has been associated with substantial morbidity and mortality. Reported morbidity rates ranges from 12 to 33%. In the largest published series of specialized centers mortality after open revascularization ranges from 2 to 15%. Although endarterectomy and antegrade or retrograde bypasses have been associated with significant rates of morbidity and mortality, open revascularization provides durable symptom relief. After open revascularization excellent clinical success rates up to 92% at 5 years follow-up have been reported. It has been considered the standard for many years. Initial technical success rate for PTAS is >90%, and morbidity and mortality rates are lower compared to surgery. However, primary patency and clinical success rates are only reasonable. On the other hand, in-stent stenoses can often be treated successfully with repeated endovascular techniques. PTAS as first-choice treatment in patients with CMI is safe, technical, successful, and will result in only 14% of the patients in conversion to open repair during longer term follow-up

12   Visceral Aneurysms

The incidence of these lesions in routine autopsy series is only 0.01–0.2%. Most commonly involved vessels include the splenic artery, hepatic artery, SMA, and CA. Nearly a quarter of the visceral aneurysms present as clinical emergencies, 8.5% will result in death. Possible risk factors are hormonal changes, high flow states, former abdominal infections, trauma, and catheterization injuries. The majority of visceral aneurysms are asymptomatic and diagnosed coincidentally at abdominal CT-scans for other indications. Risk of rupture is increased in diameters >2 cm. Endovascular treatment is preferred and consists of covered stents or embolization of the aneurysm. During the latter procedure, the outflow artery is first embolized, thereafter the inflow of the aneurysm is embolized. Before embolization of the visceral aneurysm one must be sure that the visceral artery can be occluded locally without disastrous consequences for the target organ.

13 Visceral Dissections

Most chronic dissections are asymptomatic and should not be treated. Most of the chronic dissections will resolve spontaneously. The significant majority of acute dissections occur during visceral artery catheterization, a minority will occur spontaneously. In case of persistent pain, hemodynamically significant obstructions (or occlusion) with symptoms, malperfusion of the target organ, or increase of the diameter of the false lumen the dissection must be treated. Endovascular treatment with additional stent placement is preferred. Dual platelet therapy is recommended because of the mild increased risk of distal thromboemboli.

References

1. Park WM, Cherry Jr KJ, Chua HK, Clark RC, Jenkins G, Harmsen WS, Noel AA, Panneton JM, Bower TC, Hallett Jr JW, Gloviczki P. Current results of open revascularization for chronic mesenteric ischemia: a standard for comparison. J Vasc Surg. 2002;35:853–9.
2. Kougias P, El Sayed HF, Zhou W, Lin PH. Management of chronic mesenteric ischemia. The role of endovascular therapy. J Endovasc Ther. 2007;14: 395–405.
3. Fioole B, van de Rest HJ, Meijer JR, van Leersum M, van Koeverden S, Moll FL, van den Berg JC, de Vries JP. Percutaneous transluminal angioplasty and stenting as first-choice treatment in patients with chronic mesenteric ischemia. J Vasc Surg. 2010;51:386–91.

4. Messina LM, Shanley CJ. Visceral artery aneurysms. Surg Clin North Am. 1997;77:425–42.
5. Takach TJ, Madjarov JM, Holleman JH, Robicsek F, Roushi TS. Spontaneous splanchnic dissection: application and timing of therapeutic options. J Vasc Surg. 2009;50:557–63.

Chapter 22
Endovascular Treatment
of Infrarenal Aortic Aneurysms

Eric Fishman and Peter L. Faries

The first open infrarenal abdominal aortic aneurysm (AAA) repair was performed in 1951. Dubost replaced the AAA with a thoracic aortic homograft harvested from a recently deceased 20 year old. He performed a proximal end-to-end anastomosis, and a distal right Common Iliac Artery (CIA) end-to-end anastomosis, and then an end-to-side anastomosis after an endarterectomy on an occluded L CIA in a patient who went on to live for another 8 years. The first use of synthetic material for repair of aneurysms was by Blakemore and Voorhees in 1954. They repaired 17 aortic aneurysms with Vinyon "N" cloth grafts. Open technique remained standard until the development of Endovascular Abdominal Aneurysm Repair (EVAR). In 1991, Parodi et al. performed the first EVAR in Argentina and in 1992 Parodi and Marin et al. performed the first EVAR in the USA (Fig. 22.1). Since then there has been tremendous development in stent-grafts, endovascular techniques, and management of complications which has allowed for EVAR to become the most common approach for AAA repair. Open repair is presently used mostly in patients who, for any of a variety of factors, are not candidates for

E. Fishman, M.D. • P.L. Faries, M.D. (✉)
Department of Vascular Surgery, Mount Sinai Medical Center,
5 East 98th St, 3rd Fl., Box 1273, New York, NY 10029, USA
e-mail: Peter.faries@mountsinai.org

A. Kumar and K. Ouriel (eds.), *Handbook of Endovascular Interventions*, 273
DOI 10.1007/978-1-4614-5013-9_22,
© Springer Science+Business Media New York 2013

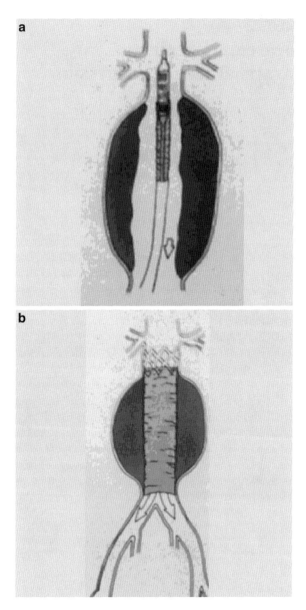

Fig. 22.1 (a) Introduction of delivery device (Schematic of Parodi JC stent—graft 1991). (b) Deployment of device (Schematic of Parodi JC stent—graft 1991)

endovascular repair. As technology advances the percentage of patients who undergo open repair is likely to become increasingly smaller.

1 Anatomy

Understanding aorto-iliac anatomy is important for the successful performance of EVAR.

Most AAA are infrarenal. However, up to 15% of AAA may have a juxtarenal or suprarenal component. Currently available FDA-approved devices can be used to treat most infrarenal AAA; however, fenestrated grafts or hybrid procedures are required to treat suprarenal AAA. In the USA fenestrated grafts are currently available only on a trial basis. Some of these devices are more readily available outside the USA.

A second anatomic factor of importance relates to the landing zone and the adequacy of the neck. A "neck" refers to the distance from the origin of the most distal renal artery and the beginning of the aneurysm. Currently most devices can treat AAA with a neck of up to 3.2 cm in diameter and 15 mm in length. The talent device is approved to treat shorter (10 mm) necks. The ideal neck is parallel, with no angulation or eccentric thrombus in the wall. 45–60° angulation is the maximum suggested by the device manufacturers (Fig. 22.2). In cases where the diameter is not uniform throughout the (conical) neck, up to a 3 mm difference in diameter is well tolerated. The presence of an accessory or duplicated renal artery may reduce the neck length. In these cases the possibility of covering an accessory renal artery and the possibility of partial renal ischemia has to be carefully considered. Other factors, which are important in terms of the adequacy of the neck, are tortuosity of the aorta and the presence and nature of thrombosis at the proximal seal zone. All devices today are bifurcated and distally the stent is landed on the iliac arteries. Distally adequate seal zones require adequate arterial length and diameter to prevent a distal type I endoleak. 20–30% of infrarenal AAA have common iliac artery aneurysms. If the common iliac arteries are short or aneurysmal, the devices may require external iliac artery deployment. In these cases the internal iliac artery or arteries may need to be embolized to prevent a type II endoleak; an internal iliac branched graft may be used in limited cases. Adequacy of

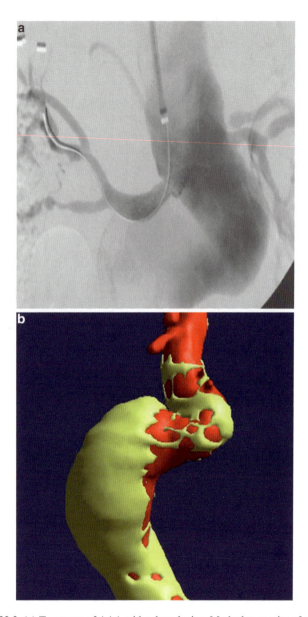

Fig. 22.2 (a) Treatment of AAA with talent device. Marked tortuosity of proximal aortic neck presented significant challenge to endovascular treatment. (b) Treatment of AAA with Talent device. CTA 3D reconstruction. (c) Treatment of AAA with Talent device. Use of proximal extension prosthesis permitted device to conform to aortic neck and prevent endoleak at proximal fixation site

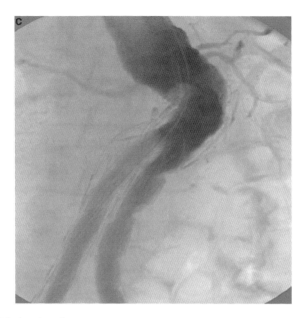

Fig. 22.2 (continued)

collateral blood supply related to previous surgical history to the colon and pelvic organs has to be taken into account. A large patent IMA may be cause for a type II endoleak and in some centers this vessel may be embolized preoperatively.

The third anatomic factor of importance relates to the access vessels. Standard deployment of stent grafts requires placement of large diameter sheaths in the common femoral arteries. Vessels of at least 6 mm are required for the current available devices. In addition, tortuosity of femoral and iliac vessels may impede passage of the device. Although the use of stiff wire may allow some straightening of these vessels, care must be taken to prevent risk of arterial rupture. Severe calcification (circumferential) of the vessels may also impede advancement of the device. Techniques such the use of an iliac conduit, may allow for passage of the device. If one iliac vessel is simply not amenable, an aorto-uni device and fem–fem bypass may be considered.

2 Disease Definition

An aneurysm is defined as a 50% enlargement of a vessel. The normal infrarenal aorta measures 2 cm on average in men and 1.8 cm in women. The normal common iliac artery measures approx 1.2 cm in men. Most AAA are fusiform as opposed to saccular which are slightly more frequent in thoracic aortic aneurysms (TAA).

In regards to etiology, more than 90% of aneurysm is degenerative. Although the term "atherosclerotic" is still commonly applied to such aneurysms, atherosclerosis per se is not a direct cause. Complex processes are associated with the pathophysiology of these aneurysms. Other causes of AAA are inflammatory or mycotic in nature. Inflammatory aneurysms that are not infectious in etiology are potentially amenable to EVAR. Mycotic aneurysms are not treated with EVAR since the focus of infection is still present. The exception is an emergency. EVAR can be used as a temporary bridge to definitive repair for ruptured mycotic aneurysms. AAA is repaired to prevent rupture which carries a high mortality rate. Size is the major factor associated with aneurysm rupture. The relationship of AAA diameter and rupture risks is described subsequently. In addition to size, the aneurysm's rate of increase over time, the patient's cigarette usage, and life expectancy play a role in the decision to operate as opposed to the decision to observe. Clinical trials have been conducted comparing observation versus repair.

3 Disease Distribution

There are 27 million AAA patients worldwide. The prevalence of AAA in the over 50 population ranges from 3% to 10% in multiple screening and autopsy studies performed in the USA and internationally. In a VA-screening study of 73,000 patients the prevalence of AAA is 4.6% among patients from ages 50 to 79. The rupture of an AAA is the 15th leading cause of death in the USA and the 10th leading cause of death in men older than 55. These numbers have steadily increased since prevalence studies were performed starting 50 years ago. The most significant risk factors for AAA are smoking, age, gender, family history, and race. Men have a two to six times higher frequency of AAA than women. Caucasians have a two to higher times frequency of AAA than non-Caucasians. Other less important risk factors are hypertension and hypercholesterolemia.

The overall mortality of patients with ruptured AAA is 80–90%. 30–50% of patients with ruptured AAA die prior to reaching the hospital. 30–40% of patients die after reaching the hospital without any intervention. There are approximately 40,000 elective AAA repair in the USA every year.

Operative mortality rates for ruptured AAA range from 40% to 50% though there is increasing evidence that mortality with endovascular repair will be lower.

4   Diagnosis

Physical examination is very limited as a form of diagnosis in this condition. The positive predictive value of physical examination is only 15%. Most AAA are found either incidentally during the course of radiologic examinations for other reasons or, more recently, from screening programs. Multiple studies of ultrasound (U/S) screening have shown benefit. Historically, most of these studies come from the UK. Today in the USA, Medicare reimburses, a one time screening for males 65 years and older. Screenings with a second ultrasound have not proved to add benefit. Routine screenings for women are not generally recommended in the USA though screenings of women with specific risk factors, such as a positive family history or a history of tobacco use are beneficial. The most common confirmatory test for physical exam results is B-mode U/S. B-mode U/S is non-nvasive, inexpensive and therefore commonly used for follow-up of small AAA. When the AAA reaches a size where repair is considered, a thin cut (3 mm) CT angiogram (CTA) is the test of choice. If a repair is indicated, the CTA is useful in deciding upon whether the repair should be open or endovascular. MRA is slightly more expensive than CTA and requires more time for imaging, but it may be used in lieu of CTA in specific circumstance such as when platinum coils from a previous embolization limits the benefit of CTA, or if the patient has an iodine dye allergy. Angiography is usually performed when a specific preoperative intervention may be required, such as pre-EVAR embolization of a hypogastric artery or the definition of renal vascular anatomy in cases where the patient has more than one renal artery. Digital subtraction angiography is rarely required at

Table 22.1 Range of potential rupture rates for a given size of abdominal aortic aneurysm

AAA Diameter (cm)	Rupture risk (%/year)
<4	0
4–5	0.5–5
5–6	3–15
6–7	10–20
7–8	20–40
>8	30–50

Brewster DC, Cronenwett JL, Hallett JW Jr, et al. (2003) Guidelines for the treatment of abdominal aortic aneurysms. Report of the sub-committee of the Joint Council of the American Association for Vascular Surgery and Society for Vascular Surgery. J Vasc Surg.37:1106–1117

present for diagnostic purposes and frequently underestimates the aneurysm diameter.

Alternative approaches such as CT without contrast, CO_2 as contrast or intravascular US (IVUS) may be utilized for preoperative planning in patients with renal insufficiency. However the EVAR procedure itself requires contrast, therefore the renal function itself must be taken into account as comorbidity when evaluating a patient for surgery.

5 Management

Repair of an asymptomatic AAA is prophylactic and elective. The decision for repair must weigh the risk of AAA rupture on the one hand with the operative risk and the patient's life expectancy on the other. A thorough discussion of each of these factors with the patient is necessary for the patient to give informed consent.

Although not ideal, the primary determinant of AAA rupture used in practice is aneurysm size. In the UK small aneurysm trial (UKSAT) annual rupture risk was found to be 0.3% (3.9 cm or smaller), 1.5% (4–4.9 cm), and 6.5% (5–5.9 cm). These finding apply mostly to men who encompassed 85% of the study population. Other studies with similar numbers document rupture rates of 10–20% (6–7 cm) and 20–40% (>7 cm). (Table 22.1) Advances in predicting the risk of rupture include models of aneurysm wall stress and finite element analysis.

Table 22.2 Life expectancy in years for patients surviving abdominal aortic Aneurysm repair by age, gender, and race

Age (yr)	Total	Male White	Black	Female White	Black
60	13	12	11	14	13
65	11	11	10	12	11
70	10	9	8	10	10
75	8	8	7	9	8
80	6	6	6	7	6
≥85	5	4	4	5	5

Rutherford's Vascular Surgery 7th Edition Page 1941

Less significant factors influencing the risk of rupture include female gender and family history, smoking (active as well as past history) and the rate of the aneurysm's expansion. Predicted rate of expansion is 10% of size per year. An expansion rate beyond 10% may assist in the recommendation for repair in smaller aneurysm.

Two major studies, The UK small aneurysm trial (UKSAT) and the aneurysm detection and management study (ADAM), have demonstrated a negligible risk of rupture in AAA less than 4 cm. These aneurysms may be followed with U/S. There was a clear benefit of AAA repair in aneurysms larger than 5.5 cm. Recommendation for follow up versus operative intervention in aneurysms 4–5.5 cm may vary according referral patterns, gender, and rate of expansion

In regards to endovascular repair, recently, two trials the CAESAR in Europe and the PIVOTAL study in the USA are in the process of studying the risk of rupture versus endovascular repair in aneurysms smaller than 5.5 cm. Operative mortality of endovascular repair is lower than for open repair and overall EVAR outcomes (in retrospective reviews) have been shown to be better in smaller AAA.

In terms of operative risk, open repair has had a steady 4% mortality rate over the last few decades. EVAR has shown an operative mortality rate of approximately 1% in multiple studies. For this reason, the decision to intervene will be different if the patient is not a candidate for endovascular repair. Given the low mortality rate for EVAR, prediction algorithms, which take into account the patient's comorbidities, have not been found to contribute significantly to the calculation of operative risk.

Calculating the life expectancy for candidates of AAA repair is not simple. Factors such as the impact of the procedure itself, the patient's comorbidities (both associated and independent from AAA), and age of the patient are all contributing factors. (Table 22.2)

6   Types of Stent Grafts

Although there a many differences across stent-grafts, there are no randomized studies comparing one device to another. The EuroSTAR database provides information in the use and long-term follow-up of a variety of devices. Use of one device versus the other may be more related to the physician's comfort with a specific device than to the technical differences among devices. However, understanding the differences among devices in terms of construction specifications, benefits and failure modes is of importance. The EVAR market was calculated at 370 million US$ in 2004 and is projected to be 1.7 billion US$ in 2012.

At present there are six FDA-approved stent graft devices in the USA. Among the Medtronic devices (Santa Rosa, CA), the Talent device has significantly replaced the use of the AneuRx device, which is no longer manufactured. Other devices in use are the Gore Excluder (W. L. Gore and Associates, Flagstaff, AZ), the Zenith (Cook, Inc. Bloomington, IN), and the Powerlink (Endologix, Irvine, CA).

6.1   The Talent Device (Fig. 22.3)

The endovascular stent graft developed by World Medical and Medtronic has been implanted in more than 15,000 patients worldwide. The Talent graft is used in two configurations: tapered/aortouni-iliac and bifurcated/aortobi-iliac. It is self-expanding and composed of a Dacron graft with a nitinol frame, which supports the graft. The proximal aortic fixation device possesses a 1.5 cm of uncovered nitinol frame proximal to the fabric portion of the device. This uncovered portion permits transrenal fixation of the device, thereby allowing the treatment of AAAs with relatively short or angulated proximal necks. The Talent device may be used for proximal aortic neck sizes up to 32 mm and for iliac implantation site diameters up to 22 mm. Deployment of the device is similar to that of the AneuRx device, although runners are not required for delivery of the Talent device. The main aortic component with the ipsilateral iliac limb is delivered through a 22 or 24-French system. The second, contralateral iliac limb module is then deployed via the contralateral femoral artery using an 18 or 20-French delivery system.

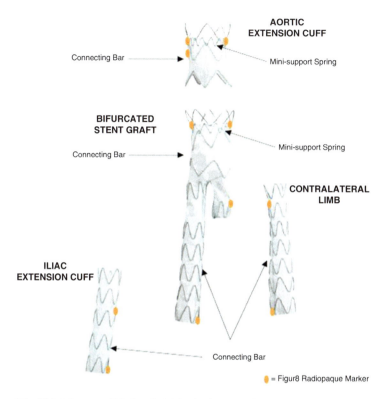

Fig. 22.3 Diagram of Medtronic Abdominal Endograft Components

6.2   The Excluder

The Excluder is a modular endoprosthesis composed of PTFE bonded to a nitinol exoskeleton. There are proximal covered flares, positive fixation anchors, and a sealing cuff. Radiopaque markers are positioned at the very end of the graft material. The device comes in aortic diameters of 23–31 mm and iliac diameters of 10–20 mm. The ipsilateral limb sheath is 18–20 Fr and the contralateral limb sheath is 12–18 Fr. The contraleral gate has a gold rim for opacification. The device is deployed with one rapid pull of the deploying cord.

6.3   The Zenith

The Zenith system from Cook is a modular bifurcated device but is also available in an aortouni-iliac configuration. It consists of woven polyester graft material supported throughout its length by self-expanding stainless steel Z-stents. The introducer tip is tapered to minimize trauma at the arterial insertion site and there are side holes at the tip to allow angiography with the system in place. The Zenith stent-graft system has a bare proximal stent that expands radially upon deployment. There are barbs on this bare stent to secure the device to the suprarenal aortic wall. The suprarenal bare stent is deployed after being released by a trigger wire, which holds it in place to avoid premature deployment. The main aortic body is deployed using an 18, 20 or 22-Fr. Sheath (inner diameter). The iliac limb is delivered using a 14 or 16-Fr. sheath (inner diameter). The Zenith device can be used in aortic necks up to 32 mm and in iliac arteries up to 20 mm. The system is designed to allow all components to be used together and as a result a greater range of anatomic sizes can be managed with the Zenith graft.

6.4   Endologix PowerLink System

The Endologix PowerLink system is a one-piece bifurcated graft comprised of polytetrafluoroethylene (PTFE) supported by nitinol. The one-piece design eliminates the risk of endoleaks seen at attachment sites in modular devices. In addition, the frame is composed of a self-expanding non-nitinol wire, which eliminates the need for sutures to hold individual stents in place. The graft is thin-walled PTFE, which may allow for downsizing of the delivery system. The PTFE fabric is sewn to the stents only at the proximal and distal ends of the device. This allows the fabric to move off the endoskeleton. Aortic necks up to 26 mm may be treated.

6.5   Other Devices

There is a small group of stent grafts, which are currently used in Europe and not available in the USA In addition to these, there is constant development of newer devices with modifications that may allow use in patients who cannot undergo EVAR with the use of current devices. These include prefabricated or in-vivo fenestrations, branched grafts and larger aortic sizes.

6.5.1 The Anaconda System (Vascutek, Terumo, Inchinnan, Scotland)

The Anaconda stent-graft system for aneurysm treatment is a fully modular system made of woven material one-third thinner than conventional graft material. The stents are made of nitinol. A unique feature is the proximal ring stent, which is composed of multiple turns of nitinol wire. The hoop strength that results from the radial force of this ring stent allows the proximal end to anchor to the aortic wall. Because of the saddle configuration of the proximal ring stent, the device can be placed so that the graft is situated at and above the renal ostia while the renal ostia themselves are uncovered. A system of magnets is used to aid in cannulating the main body of the graft in order to position the contralateral limb in place.

6.5.2 Trivascular Enovus and Ovation (Trivascular Corporation, Santa Rosa, CA, USA)

The Trivascular graft employs a novel technology to provide support to the vascular graft material. Rather than employing metallic stents along the length of the graft material, the device contains longitudinal channels that spiral along the course of the graft. After the device has been positioned within the vascular system, the channels are filled with a synthetic polymer that, when it subsequently hardens, provides radial and longitudinal support to the graft material. In eliminating stent support along the length of the graft, the profile of the device has been lowered considerably. As a result, the device may be deployed through a 14-French system. This reduction in the diameter of the delivery system may ultimately allow for percutaneous application of this endovascular technology.

6.5.3 Incraft (Cordis)

The Incraft device has recently started a phase II trial. The devices uses an integrated sheath of braided construction which allows for a small profile of 13 french. This ultra-low profile may allow for use in a wider group of patients. The INNOVATION TRIAL is in progress in Germany and Italy at this time.

6.5.4   Endurant (Medtronic)

The Endurant device is used in Europe at present time. The device is undergoing evaluation in the USA for FDA approval. The device has increased flexibility and smaller profile with 18–20 French for the main device and 14–16 French for the contralateral iliac limb. The delivery system is hydrophilic with an inner nitinol in delivery device for support. Proximally, the device has suprarenal bare stent and covered M-shaped stent for increased radial force and improved proximal fixation. There is availability of straight, tapered, or flared limbs for variable iliac anatomy.

6.5.5   Aorfix (Lombard UK)

The Aorfix device is designed for complex proximal aortic neck with an angulation of up to 90°. The fishmouth design contributes to effective sealing. This device has been used in small group of patients in Europe, Russia, and Brazil.

6.5.6   Aptus (Aptus Endosystems INC.)

The Aptus device uses helical endostapling technology for independent endograft fixation. This device is being used on a trial basis in Europe, where it is used in primary or secondary intervention for complex necks.

6.5.7   Nellix (Nellix Endovascular)

The Nellix device uses a fully contained, polymer filled (PEG based) endobag, which conforms to aneurismal sac and theoretically reduces likelihood of endoleak. This device is being used investigationally in New Zealand and California.

7 Stent Graft Design

Stent grafts must create a seal for successful treatment of AAA to take place. One of the factors, which may prevent this seal, initially or in the long term, is migration of the graft distally. Other distal components may also become separated from the normal aortic wall by forces created by the pulses pressure of blood flow. There are different methods of fixation to prevent migration.

Positive fixation refers to the use of anchoring devices such as barbs or hooks which embed into the aortic wall, which may provide high fixation force and prevent migration. Of note, some circumstances such as proximal neck calcification may prevent embedding of barbs. The, proximal covered flares and sealing cuffs may provide further apposition. Stent stiffness along the length of the graft may use a good seal in the iliac arteries to prevent migration of the proximal end of the device. Radial force may keep the device in place.

Suprarenal fixation in which a bare stent extends proximal to the renal arteries may provide a theoretical advantage to prevent migration.

Radio-opaque markers are present in different forms in all devices. It's important to be aware of the different relationship of these markers to the actual end of the stent-graft (which is not radio-opaque). In this manner deployment, proximally and opening of the contra-lateral gate will be performed in the exact location and angle desired.

Since the initial development of stent grafts, there has been significant improved in ease of the deployment mechanism. Although a device may be more "simple" to deploy, the only real important factor in successful deployment is the understanding of device function. Each device has a different type, use, and profile of sheath. Each sheath has a different type of valve and may or may not allow for injection of contrast through the device at time of deployment. Improved flexibility and trackability of devices has reduced injury to the access arteries. In the future an even lower device profile may allow for percutaneous access to the femoral vessels. It's important to keep in mind that as devices evolve in minor characteristics, we must renew our long-term follow-up to confirm the improvement of EVAR results.

8   Intervention: Technique and Pitfalls

We perform all procedures in the operating room, where the utmost sterility and nursing as well as instrument access is present in case of the need for conversion to open repair. Anesthetic technique is mostly based on the surgeon's preference. The primary choice is between spinal anesthesia with mild sedation or general anesthesia. Exceptions are severe pulmonary disease where spinal anesthesia may be a better option and situations when the need for iliac conduit makes general anesthesia the better choice. We have used local with sedation, at least initially, in cases of aneurysm rupture.

Historically access to the femoral vessels has been performed in an open manner. With rare exceptions we perform a transverse incision above the femoral crease. This may prevent slightly the rate of wound complications. More recently the availability of closure devices, such as the Proglide device with the preclose technique, has allowed us to perform a percutaneous access in certain group of patients. CTA characteristics of femoral vessels (occlusive disease; calcification), U/S and micropuncture-guided access and body mass index (BMI) of patients are important factors to consider when utilizing percutaneous access.

If CTA evaluation of the external or common iliac arteries shows severe tortuousity, circumferential calcification, or severe occlusive disease, a few maneuvers may be considered. If the anatomy is considered prohibitive in terms of femoral access, an iliac artery conduit using a retroperitoneal incision may be used. The anastomosis is performed in an end-to-side fashion with a 10-mm graft. After placement and deployment of the stent graft, the conduit stump may be over-sewed or may be anastomosed to the common femoral artery in an end-to-side fashion. This maneuver may allow for increased flow in cases of severe occlusive iliac disease or more importantly for the possibility of need for re-intervention in the future. In our institution, in specific groups of patients, we may perform an internal endoconduit. This procedure requires deployment of a covered stent (to prevent iliac artery rupture) with subsequent angioplasty to allow for a sufficient diameter. Sewing an 8-mm PTFE graft to the distal end of the covered stent may allow for anastomosis to the common femoral artery at the end of the procedure. After access is acquired, stiff wires will be required for delivery of the device. This type of wire will straighten a tortuous iliac artery and allow for easier delivery of the device. Stiff wires must be inserted with the use of catheters to prevent arterial injury or plaque disruption. Initially a stiff wire is placed through the side of the main limb to the level of the descending thoracic aorta. A pigtail is placed right above the renal arteries (L1–L2).

Prior to starting to deploy, is important to plan the orientation of the contralateral gate, for ease of access of the gate. For proximal deployment, a magnified view is used. Parallax is avoided by centering the gantry over the renal arteries. Cranio-caudad angulation of the gantry is important to compensate for the possible anterior angulation of the aortic neck. In the same fashion visualizing the take-off of the lowest renal artery at right angle will allow for exact deployment (within 2 mm of lowest renal artery). This will limit the risk of type I endoleak in short necks and minimize the risk for device migration in the long-term.

In terms of deployment, the Cook Zenith and Medtronic Talent devices use a slow deployment. For these devices we begin with deployment 1–2 cm proximal to intended deployment site. For the Gore excluder, rapid deployment, the device is placed at the exact site of intended placement. For the Gore or Medtronic device the main device is deployed until the ipsilateral limb is open. In specific cases the ipsilateral limb may remain constrained to allow ease of contralateral gate access. For the Cook device the ipsilateral limb remains constrained. At this point the contralateral gate maybe accessed or deployment of the suprarenal fixation may be done first.

For access of the contra-lateral gate, putting the main device up the more tortuous iliac (if safe from the profile standpoint), may allow for a straight shot at time of cannulation. For the Medtronic and Gore device the limbs may be crossed or parallel depending on the angles of the iliac in question. For the Cook device crossing the limbs is not recommended.

Access of the contra-lateral gate is successful in 99% of cases. In case of inability to access the gate, conversion to an aorto-uni device with a femoral–femoral bypass is performed. To access the contralateral gate, an angle glidewire and catheters of different angles may be used. If unsuccessful the wire may be snared from the main limb (up and over), or using brachial access. Deployment of the iliac limbs must be performed with maximum coverage (as close to hypogastric as possible) to prevent migration and a distal type I endoleak in the future. After complete deployment of the device, a compliant balloon is used to complete apposition of the graft to the aortic wall. Care must be taken to avoid inflating the balloon in the uncovered distal iliac arteries in order to prevent arterial injury or rupture. Completion arteriography is performed with an overall image and magnified proximal and distal views. Endoleaks must be ruled-out, patency of renals and hypogastric must be evaluated and exact landing of the device proximally and distally must be confirmed.

For treatment of a proximal type I endoleak, after using the balloon for a second time, a proximal cuff and, if necessary, a large (uncovered) Palmaz stent may be used (Chap. 17—Endovascular treatment of symptomatic abdominal aortic aneurysms). This sometimes requires extending the coverage proximally at or above the renal arteries. To preserve the renal arteries the chimney graft technique has been suggested.

8.1 Chimney Stent

This is a stent placed parallel to the aortic stent graft to maintain flow to the visceral side branches including the renal arteriesm which were overstented to ensure an adequate seal. Depending upon the extent to which the stent graft is deployed, this might require stenting of the superior mesenteric artery (SMA), one or both renals.

Typically covered stents are used; however, uncovered stents can also be used in certain circumstances. Both can be either balloon expandable or self expanding, depending upon the need, whether the need is for radial strength or flexibility respectively.

In preplanned procedures, a juxta-aneurysmal branch is cannulated in an antegrade fashion by brachial artery access. A hydrophilic glidewire is used to cannulate the branch. This is exchanged for a stiff wire such as an Ampltaz Super Stiff (Boston Scientific, Natick, MA, USA). Over this a long sheath with a stent is introduced into the side branch. The aortic stent graft is then released, and the renal stet is deployed in the side branch as a chimney stent.

For a distal type I endoleak, limb extensions may be used. If the size of an ectatic common iliac artery does not allow for a proper seal, intra-op embolization of the hypogastric artery with limb extension into the external iliac artery may be performed. Newer branched devices are being developed to preserve flow into the internal iliac. They are not FDA approved yet. A femoral–femoral bypass, or external-to-internal iliac bypass may be performed to preserve flow to the pelvis; although there is good evidence that preoperative, early embolization of one or both hypogastric arteries is well tolerated.

9   Complications and Management

(a) **Endoleaks**: These are described in detail in Chap. 23 — Endoleaks — Types and Management (Figs. 22.4 and 22.5).

(b) **Renal Artery Occlusion**: Renal artery occlusion is primarily caused by a deployment issue. Awareness of parallax, renal artery angle, distance of covered graft to opacified markers is of paramount importance. If partial renal artery coverage is diagnosed at time of procedure, attempt at stenting through brachial artery access should be considered.

(c) **Graft Limb Occlusion**: With the recent modifications of using short evenly distributed stents within the limb grafts, and adequate preoperative measurement, limb occlusion is uncommon. However, close early postoperative clinical surveillance must take this potential complication into account. In case of suspicion of this, the patient should undergo a rapid CT angiogram.

(d) **Stent-Graft Infection**: Prevention requires keeping strict sterile surgical technique. Reported stent graft infection is low at less than 0.5%. However, if this does develop, this requires explantation of part or all of the graft.

(e) **Pelvic Ischemia**: Occlusion of one or both internal iliac arteries may lead to pelvic ischemia. Buttock claudication is the most common consequence; at approximately 30% of patients with bilateral hypogastric artery occlusion. 50% of these patients' symptoms will usually resolve within 6 months, other patients' symptoms may improve. Other potential consequences of internal iliac artery occlusion are erectile dysfunction, buttock necrosis, ischemic colitis, colon necrosis, and spinal ischemia. Previous colonic surgery where the SMA does not provide collaterals to the colon and diseased profunda femoris artery with decreased pelvic collaterals are some of the risk factors. At our institution we embolize one side, wait 2 weeks looking for signs of ischemia of pelvic ischemia and then wait another 2 weeks prior to EVAR. In specific cases we perform routine sigmoidoscopy the day after surgery.

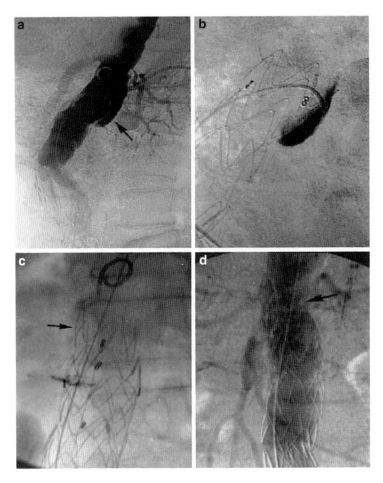

Fig. 22.4 As in the figure

(f) **Complications of Vascular Access**: Rupture of the iliac artery at time of the delivery of the device is potentially catastrophic and maintaining wire access when starting the closure of the artery may be life saving. Alternatively, in case of suspicion an angiogram with the sheath tip just inside the arteriotomy site can be done. We routinely mark pulses or Doppler signals prior to starting the procedure. A dissecting flap of a diseased access artery or embolization may cause distal vessel occlusion.

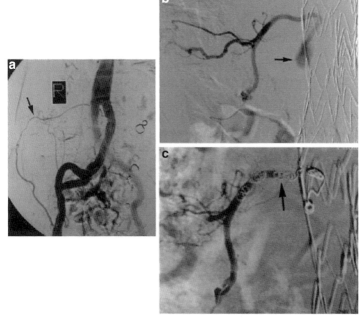

Digital subtraction angiogram of collateral branch endoleak treatment. A, Flush aortogram demonstrates that the type II endoleak originates from collateral communication between the circumflex iliac and lumbar arteries *(arrow)*. B, Selective injection of the lumbar artery demonstrates contrast material collecting in the aneurysm sac *(arrow)*, confirming location of the endoleak. C, Cessation of aneurysm perfusion is seen after deployment of embolic coils *(arrow)* at site of origin of the lumbar artery from the aneurysm sac.

Peter L. Faries PL, Marin ML, et al (2002)
Management of endoleak after endovascular aneurysm repair: cuffs, coils, and conversion
Journal of Vascular Surgery 37, 6, 1155-1161

Fig. 22.5 As in the figure

10 Follow-up Protocol

At this time, there is wide institutional variability in terms of EVAR follow-up. Initial rigorous follow-up with contrast-enhanced CT was required to confirm ongoing procedural success. Many institutions still used the initial protocol of a 1-month, 6-months, 1-year, and then yearly CTA. A CTA with a non-contrast phase, an early phase (type I and III endoleaks), and late phase (type II endoleaks) with 3D reconstruction. Recent studies have shown that up to 25% of endoleaks may not be adequately characterized by CTA. To distinguish the source of the endoleak, a duplex U/S (with or without contrast) or a time resolved MRA (dynamic 3D) may be helpful. MRA will not be useful in stents made with stainless steel.

After initial 1-month and 12-month follow-up with CTA some institutions advocate follow-up with a duplex U/S. A CT without IV contrast can also be used and is accurate in terms of aneurysm size growth. U/S is being used in many institutions as part of the follow-up protocol in attempts to minimize the use of CT or MR. However, U/S is operator dependent and may not be as accurate in obese patients. Further studies are required to clearly determine a standard multi-institutional protocol.

11   Outcomes

EVAR has replaced Open AAA repair as the procedure of choice in treatment of infrarenal abdominal aortic aneurysm. This is based on the fact that in both level I randomized trials (EVAR I and DREAM) and both major registries (EuroSTAR and Lifeline), as well as in industry-supported studies the 30-day mortality was 1.5% in average, and the 30-day mortality for open repair is 4.5–5%. Questions of whether or not this benefit will hold up over the long term are difficult to answer at the present time. Although the overall mortality curves meet around the 2-year mark and aneurysm related death meet at the 4-year mark. In addition, in some of the studies, there may have been an implicit bias against EVAR since healthier patients were more likely to undergo open repair while patients who were less healthy and were not candidates for open repair underwent EVAR.

One of the questions that have arisen has been whether EVAR requires more re-interventions and more readmissions to the hospital and whether this explains the potential loss of benefit when compared to open surgery. However in a recent study, readmission and operations for complications of open surgery (such as bowel obstruction 9.7% and abdominal wall hernias 14.2%) were taken into account. The study demonstrated that EVAR patients did well in terms of long-term re-interventions.

References

1. Parodi JC, Palmaz JC, Barone HD. Transfemoral intraluminal graft implantation for abdominal aortic aneurysms. Ann Vasc Surg. 1991;5:491–9.
2. Lederle FA, Wilson SE, Johnson GR, et al. Immediate repair compared with surveillance of small abdominal aortic aneurysms. N Engl J Med. 2002;346: 1437–44.
3. The UK Small Aneurysm Trial Participants. Mortality results for randomized controlled trial of early elective surgery or ultrasonographic surveillance for small abdominal aortic aneurysms. Lancet. 1998;352:1649–55.
4. EVAR trial participants. Endovascular aneurysm repair versus open repair in patients with abdominal aortic aneurysm (EVAR trial 1): randomized controlled trial. Lancet. 2005;365:2179–86.
5. Prinssen M, Verhoeven EL, Buth J, et al. Dutch Randomized Endovascular Aneurysm Management (DREAM) Trial Group. A randomized trial comparing conventional and endovascular repair of abdominal aortic aneurysms. N Engl J Med. 2004;351(16):1607–18.
6. Schermerhorn ML, O'Malley AJ, Jhaveri A, et al. Endovascular vs. open repair of abdominal aortic aneurysms in the Medicare population. N Engl J Med. 2008;358:464–74.
7. Cao P. CAESAR trial collaborators. Comparison of surveillance vs. aortic endografting for small aneurysm repair (CAESAR) trial:study design and progress. Eur J Vasc Endovasc Surg. 2005;30:245–51.

Chapter 23
Endoleaks-Types and Management

Dustin J. Fanciullo and Karl Illig

Since the dawn of the endovascular era, it has been apparent that in a substantial minority of cases, all flow cannot be excluded from the aneurysm sac (at least acutely)—this situation is termed an "endoleak."

1 Anatomy

With improvements in both technology and surgeon experience, a greater percentage of aneurysms are now being successfully treated with endovascular stent grafts. To help ensure optimal outcomes, preoperative surgical planning is of crucial importance. Several factors can help predict the likelihood of potential endoleaks.

D.J. Fanciullo, M.D.
Division of Vascular Surgery, University of Rochester, Rochester, NY, USA

K. Illig, M.D. (✉)
Division of Vascular & Endovascular Surgery, University of South Florida,
South Florida, FL, USA
e-mail: killig@health.usf.edu

A. Kumar and K. Ouriel (eds.), *Handbook of Endovascular Interventions*,   297
DOI 10.1007/978-1-4614-5013-9_23,
© Springer Science+Business Media New York 2013

1.1 Aorta

There are several key considerations with regard to the aorta and proximal neck when planning for an EVAR. These include the following:

1. Length of the proximal neck—current commercially available stent-grafts require between 1.0 and 1.5 cm of healthy infrarenal proximal neck length to ensure adequate seal and encourage apposition between the graft and aortic wall.
2. Diameter of the proximal neck—the largest commercially available stent grafts have diameters of 36 mm. Most companies suggest a 10–20% oversizing of their grafts to allow for apposition. As such, the largest treatable neck diameters are in the range of 32 mm.
3. Aneurysm morphology—proximal neck angulation of >40° and reverse conical shaped necks are associated with a higher likelihood of endoleak
4. Mural thrombus and calcification—both mural thrombus and aortic calcification are associated with higher rates of endoleak. Thrombus extending for more than 90° of the luminal circumference has been identified as a risk factor. Heavily calcified plaque increases the risk of poor apposition and stent migration, thereby contributing to endoleak formation.

1.2 Iliac

The iliac arteries typically serve as the distal landing zone for aortic stent grafts. As was the case with the proximal neck, a distance of 1.0–1.5 cm is advisable to promote apposition of the graft and arterial wall. The stent graft must also be sided appropriately according to the diameter of the common iliac vessel. If an adequate landing zone cannot be achieved or if the common iliac diameter is too large, the stent graft may be extended into the external iliac artery. However, this might necessitate embolization of the ipsilateral hypogastric (internal iliac) artery to prevent a Type II endoleak.

1.3   Lumbar and Mesenteric Vessels

While these vessels are often chronically occluded, they remain patent in approximately 25% of patients with abdominal aneurysms. After the graft is implanted, the pressure in the sac drops to virtually zero and therefore the flow is reversed. In this situation, a subtle "puddling" of contrast is seen, usually late in the run. If a single vessel is patent, there is nowhere for the blood to go and the Type II leak will thus thrombose in days to weeks. If, however, two or more vessels are patent with a pressure gradient between them, flow (and therefore the leak) will in theory persist. Whether or not this will occur has not been predictable. A hypogastric or left subclavian artery can produce a Type II endoleak in the same fashion in appropriate cases.

2   Disease Definition

An endoleak is defined as the persistence of blood flow into the native aneurysm sac despite the presence of an endograft. In general, leaks come from one of four sources: retrograde flow through native vessels originally supplied by the aorta (inferior mesenteric, hypogastric, subclavian, or lumbar/intercostal arteries), from an incomplete seal proximally or distally, or from defects in materials or separation of components of the device. In all cases, the significance of the leak occurs from continued pressurization of the sac with resultant risk of rupture despite the endograft. However, this risk varies highly according to the type and timing of the leak. It should be emphasized that the term "endoleak" is frequently misinterpreted to mean actual leakage of blood *outside* the sac (i.e., rupture). Although the term is unfortunate, it is here to stay and the endovascular surgeon must be aware of this misperception and be prepared to relieve the anxiety caused by this in both patients and nonsurgeons alike.

3   Disease Distribution

Type II endoleaks are seen acutely after 25% of repairs. Early Type I endoleaks, by contrast, simply mean that the repair was not successful and mandate immediate treatment. Late Type I endoleaks usually result from proximal graft dislodgement and are devicedependent. They too require correction in essentially all cases. Type III endoleaks are rare but relatively easy to fix, while Type IV endoleaks are very rarely seen with modern devices. Type V endoleaks, or more appropriately, "endotension," remain a difficult problem by contrast, with no single solution.

4 Endoleak Classification

Endoleaks are classified (defined) by their time of occurrence and pathophysiology.

A. Time of Occurrence

    1. Primary—endoleak noted during the perioperative (i.e. <30 day) period

    2. Secondary—endoleak observed after the initial perioperative period

B. Pathophysiology (Anatomic Source)

    1. Type I—continued perigraft flow of blood due to inadequate seal between graft and aortic wall:

       (a) Type I-a—inadequate seal at **proximal** attachment site

       (b) Type I-b—inadequate seal at **distal** attachment site

       (c) Type I-c—persistent flow of blood **around an iliac occluder** plug when used in conjunction with an aorto-uni-iliac prosthesis

    2. Type II—retrograde perfusion of aneurysm sac through a pre-existing, named vessel:

       (a) Type II-a—perfusion via the inferior mesenteric artery (IMA) (Fig. 23.1).

       (b) Type II-b—perfusion from lumbar arteries

    3. Type III—perfusion resulting from a defect within the graft:

       (a) Type III-a—between the components of a modular graft

       (b) Type III-b—tear or other disruption within graft fabric

    4. Type IV—generalized, diffuse leakage due to fabric porosity

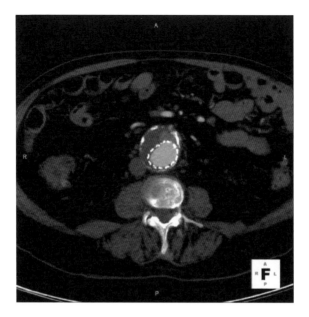

Fig. 23.1 Type II endoleak

    5. Type V—persistent pressurization or enlargement of the aneu-
       rysm sac without demonstrable flow or endoleak. Because no
       flow can be visualized (by definition), the best term for this
       situation is "endotension."

5 Diagnosis

As an endoleak creates continued pressurization of the aneurysm sac,
the potential for rupture still exists. Because the chance of this varies
according to the type and timing of the leak (as leaks can occur late),
routine follow-up with imaging of the aneurysm repair remains the
standard of care.

5.1 Clinical Follow-up

No standardized algorithm exists. Most often, patients undergo initial
postoperative imaging and clinical evaluation approximately 1 month

after their surgery. Subsequent imaging and evaluation is performed are 6 and 12 months, and if all is well, annually thereafter. If an abnormality such as a newly diagnosed endoleak, persistent endoleak, or aneurysm sac enlargement is detected during routine surveillance, further evaluation is necessary.

5.2 Imaging Modalities

The goal of postoperative imaging is to assess the size of the residual sac and to identify or exclude the presence of an endoleak. Each can be accomplished by computerized tomography (CT), magnetic resonance (MR) scanning, or ultrasound (USG). Angiography is frequently used to look for (and treat when applicable) the source of an endoleak. However, it cannot assess the sac size and is obviously much more invasive; therefore, it is not used for routine postoperative surveillance.

5.2.1 Computerized Tomography

Often combined with postprocessed vessel reconstruction (CT angiography CTA), this is the primary study used for postoperative surveillance because of its high resolution. CTA is felt by most to be the most sensitive test for detecting endoleaks when compared to both USG and conventional angiography. Other advantages include safety, availability, reproducibility, accuracy, lack of operator dependence, ease of interpretation, and rapid acquisition times. Importantly, however, significant disadvantages exist. CTA requires that the patient be exposed to a not-insignificant dose of ionizing radiation on an annual basis for life. Further, it requires a relatively high dose of intravenous contrast dye with risks of allergic reaction and nephrotoxicity; the latter effect having been shown to be associated with cumulative renal damage over time. Other disadvantages include difficulty in discerning calcifications from contrast and the directionality of blood flow from an endoleak. Further, subtle late leaks are poorly visualized. Finally, the cost of a CT scan is greater than other available imaging modalities. Timing the scan (i.e., precontrast, and postcontrast) can help to identify fixed calcium and late endoleaks;

however, the radiation dose needed is obviously greater. Overall, CT and CTA provide the highest resolution but have significant drawbacks to their use.

5.2.2 Magnetic Resonance Angiography

Recent data suggest that magnetic resonance angiography (MRA) is as sensitive at detecting endoleaks as CT. While appealing due to the elimination of nephrotoxic contrast agents (in most situations) and radiation, the disadvantages of MRA are significant enough to preclude its routine use for postoperative surveillance. First, grafts made of stainless steel (Cook Zenith, Bloomington, IN) are in theory not compatible, although empirically no adverse events have been seen in such patients undergoing early or late MR scanning. Further, many patients are unable to undergo MR scanning due to preexisting implants. Most clinicians feel that MR does not image the central vascular system as well as other imaging modalities. Finally, MR suffers from the well-known drawbacks of longer acquisition time and patient dissatisfaction (noise and claustrophobia), further limiting its role for widespread routine surveillance in this situation.

5.2.3 Ultrasonography

Although reports vary extensively regarding the sensitivity in which ultrasonography (USG) can detect endoleaks (43–100%), it has many advantages that make it an ideal screening tool. Foremost, it is a safe, noninvasive, inexpensive tool that is highly reproducible given the proper environment. No contrast is needed and there is no exposure to radiation. However, the examination does take longer to complete and is subject to a greater degree of operator/interpreter variability. Also, patient variables such as body habitus, fasting status, and bowel gas can make the exam less accurate. Patients therefore should be instructed to fast before the exam, and lower frequency (3–5 Hz) scan heads should be utilized to allow for deeper penetration. Finally, it should be obvious that if USG results are to be reliably trusted, they should be obtained by a very experienced, accredited laboratory with rigorous quality control and internal verification of results.

Some argue that USG is less sensitive than CT in detecting endoleaks. This may or may not be true, but it has been pointed out by many that if a sac is shrinking, the presence of a Type II endoleak per se is not critical. Ultrasound is highly accurate for determining sac size, and thus an increasing number of clinicians and investigators are relying primarily upon USG for routine postoperative follow-up, resorting to CT (and/or angiography) only if a problem is identified by USG.

5.2.4 Conventional Angiography

Because of the risks and expense of arterial access, this is the most invasive imaging modality used in the detection of postoperative endoleaks. In addition, it too requires radiation and the administration of a contrast agent (although with selective catheterization, the operator has more control of the actual dosage used and can limit the amount when mitigating factors exist). It cannot determine the sac size and has been shown to be **less** sensitive in detecting endoleaks. For all of these reasons, it is not used as a postoperative surveillance tool. However, if an endoleak is detected, angiography is necessary if intervention is planned and as such should be viewed as more of a **therapeutic rather than diagnostic** tool.

6   Management (Fig. 23.2)

There is no universally accepted protocol for the detection and management of endoleaks after aneurysm repair, in part because situations differ. It is agreed that these patients require lifelong surveillance, partly because EVAR has "only" been performed for approximately 15 years. As such, vascular surgeons are still dealing with early generation devices, and despite, their theoretical attractiveness, newer generation devices have a short, empiric track record. As described above, we evaluate patients at 1, 6, and 12 month intervals during the first postoperative year. If the patient's course is uneventful, they are then evaluated on an annual basis. At each evaluation, we obtain fasting USG only (along with clinical examination). Provided no endoleak is seen and the sac is not enlarging, we continue this protocol indefinitely. If a Type II leak is seen early, we observe and recheck the patient in 6 months. If a Type I or III leak is seen at any time during follow-up or if the sac is not shrinking with an associated Type II endoleak a year out from surgery, we will either obtain a CT scan

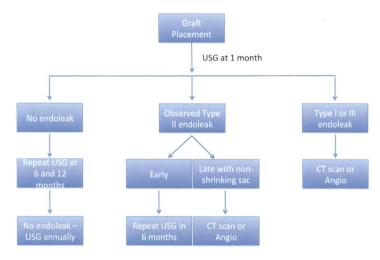

Fig. 23.2 Endoleak management algorithm

(if the situation is not clear-cut) or proceed directly to a confirmatory and therapeutic angiography if the source of the leak is readily evident. In general, a guiding principle is that intervention should be performed to reduce the risk of death by rupture and not for the presence of an endoleak per se.

7 Treatment Options

A. Endovascular Intervention

1. Coil embolization (including with glue)
2. Graft modification (proximal cuff)
3. CT guided sac injection

B. Laparoscopic Intervention

1. IMA clipping
2. Lumbar clipping

C. Open Repair

1. Proximal cuff modification
2. Conversion to open repair

8 Intervention: Technique and Pitfalls

As with any interventional procedure, consideration should be given to the patient's renal function. If appropriate, patients should undergo preoperative renal protective measures per hospital protocol. During the procedure, patients should also be systemically anticoagulated. Full anticoagulation is not typically necessary.

8.1 Type I

Ideally, no patient should leave the operating room with a Type I endoleak, although, in practice, this rule is occasionally broken. In these rare situations (usually in cases where the risks of alternative treatment are extremely high), we will follow small, persistent leaks for a short period of time—typically at 2 to 3 month intervals. Any enlargement of the sac or increase in volume of such an endoleak would mandate prompt treatment. Use grafts with active proximal fixation and be aggressive about landing such grafts at the renal orifices (or, in specific cases, even allowing for slight overlap). Treatment of a Type I endoleak in this case would be modification of a commercially available device to create a fenestrated graft or conversion to open repair. Anecdotal reports exist of wrapping a proximal cuff around the (balloon supported) device, but experience in this regard is lacking.

In our experience, we have never seen a late Type I endoleak after implantation of a suprarenally fixed device into healthy aortic neck. Most commonly, this is seen in the setting of an older device without active fixation or in the case of a newer device theoretically supported from below. In both cases, the device itself has usually slipped or migrated a fair amount distally and an adequate proximal cuff can be found. In this setting, a proximal extension cuff or a type I endoleak-specific device (Cook Renu, Bloomington, IN) can be used—it must be stressed that attention must be paid to the flow divider of the existing device. If no proximal seal zone is present, conversion to open repair is usually the only option; commercially fenestrated devices are currently under investigation. It should be noted that proximal Type I endoleaks (Type I-a) are highly device specific; occurring less frequently with suprarenal fixation and most frequently (including frank graft dislodgement and distal migration) with grafts that depend solely on friction for seal and positioning.

Type I-b endoleaks (arising distally) can usually be treated relatively easily. Extension to the external iliacs will usually solve the problem, although the hypogastric should usually be occluded (with coils, for example) to avoid a secondary type II endoleak. At times, these can be due to improper graft sizing but calcium and thrombus can also prohibit appropriate seal as described earlier. In these cases, a balloon-expandable stent with high radial force can solve the problem and create a strong, durable seal.

8.2   Type II

Typically, these are the easiest to deal with as they are usually benign. Approximately 25% of patients will have an immediate type II leak no matter which device is used. We follow such leaks for up to 6–12 months if the sac is not enlarging and lifelong if the sac is shrinking. Sacs typically enlarge slightly at 1 and 6 months; this is probably due to the expansive effect of sac thrombosis. However, if the sac has dramatically enlarged by 6 months, we will consider intervention. Type II leaks usually arise from the IMA (anterior leaks) or lumbar arteries (posterior) and, as such, are often accessible using catheter-based techniques. An IMA that is patent and thus the source of an endoleak can often be accessed via branches of the hypogastric or superior mesenteric arteries; selective cannulation and visualization of these vessels are needed followed by microcatheter techniques for access. Similarly, most significant lumbar vessels are fed by ascending branches of the hypogastric arteries. Once sufficiently distal, coil or glue embolization is straightforward. Although two vessels (one for blood supply and the other for drainage) are often present, only one needs to be treated as elimination of the pressure gradient will allow the other to quickly thrombose. Finally, if an IMA (or *clearly* defined lumbar) is the source of the leak but cannot be accessed using catheter-based techniques, laparoscopic clipping can be utilized and is fairly straightforward.

8.3   Type III

These endoleaks are quite rare and almost always apparent at implantation, although late component separation can occur. The problem here is diagnosis. Once made, repair should be straightforward. If the components are substantially joined, relining with the appropriate secondary component is easy, but consideration can also be given to conversion to an aortouni-iliac configuration with occlusion of the problem segment.

8.4   Type IV

By definition, these endoleaks are seen at the time of implantation only and newer generation devices have essentially eliminated this entity. If felt to be present, they should be treated as endotension (see following).

8.5   Type V

These "endoleaks" or endotension, by definition, refer to the situation in which the sac is enlarging (or pressure is elevated), but no contrast leak can be seen (a Type IV endoleak technically should only be diagnosed if actual contrast is seen outside the graft but no Type I, II, or III source is present). This was originally seen with the first-generation Gore Excluder device (Flagstaff, AZ), but the problem was recognized and the graft underwent subsequent modification. Management is unclear. There have been reports of sac rupture in this situation, but morbidity and mortality are much lower than rupture after an unrepaired aneurysm. Some advocate opening the sac, removing the contents, and wrapping the residual tissue around the graft (often with a chemical sealant). This technique has the advantage of definitively identifying and treating any other type of endoleak. Most, however, simply "reline" the graft with a newer device. Again, because of the physical configuration of an endograft, it is usually easiest to convert to an aortouni-iliac configuration with occlusion of the contralateral limb.

8.6   Graft Explantation

Occasionally, endografts must be explanted. We strongly suggest elective supraceliac aortic control in this situation with exposure of the aneurysm sac to the level of the renal arteries. In most situations, such explant is being performed for a persistent Type I endoleak with a large sac and no proximal neck (i.e., the graft literally falls out of position or is bunched within the sac already). Grafts with suprarenal fixation will rarely be loose proximally. Even in this situation, most of the barbs will be well incorporated into the suprarenal tissues and any attempts to remove all metal will be dangerous. In this regard, it is best to use wire cutters to remove the graft while leaving the barbs in place, after which a conventional graft can be easily sewn in place.

9 Complications and Management

The complications of intervention for endoleaks are the complications inherent in interventional angiography and are covered throughout this book in detail. The major "complication" unique to such intervention is persistence of the leak, which can be quite troubling, or even continued sac enlargement.

A. If the endoleak persists, the diagnostic algorithm should be repeated. The question that needs to be answered was whether or not the source of the leak was properly identified. For example, what was felt to be a blush from a lumbar creating a Type II leak might, in fact, have been bowel gas and the original Type III leak persists. We find it useful in this situation to occlude various parts of the system during angiography—for example, balloon occlusion of one limb of the graft while injecting contrast will effectively rule out a Type I-b or III leak from this area, thereby narrowing the possibilities. No single algorithm can be described and the clinician must be persistent and use all available tools (including input from another physician) to solve this puzzle.

B. We have noticed anecdotally that sacs sometimes do not shrink even after an endoleak has been fixed. In this situation, aggressive attention should be paid to sac size over time and the presence of subtle persistent leaks. If no leak can be documented using all available imaging techniques (including good quality CT scanning), the sac can be safely observed.

10   Outcomes

As we are not covering all involved vessels, Type II endoleaks are inevitable. Type I and III endoleaks can be eliminated by performing EVAR on perfect candidates only, but then many patients who would benefit will be excluded. In practice, a balance is sought between perfect cases and "pushing the envelope," knowing that a certain rate of such endoleaks will inevitably occur. Having said this, Type IV leaks are of no clinical concern and Type V leaks are probably missed Type I, II, or III endoleaks.

Overall, early or primary endoleaks are seen in as many as 25–44% of all cases. Fortunately, most of these are Type II endoleaks and, as such, as many as 60–70% resolve within the first postoperative month. Historically, 10–18% of all patients undergo a secondary intervention at some point during the course of follow-up and approximately 92% of endoleaks are repairable via catheter-based intervention; these rates may be even better today. At present, overall clinical success rates of endovascular aneurysm repair approach 95%.

References

1. White GH, Yu W, May J, et al. Endoleak as a complication of endoluminal grafting of abdominal aortic aneurysms: classification, incidence, diagnosis, and management. J Endovasc Surg. 1997;4:152–68.
2. Brewster DC, Jones JE, Chung TK, et al. Long-term outcomes after endovascular abdominal aortic aneurysm repair: the first decade. Ann Surg. 2006;244: 426–38.
3. Faries PL, Cadot H, et al. Management of endoleak after endovascular aneurysm repair: cuffs, coils, and conversion. J Vasc Surg. 2003;37:1155–61.
4. Hiatt MD, Rubin G. Surveillance for endoleaks: how to detect all of them. Semin Vasc Surg. 2004;17:268–78.
5. Laheij RJ, Buth J, Harris PL, et al. Need for secondary interventions after endovascular repair of abdominal aortic aneurysm: Intermediate-term follow-up results of a European collaborative registry (EUROSTAR). B J Surg. 2000;87:166–73.

Chapter 24
Endovascular Treatment of Iliac Artery Lesions

Wei Liang and Jiwei Zhang

1 Anatomy

The common iliac artery (CIA) originates from the distal abdominal aorta at the level of the fourth lumbar vertebra. The CIA subsequently divides into the internal iliac artery (IIA) and the external iliac artery (EIA). The IIA supplies the pelvis, which includes parts of the rectum, the sexual organs, and the buttocks. The EIA, which continues as the common femoral artery (CFA), supplies the blood to the legs. The diameter of the CIA and the EIA ranges from 7 to 10 mm, and from 5 to 7 mm, respectively.

Variations and Special features

(a) CIA origin: Most commonly in the fourth lumbar vertebra, but sometimes in the level of the third or fifth lumbar vertebra.

(b) The branches of IIA: Historically described as having posterior and anterior divisions. The posterior division consists of the superior gluteal, iliolumbar, and lateral sacral arteries. The anterior division includes the obturator, middle hemorrhoidal (or rectal), inferior hemorrhoidal (or rectal), vesical, internal pudendal, and inferior gluteal arteries. The anterior division also gives rise to the

W. Liang (✉) • J. Zhang, M.D. (✉)
School of Medicine, Renji Hospital,
Shanghai Jiaotong University, Shanghai, China
e-mail: weiliang3003@163.com; zhangjiwei001@sina.com

A. Kumar and K. Ouriel (eds.), *Handbook of Endovascular Interventions*, 311
DOI 10.1007/978-1-4614-5013-9_24,
© Springer Science+Business Media New York 2013

deferential or uterine arteries in male or female patients, respectively.

(c) Persistent sciatic artery: Seen in less than 0.1% of individuals, this large vessel arises from the anterior division of the internal iliac artery, passes through the sciatic notch, and runs posterior to the femoral head. It then continues in the posterior aspect of the thigh to become the popliteal artery. In patients with this anomaly, the external iliac continues as the profunda femoris, and the superficial femoral artery is absent. Because of its posterior location, the sciatic artery is subject to trauma by the femoral head when the patient is seated. Traumatic aneurysms in the vessel are common and can be a nidus for thromboembolic events, including acute thrombosis of the aneurysm or distal thromboembolic occlusion.

2 Disease Definition

2.1 *Iliac Artery Stenosis*

The narrowing of the iliac artery lumen causes the ischemia of the lower limb. Atherosclerosis is responsible for almost all the iliac artery stenosis. Other rare reasons include cystic adventitial disease and fibromuscular dysplasia.

2.2 *Iliac Artery Aneurysm*

Iliac artery aneurysm is defined as a focal dilatation at least 50% larger than the expected normal arterial diameter. Isolated iliac artery aneurysms are rare. Of all aortoiliac aneurysms, only 0.6% were isolated to the iliac arteries. Most of them are true aneurysm, which are caused by atherosclerosis.

3 Disease Distribution

There are three distinct patterns

Type I, atherosclerosis involves exclusively the distal abdominal aorta and the CIA. It is present in about 5–10% of patients with PAD and is more frequently encountered among women.

Type II, atherosclerosis involves the infrarenal aorta, CIA, and EIA, and may extend into the CFA. It is present in 35% of patients with PAD.

Type III, atherosclerosis involves the infrarenal aorta, iliac, femoral, and popliteal arteries as well as the infrapopliteal circulation. It is present in 55–60% of patients with PAD.

Among the iliac artery aneurysm (IAA), the incidence of CIA and IIA aneurysms are 70–90% and 10–30% respectively. The most common site for IAAs is the common iliac artery, with the external iliac the most rarely affected. There is significant male predominance (male-to-female ratios of 5:1 to 16:1). Approximately 50% are bilateral.

4 Classification-TASC

According to the TASCII classification iliac artery stenosis can be classified into four types:

4.1 Type A

Unilateral or bilateral stenosis of CIA, unilateral or bilateral single short (≤3 cm) stenosis of EIA (Fig. 24.1)

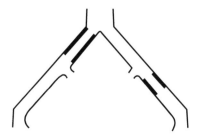

Fig. 24.1 Type A lesions
• Unilateral or bilateral stenoses of CIA
• Unilateral or bilateral single short (≤3 cm) stenoses of EIA

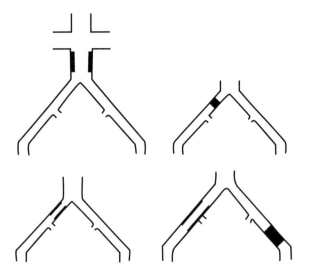

Fig. 24.2 Type B lesions
- Short (≤3) cm stenosis of infrarenal aorta
- Unilateral CIA occlusion
- Single or multiple stenosis totaling 3–10 cm involving the EIA not extending into the CFA
- Unilateral EIA occlusion not involving the origins of internal iliac or CFA

4.2   Type B

Short (≤3 cm) stenosis of infrarenal aorta, unilateral CIA occlusion, single or multiple stenosis totaling 3–10 cm involving the EIA not extending into the CFA, unilateral EIA occlusion not involving the origins of internal iliac or CFA (Fig. 24.2)

4.3   Type C

Bilateral CIA occlusions, bilateral EIA stenosis 3–10 cm long not extending into the CFA, unilateral EIA stenosis extending into the CFA, unilateral EIA occlusion that involves the origins of internal iliac and/or CFA, heavily calcified unilateral EIA occlusion with or without involvement of origins of internal iliac and/or CFA (Fig. 24.3)

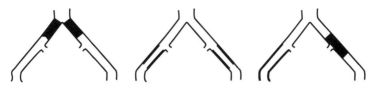

Fig. 24.3 Type C lesions
- Bilateral CIA occlusions
- Bilateral EIA stenoses 3–10 cm long not extending into the CFA
- Unilateral EIA stenoses extending into the CFA
- Unilateral EIA occlusion that involves the origins of internal iliac and/or CFA
- Heavily calcified unilateral EIA occlusion with or without involvement of origins of internal iliac and/or CFA

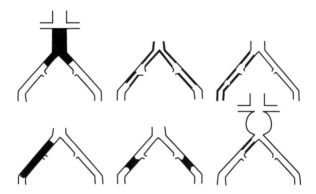

Fig. 24.4 Type D lesions
- Infra-renal aortoiliac occlusion
- Diffuse disease involving the aorta and both iliac arteries requiring treatment
- Diffuse multiple stenoses involving the unilateral CIA, EIA, and CFA
- Unilateral occlusions of both CIA and CFA
- Bilateral occlusions of EIA
- Iliac stenoses in patients with AAA requiring treatment and not amenable to endograft placement or other lesions requiring open aortic or iliac surgery

4.4   Type D

Infra renal aortoiliac occlusion; Diffuse disease involving the aorta and both iliac arteries requiring treatment; Diffuse multiple stenosis involving the unilateral CIA, EIA and CFA, Unilateral occlusions of both CIA and EIA, Bilateral occlusions of EIA, Iliac stenosis in patients with AAA requiring treatment and not amenable to endograft placement or other lesions requiring open aortic or iliac surgery (Fig. 24.4)

5 Diagnosis-Clinical and Laboratory

Iliac artery stenosis may be asymptomatic, or cause, intermittent claudication, critical limb ischemia (CLI) or blue toe syndrome. Acute ischemia may result from thrombosis in a lesion or from embolism. Buttock/thigh claudication is typically associated with iliac disease, whereas CLI is due to multilevel disease. Impotency results from disease in the internal iliac circulation. Blue toe syndrome results from cholesterol crystals or microemboli of thrombus/atheroma embolizing into the foot vessels from proximal ulcerating lesion. On palpation of the outflow femoral artery, one finds the presence of weak or absent pulsation.

Iliac artery aneurysms (IAAs) may be asymptomatic, or cause symptoms in the pelvis due to their size. Chronic pain is caused by nerve root (sciatica) or visceral compression. Large aneurysms may cause urologic obstruction and the symptoms of iliac vein compression. Severe pain in the pelvic area with symptoms of shock suggests the occurrence of IAAs rupture. Usually, these aneurysms cannot be palpated due to their deep location in the pelvis.

Laboratory tests of blood lipid and glucose may be abnormal in some arteriosclerosis patients. Rapid reductions of the value of hemoglobin and hematocrit indicate IAA rupture.

6 Diagnostic Imaging: USG/CT/MRI/Diagnostic Angiography

Ultrasound in occlusive disease allows the delineation of the nature and severity of stenosis prior to angiography.

CT angiography is an important noninvasive tool for the diagnosis of iliac artery disease. Compared with the MR angiography, CT scan has the advantage to provide the detail of the extent of calcification of the vessels. It is currently the gold standard for imaging the iliac artery.

MR angiography is an alternative to CT angiography and has the benefit of not exposing the patient to radiation or nephrotoxic contrast agents.

Diagnostic angiography has been considered the gold standard for evaluating the iliac artery disease. It is unnecessary at the present time unless the above modalities have been unable to delineate the pathology adequately. It has the advantage of being able to be combined with an intervention at the same setting.

7 Management

7.1 Iliac Artery Stenosis

Indications for treatment

1. Lifestyle limiting claudication
2. Limb-threatening ischemia
3. Blue toe syndrome
4. As a precursor to renal transplantation
5. Vasculogenic impotence

7.2 Iliac Artery Aneurysm

Indications for Treatment

1. Symptomatic aneurysm of any size
2. At the time of repair of abdominal aortic aneurysm
3. Elective repair should be considered for IAAs 3.5 cm or larger in good-risk patients.

8 List of Open Operative Choices

8.1 Iliac Artery Stenosis

1. Direct anatomic reconstruction
   (a) Iliac artery endarterectomy with or without patch angioplasty
   (b) Aorto-iliac or ilio-femoral artery bypass

2. Extra-anatomic bypass
   (a) Femoro-femoral or axillo-femoral bypass

8.2   Iliac Artery Aneurysm

1. Open aneurysmorrhaphy with graft insertion, with or without internal iliac reimplantation For lesions related to CIA or/and EIA
2. Open ligation of IIA, For solitary IIA aneurysm, if graft interposition is not possible.

9   Intervention-Techniques

9.1   Iliac Artery Stenosis

Before the intervention, the patient should take Aspirin 100 mg/day orally for at least 5 days. During the procedure the patient is given intravenous heparin 100 units/kg.

9.1.1   Access

Contralateral common femoral artery (CFA) puncture with placement of a 6-Fr sheath is done. This is useful in iliac artery occlusions, which are best recanalized in an antegrade fashion. For stenotic lesions an ipsilateral CFA puncture with 6-F sheath is made for lesion traversal and possible stenting. Brachial artery puncture is seldom required unless thrombolysis or antegrade recanalization is needed.

9.1.2   Crossing the Lesion

It is performed with a curved catheter and a hydrophilic wire to cross the lesion from the contralateral puncture with antegrade recanalization. If it is difficult, or the lesion is located in the proximal part of the CIA, an ipsilateral retrograde recanalization should be used. However, an antegrade recanalization is required when the femoral artery is also involved. The brachial puncture can be used in the situation of bilateral iliac artery stenosis and the need of antegrade recanalization. The iliac lesion should be imaged by injection of contrast and then crossed, preferably under road map conditions, with a guidewire.

9.1.3   Thrombolysis

Thrombolysis is performed when the wire easily passes the lesion especially in cases with acute ischemic symptoms. The brachial artery is the usual access to insert a thrombolysis catheter for the iliac artery thrombolysis.

9.1.4   Percutaneous Transluminal Angioplasty (PTA)

After initial traversal of the lesion, balloon angioplasty is performed. It would make sense to measure the diameter of the iliac artery before choosing an appropriate-sized balloon. In males the common iliac artery is approximately 7–9 mm and the external 6–7 mm in diameter. Vessels in women are approximately 1 mm smaller. The size of balloon should be 1–2 mm smaller than the diameter of the target artery, being especially mindful of this in lesions involving the external iliac artery. The duration of inflation is variable, and we typically inflate the balloon for 1–2 min after the waist is gone.

9.1.5   Stent

Balloon expandable stents are used for common iliac artery ostial lesions that require extra radial force and very precise placement so that they do not overhang the contralateral iliac artery. Self-expanding stents are preferred elsewhere because of their ability to conform to the natural curve of the iliac artery. The diameter of stents should be oversized 10–20% of the target vessel. A cover stent is kept at hand if a perforation/rupture occurs.

9.2   Iliac Artery Aneurysm

9.2.1   Access

An ipsilateral CFA is usually exposed surgically and CFA punctured for placement of a large sheath. Contralateral CFA is exposed if the internal iliac artery has the lesion and requires embolization.

9.2.2 Embolization of Internal Iliac Artery

If an internal iliac artery aneurysm exists, coil embolization is performed from a contralateral CFA puncture. It is important to target the distal outflow first, and this includes specific vessels or branches. The size of the coil has to be compatible with the diameter of the artery to be occluded, oversizing these by about 10–15%. It must be ensured that the contralateral internal iliac artery should be patent to minimize the risk of pelvic ischemia.

9.2.3 Stent-Graft Stent

The straight stentgraft can be used if the proximal neck is more than 2 cm. The size of stent is 10–20% larger than the normal vessel. If there is not enough proximal neck, and the aneurysm is too close to the aortic bifurcation, a bifurcated aortoiliac stentgraft is needed. Alternative endovascular treatment is an aorto-uni-iliac stentgraft, with blockage of the contralateral common iliac artery and placement of a femoral-femoral bypass. Iliac branch devices (IBDs) are now available to exclude iliac aneurysms and preserve the internal iliac artery.

10 Postprocedure Management and Follow-up Protocol

10.1 Iliac Artery Stenosis

1. Modification of atherosclerotic risk factors includes the following:
   (a) Smoking cessation
   (b) Weight reduction
   (c) Blood pressure control
   (d) Hyperlipidemia control
   (e) Blood glucose control

2. Antiplatelet drug therapy:
   (a) Clopidogrel 75 mg/day for 3–6 months with ASA (Aspirin) 75–100 mg/day
   (b) Followed by Aspirin 100 mg/day for lifetime

3. Follow-up protocol—Evaluate by:
    (a) Change of foot ulcer
    (b) ABI improvement
    (c) Checking patency of revascularization with duplex

10.2   Iliac Artery Aneurysm

1. Modification of aneurysm risk factors:
    (a) Control of blood pressure

2. Follow-up protocol
    (a) Check for exclusion of aneurysm
    (b) Check for endoleak
    (c) Check at 1, 3, 6 and 12 months postprocedure and then annu-
        ally thereafter depending upon the findings of previous scans

11   Complications and Management

11.1   Iliac Artery Stenosis

According to the area where the complication occurs, these can be
divided as:

(a) Access site complications
    1. Hematoma and false aneurysms
    2. Arteriovenous fistula
    3. Access vessel thrombosis

(b) Target site complications
    1. Acute closure: The acute occlusion of the treatment site is usu-
       ally due to dissection and acute thrombosis. The patient should
       be sufficiently anticoagulated to limit thrombus formation and
       the dissection should be managed with a stent.
    2. Rupture: Is more common in the external iliac artery than the
       common iliac artery. The first intervention is inflating a bal-
       loon across or proximal to the tear to stop the bleeding and a
       covered stent is then placed across the tear.

3. Stent infection: Initial trial of antibiotics is attempted in the very early stages, but a low threshold for explant of the stent with extraanatomic bypass done for limb salvage.
4. Distal complications: Embolization of plaque is sometimes seen. If symptomatic, the embolectomy may initially be attempted as a percutaneous aspiration thromboembolectomy especially in the more distal embolizations. If unsuccessful, open thromboembolectomy often has to be done.

11.2   Iliac Artery Aneurysm

(a) Access site complications: As above

(b) Target site complications:
   1. Endoleak: These are related to back bleeding from side branches (Type II) or from the proximal / distal segments of the stent (Type I). Embolizaton is usually successful in Type II, however the type I endoleak often requires an extension with an additional stent.
   2. Graft thrombosis: Excess folding of the stentgraft can occlude blood flow in the lumen of a graft and cause the graft thrombosis. Others include the runoff vessel stenosis and kink of the graft. Using catheter thrombolysis and then stent within the vessel or graft can treat this complication.
   3. Internal iliac artery ischemia: Buttock claudication, erectile dysfunction, bladder dysfunction and sacral ulceration can result from internal iliac artery embolization, especially occlusion of bilateral internal iliac artery. At least, one internal iliac artery should be reconstructed to treat the syndrome.

12   Outcomes

12.1   Iliac Artery Stenosis

The change in quality of life after iliac intervention for claudication has shown significant and durable improvement following intervention, persisting to last follow-up at three years.

The technical and initial clinical success of PTA of iliac stenosis exceeds 90% in all reports in the literature. The technical success rate of recanalization of long-segment iliac occlusions is 80–85% with or without additional thrombolysis. The periprocedural complications range 0–5.7% with low to no operative mortality.

5-year patency rate can be more than 70% after iliac artery stenting. Factors negatively affecting the patency of such interventions include quality of runoff vessels, severity of ischemia and length of diseased segments. Female gender has also been suggested to decrease patency of external iliac artery stents. A meta-analysis of the results of angioplasty and stent placement concluded that compared to angioplasty, stents have an improved technical success rate, a similar complication rate, and a 39% reduction in the risk of long-term failure.

12.2   Iliac Artery Aneurysm

The perioperative mortality of elective endovascular management of asymptomatic iliac artery aneurysms ranges between 0 and 4%. The overall incidence of such perioperative complications ranges from 10% to 23%. The most common complication is an anastomotic endoleak occurring in 4% of patients (range, 0–7%) and associated with 50% rupture rate. Others include graft thrombosis, distal arterial embolization, internal iliac artery ischemia, access site complications including and infection, hematoma, and pseudoaneurysm. Good mid-term results can be obtained with endovascular repair of IAAs.

13   Flowchart Summarizing the Role of Medical Treatment

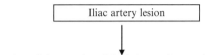

Evaluation of the severity of the lesion and generalized situation

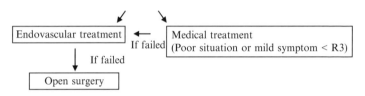

References

1. Norgren L, Hiatt WR, Dormandy A, et al. Inter-society consensus for the management of peripheral arterial disease (TASC II). J Vasc Surg. 2007;45:S5–S67.
2. Sandhu RS, Pipinos II. Isolated iliac artery aneurysms. Semin Vasc Surg. 2005;18:209–15.
3. Ghosh J, Murray D, Paravastu S, et al. Contemporary management of aorto-iliac aneurysms in the endovascular era. Eur J Vasc Endovasc Surg. 2009;37:182–8.
4. Bosch JL, van der Graaf Y, Hunink MG. Health-related quality of life after angioplasty and stent placement in patients with iliac artery occlusive disease: results of a randomized controlled clinical trial. The Dutch Iliac Stent Trial Study Group. Circulation. 1999;99:3155–60.
5. Bosch JL, Hunink MG. Meta-analysis of the results of percutaneous transluminal angioplasty and stent placement for aortoiliac occlusive disease. Radiology. 1997;204:87–96.

Chapter 25
Femoral Artery: CFA, SFA, Profunda Femoris Artery Lesions

Martin Schillinger and Erich Minar

1 Anatomy

The femoral artery has its origin from the external iliac artery at the level of the inguinal ligament and continues at the popliteal fossa as the popliteal artery.

- Until its first major bifurcation, the vessel is referred to as the common femoral artery (CFA). The CFA then splits into the deep femoral artery (DFA) (profunda femoris) and the superficial femoral artery (SFA); this bifurcation has a lot of variations and usually is situated slightly below the level of the femoral head. Based on these anatomic prerequisites, the femoral head is an acceptable bony landmark to localize the CFA, and puncture of this artery typically should be done in the level of the lower or middle third of the femoral head.

M. Schillinger, M.D. (✉)
Department of Internal Medicine, Vienna Private Hospital,
Pelikangasse 15, Vienna, 1090, Austria

Department Angiology, Medical University of Vienna,
Waehringer Guertel 18-20, A 1090, Vienna, Austria
e-mail: m.schillinger@imed19.at

E. Minar, M.D.
Department Angiology, Medical University of Vienna,
Waehringer Guertel 18-20, A 1090, Vienna, Austria

A. Kumar and K. Ouriel (eds.), *Handbook of Endovascular Interventions*,   325
DOI 10.1007/978-1-4614-5013-9_25,
© Springer Science+Business Media New York 2013

- The DFA has several side branches including the medial and lateral circumflex femoral artery and several perforating branches which may join the distal SFA or the popliteal artery at the supragenicular level. These arteries may considerably vary in diameter and capacity and are the most important collaterals in patients with occlusion of the SFA.
- The superficial femoral artery (SFA) is the longest artery of the body and arises at the femoral bifurcation, the distal third dives through the adductor channel and then feeds the popliteal artery at the proximal edge of the popliteal fossa. The definition for the femoropopliteal conjunction varies depending on the imaging modality. Anatomically, the beginning of the popliteal artery is defined by the distal end of the adductor channel, the tendinous hiatus. Mechanically, the superficial femoral artery is fixed between two hinge points—the hip and the knee. Due to the movement of the leg, several forces are effective in the SFA including bending, compression, elongation, and torsion. This is particularly important when stents are implanted since these forces have a considerable impact on the integrity of stents and may lead to fractures of the implants.

2 Disease Definition

Chronic obstructive lesions of the femoral artery are due to

(a) Atherosclerosis in >95% of the patients
(b) Inflammatory diseases, such as arteritis, may affect the femoral segment. The most frequent being thrombangitis obliterans and giant cell arteritis, which has to be considered as a differential diagnosis mainly in young smokers. The following chapter covers only atherosclerotic disease since therapeutic principles of arteritis are completely different to those in atherosclerosis. Briefly, in patients with arteritis in the acute phase, vascular surgical and endovascular therapies have very high failure rates.

3   Disease Distribution

Disease distribution follows a typical pattern: the male to female ratio is approximately 4:1, although females keep up due to changes in smoking habits. Smoking is considered the most important risk factor for SFA occlusions. In contrast, the DFA is most frequently affected in patients with diabetes mellitus (40% as compared to 10% in non-diabetic patients).

The SFA frequently is affected at an early stage of peripheral artery disease and is the most frequent artery affected in patients with single-level peripheral artery disease. In contrast, the deep femoral artery usually remains disease free, unless the patient is a diabetic, and serves as the most important collateral vessel. Patients with SFA occlusion and strong DFA collaterals may even walk pain free. Preservation of the DFA therefore is one of the main treatment goals. The CFA usually gets affected at rather late stages of the disease, and most lesions are heavily calcified and frequently do not respond well to endovascular therapies.

4   TASC Classification

The current TASC II classification of femoropopliteal lesions is displayed in Fig. 25.1. Disease of the CFA is included in the aorto-iliac segment. Involvement of the CFA classifies a lesion automatically as TASC C or TASC D, suggesting surgery as the preferred treatment option. Obviously, this classification does not include disease of the DFA. Briefly addressing the TASC document, this classification is very helpful in classifying lesions and in defining a common language between different medical disciplines, but it is hardly helpful in defining indications for an endovascular or open surgical approach. Furthermore, the TASC document includes only a morphological classification of lesions but does not address the clinical background, i.e., whether a patient is treated for intermittent claudication or critical limb ischemia.

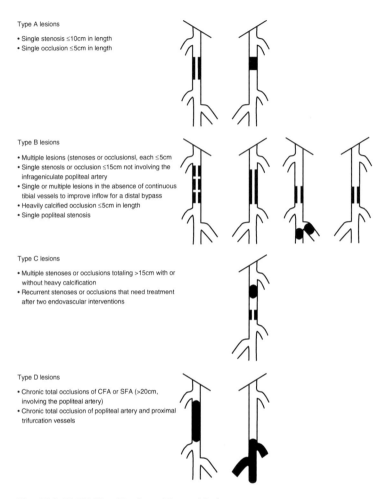

Fig. 25.1 TASC Classification of femoral lesions

5   Diagnosis: Clinical and Laboratory

The diagnosis of femoral artery disease can be made clinically in vast majority of patients. Typical symptoms include intermittent claudication of the calf and limitation of the walking distance. Patients with CFA lesions may also report thigh claudication. Some patients with SFA obstructions and strong profunda collateral describe a "walking-through-phenomenon": claudication starts after a certain distance at the beginning of the exercise but then disappears during further exercise, and patients are then able to walk pain free for hours.

Occlusion of the SFA in patients with poor collaterals as well as in patients with multi-level disease leads to critical limb ischemia. In patients with single-level disease, even acute occlusion of the SFA frequently causes only an incomplete ischemia, whereas acute occlusion of the entire femoral axis by embolic obstruction of the CFA or both the SFA and DFA always results in symptoms of acute complete ischemia, acutely endangering patient's limb and life.

Clinical investigation in patients with isolated femoral disease typically reveals a strong pulse at the levels of the groin and a diminished or absent pulse in the popliteal fossa. Auscultation may reveal a bruit of the affected vessel. However, interpretation of vascular bruits remains difficult since harmless plaques particularly in the CFA may cause loud bruits, whereas complete occlusions remain silent.

Despite ongoing scientific efforts, there is still no laboratory test which helps to identify patients with peripheral artery disease. Nevertheless, certain laboratory parameters are helpful when treating these patients:

- Traditional risk factors: blood lipids, blood glucose, glycated hemoglobin—to assess the necessity and dosage of adjunctive pharmacological therapy.
- Renal function parameters: creatinine—to assess the risk of contrast administration and decide upon renal protective measures before, during, and after an intervention.
- Thyroid parameters: TSH—to assess the risk of iodinated contrast administration.
- Muscle encymes: creatin kinase and myoglobin—to detect and assess the extent of ischemia of the muscle in patients with acute complete ischemia.
- Inflammatory parameters: C-reactive protein, leucocyte count—to identify and assess the extent of inflammation and infection in patients with chronic critical limb ischemia.

Further diagnostic testing should include the following:

(a) Measurement of the ankle brachial index (ABI) at rest, and optionally ABI after exercise in patients with inconclusive findings at rest.
(b) Toe pressures have to be measured in patients with diabetic medial sclerosis.

(c) Oscillography is a useful and quick screening method, which also nicely uncovers the presence of medial sclerosis and can be done in addition to ABI measurements.

6   Diagnostic Imaging

6.1   Duplex Ultrasound Investigation

The femoral segment is the ideal segment for duplex ultrasound investigations. The diagnostic accuracy in skilled hands is about 90%; it is noninvasive and risk free and is an excellent tool to plan endovascular interventions in the entire femoral segments. In our practice, duplex sonography is the only required imaging method for isolated femoral interventions. Furthermore, duplex ultrasound can be used for evaluation of stents or bypasses in the femoral area. Using the peak velocity ratio (PVR: ratio between the maximum systolic flow within the stenosis compared to the systolic velocity in the pre-stenotic segment), an estimation of the degree of stenosis can be given, which nicely corresponds to angiography. Usually, a PVR of 2.4 or 2.5 is considered indicative of a flow-limiting stenosis with a degree of at least 50%. Limitations of duplex ultrasound are as follows:

(a) Excessive calcifications
(b) Very obese patients with limited ultrasound visibility
(c) In patients with proximal flow limitation assessment of the distal vessel can be difficult. Therefore, prior to surgery, advanced imaging methods should be used particularly to assess the distal landing zone of the bypass graft. In the context of bypass surgery, duplex ultrasound also plays an important role in assessing the ipsilateral and contralateral vein situation and suitability as a bypass vessel. A well-trained ultrasound team therefore is mandatory.

6.2   MR Angiography with Gadolinium

(contrast-enhanced magnetic resonance angiography—ce-MRA) can be considered as the new gold standard for evaluation of the lower limb arteries. The diagnostic accuracy particularly in the femoral segment is above 95%, the diagnostic accuracy is not affected by calcification and it can be used to plan endovascular as well as surgical interventions. Nevertheless, there are some limitations of ce-MRA: it tends to overestimate the degree of stenosis—short high-grade stenoses are frequently displayed as complete occlusions. Furthermore, ce-MRA has to be carefully used in patients with severe renal dysfunction due to the risk of nephrogenic fibrosis. In patients with stents, artifacts usually make the interpretation of the remaining lumen problematic. Finally, general contraindications for MR like pacemakers or metal implants have to be considered. In clinical practice, a certain percentage (approximately 5%) of the patients therefore is not suitable for MRA.

6.3   CT Angiography

In contrast to the predominant role of CTA for assessment of aortoiliac disease, heavy calcification frequently limits the usefulness of CTA for assessment of the femoral segment. CTA has the definite advantage of adequately assessing stents and instent-restenosis, but has problems with calcification, includes the use of iodinated contrast administration and radiation.

6.4   Angiography (Digital Subtraction)

This method remains the most accurate way of assessing the vasculature and has to be done routinely immediately before all endovascular interventions. Femoral angiography can be done via an ipsilateral antegrade access by direct puncture of the CFA at the level of the femoral head, by contralateral access via retrograde puncture of the contralateral CFA and an over-the-bifurcation approach or alternatively via a left (preferred) or a right transbrachial or transradial access. Contrast injection can be done manually in doses of 5–10 ml (diluted) contrast, which is the preferred way for selective injection, or via an automated flush injection to the distal aorta, when bilateral overview angiograms are acquired. The usual dosage for an automated overview angiogram to the distal aorta using a pig-tail catheter is 20 ml contrast injected within 10 s.

7 Management

The clinical stage of peripheral artery disease is categorized using the Rutherford–Becker (1–6) or Fontaine (I–IV) classifications. Femoral artery disease should be treated only in symptomatic patients with either intermittent claudication (Rutherford 3) or symptoms of critical limb ischemia (Rutherford 4: ischemic rest pain; Rutherford 5: minor tissue loss; Rutherford 6: major tissue loss). The only exception is patients after peripheral bypass surgery with asymptomatic high-grade stenosis of the bypass or its proximal or distal anastomosis. These patients also have to be treated in an asymptomatic stage to preserve the function of the bypass graft and prevent graft thrombosis; all other patients should be treated only when symptomatic.

Clinical Indications

- In patients with intermittent claudication, the indication for treatment is improvement of symptoms, improvement of the walking distance and quality of life. Patients with intermittent claudication have an excellent spontaneous prognosis with respect to limb salvage. Therefore, it has to be clearly stated that in these patients, interventions (or operations) are not necessary to preserve the limb. Patients have to be informed that any intervention at this stage is a "life-style indication." Nevertheless, considering that intermittent claudication can be a severe burden and may lead to a significant reduction in the quality of life, revascularisation also is justified in patients with severe intermittent claudication. Furthermore, improvement of the walking distance and increase of the exercise capacity also help to improve cardiovascular risk profile.
- In patients with critical limb ischemia, revascularisation is mandatory and has to be attempted in almost all patients. Amputation rates in patients with critical limb ischemia with and without successful revascularisation are 5–10% versus 40–75% indicating the huge benefit of revascularisation in these patients. Therefore, in patients with critical limb ischemia, the indication for revascularisation is limb salvage. Exceptions to this rule are patients with permanent paraplegia as well as patients with extensive irreversible tissue necrosis, where primary amputation might be an adequate treatment option.

Indications by Morphology and Location of the Disease

- As mentioned above, the CFA traditionally is "surgeon´s territory." Results of endarterectomy of isolated CFA lesions are clearly better than any endovascular treatment of this segment; therefore, endovascular therapy of the CFA is reserved for selected patients. This includes patients who are unfit for surgery due to general medical conditions, patients with hostile groins (skin infections, very obese patients) as well as patients who are undergoing simultaneous revascularisation procedures of the SFA or DFA. Generally, we try to avoid stenting of the CFA to keep the surgical option. Stenting of the CFA can be done using self-expanding stents and stents later can be even re-punctured for an ipsilateral groin access, but if the stent fails in the CFA a surgical procedure can become very complex.
- Indication for endovascular DFA interventions is exclusively given in patients with chronic SFA occlusions to improve the collateral flow when the SFA cannot be reopened.
- SFA interventions are done for lesions of any length and grade. Today, the decision for medical treatment, endovascular or surgical treatment will not only depend on the length and morphology of the lesion, but mainly on the clinical stage and patient's comorbid conditions.

8 List of the Open Operative Choices

- Thrombendarterectomy with or without patch of the CFA/DFA/SFA origin
- Bypass surgery including femoral-femoral, femoral-popliteal (P1, P3), femoral-crural, femoral-pedal, iliaco-femoral, or ilaco-crural bypass operation. Bypass materials include vein grafts, which have the best patency, or alternatively prosthetic grafts, which are mainly used for supra-genicular anastomosis. Alternatively, hybrid grafts with a prosthetic body and a venous cuff for the distal anastomosis can be used, particularly, for below the knee anastomosis.
- Remote endarterectomy with or without endovascular stent support.

9   Intervention: Technique and Pitfalls

9.1   Patient Preparation

Patients receive therapy with aspirin (100 mg) and clopidogrel (75 mg) in preparation for stent implantation. If clopidogrel is started less than 7 days before the intervention, a loading dose with 300 mg is administered 1 day pre-procedure or 600 mg at the day of the procedure. Patients should be well hydrated. During the intervention, we administer 2.000–5.000 IU (rarely 7.000) unfractionated heparin, depending on the length of the intervention. ACT monitoring is not routinely used at our institution.

9.2   Access to the Lesion

Generally, we prefer the contralateral crossover approach (Fig. 25.2) due to the following reasons: First, arterial closure devices are safer to use after retrograde puncture than after antegrade puncture. Second, the use of an ipsilateral compression bandage after the procedure may reduce the flow in the treated area and thereby increase the risk of early thrombotic occlusions. Third, in patients with puncture-site-associated complications like pseudoaneurysms, treatment of the complication (e.g., by prolonged compression) may endanger a good result in the ipsilateral limb again through flow disturbances. Nevertheless, in the era of four french compatible devices, the antegrade approach has gained importance again (Fig. 25.3). Also, the antegrade approach has certain advantages with respect to wire steer-ability, push-ability, and backup and therefore might be preferred in patients with very complex lesions. Furthermore, in patients with severe kinking or atherosclerotic disease of the pelvic arteries, the crossover approach might not be suitable and therefore antegrade access can be the adequate strategy in these patients. There is certainly no general recommendation suitable for all patients, but in clinical practice in patients where both access routes are feasible, the following rule has proven useful: if four french systems can be used, the antegrade access is suitable, if six french systems are planned, we prefer the crossover access.

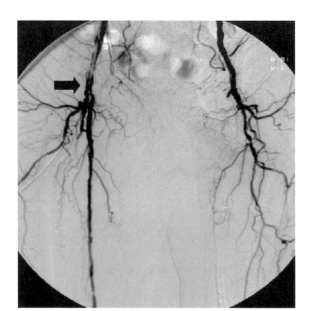

Fig. 25.2 Crossover approach using a 6-french sheath

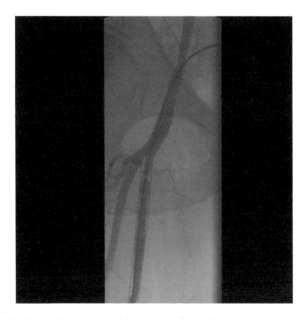

Fig. 25.3 Antegrade puncture of the common femoral artery

CFA and DFA lesions are routinely accessed via a contralateral femoral approach using a six french crossover sheath. Very recently even four french crossover sheath have become available. In patients with contralateral obstructions or bilateral disease, we use a left transbrachial approach and a 90-cm long hydrophilic sheath to access the lesions. Today in our institution, many SFA lesions are also approached from the contralateral groin. However, in patients with short (TASC A) lesions, which are located at least 3–5 cm distal of the femoral bifurcation, the ipsilateral antegrade puncture using a 4-french sheath is a feasible alternative.

Very rarely, alternative access routes like the popliteal puncture can be used after failed revascularisation procedures from a groin access. The popliteal approach is safe in experienced hands, but should be done under ultrasound or angiographic guidance (using an additional groin access to inject contrast and locate the popliteal artery by road-map or overlay technique). Blind puncture of the popliteal artery bears a considerable risk of bleeding after failed punctures and occurrence of AV fistulas. The puncture should be done in the supragenicular (P1) segment to avoid puncture of the vein (which is overlaying the artery in the P2 segment).

9.3 Placement of the Sheath

The sheath should be placed as close to the target vessel as possible. For SFA interventions we place the sheath to the CFA to allow collateral contrast flow via the DFA, which is particularly helpful when treating chronic occlusions.

9.4 Pre-Procedure Angiograms

We routinely perform an inflow angiogram only in patients when a pre-procedure ce-MRA is not available or when pelvic lesions are treated within the same session. Otherwise we start the angiographic evaluation at the level of the CFA including the DFA and the entire femoropopliteal segment. We then perform complete tibioperoneal run-off images as well as images of the foot. All angiograms are performed pre- and postprocedure, but routinely only in one plane. The target segment usually is evaluated in two planes pre- and postprocedure. Exceptions to this rule are patients with severe renal dysfunction. In these patients, only the target segment is evaluated pre- and post-procedure, and the run-off is checked clinically and by duplex ultrasound.

9.5 Recanalisation Wires and Techniques

Our standard wires are a 0.035 Terumo glide wire (stiff version) and a 0.018 hydrophilic wire (0.018 control wire, Boston Scientific). Using these wires more than 90% of the lesions can be crossed. In patients with very rigid or calcified lesions, these wires can be prepared to improve success rates. Routinely, we perform recanalisation using a wire supported by a catheter—with the catheter closely following the tip of the wire. Either a diagnostic catheter (multi-purpose) or a balloon catheter can be used.

- *Intraluminal Recanalisation.* Whenever possible we intend intraluminal recanalisation. This is mandatory not only in all CFA, DFA, and SFA stenosis but also should be anticipated in patients with occlusions. Frequently, occlusions contain micro-channels which allow relatively easy passage of a wire even through long segments. In these patients, we prefer the 0.018 Boston Scientific control wire with a hydrophilic tip, which very smoothly crosses these lesions. However, in heavily calcified chronic total occlusions, this technique will frequently fail.
- *The Wire-Loop Technique.* The wire-loop technique (Fig. 25.4) for subintimal passage (Bolia technique) helps to pass complex occlusions in the subintimal space. Using a 0.035 hydrophilic Terumo wire, the tip is entered the subintimal space proximal of the occlusion. Then a loop is formed and the wire thus can be advanced in the subintimal space. Usually, the wire should be supported by a catheter (diagnostic or balloon). The length of the loop should be kept under control, particularly in the phase of re-entry to the true lumen. A short loop usually is helpful to re-enter at the distal end of the occlusion. Theoretically, the loop should re-enter the true lumen by itself as soon as the occlusion has been passed. However, especially when the distal arterial segment is also diseased, re-entry can be complicated or impossible resulting in a dissection and prolongation of the treated segment.

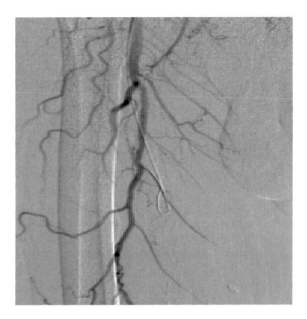

Fig. 25.4 Wire loop technique for subintimal passage of a chronic total occlusion

- *Difficult Re-Entry*. We always intend to re-enter the true lumen immediately at the distal edge of the occluded segment to avoid any propagation of the treated segment. If the loop does not re-enter at the distal edge of the occlusion, various support catheters with different shapes (multi-purpose, head-hunter, JR-4) can be used to redirect the tip of the wire to the true lumen. Contrast injections in various planes are helpful to locate the true lumen. Alternatively, the reverse "bad" end of the Terumo wire can be used to puncture the true lumen or the tip of the 0.018 Boston control wire can be cut to a needle-like instrument and be used as a puncture device. Both techniques are off-label and can lead to severe bleeding complications. Recently, re-entry devices have been released like the Outback catheter (Cordis) (Fig. 25.5), which helps to re-enter the true lumen in almost all cases of previously failed recanalisation procedures. This device includes a small puncture needle which can be directed to the true lumen using a marker system, and then a 0.014 wire is entered to the lumen via the needle and allows balloon dilatation and stenting (Fig. 25.5). Usually, the 0.014 wire has to be exchanged to a more stable wire after an initial balloon dilatation.

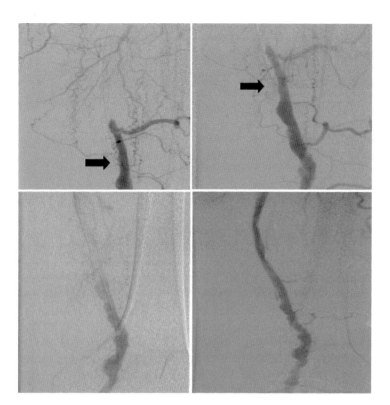

Fig. 25.5 True lumen re-entry using the Outback catheter (Cordis) in a patient with a long segment superficial femoral artery occlusion

- *Treating Bifurcated Lesions*. Treating lesions at the femoral bifurcation includes the risk of plaque shift. Therefore, depending on the plaque load in the SFA and DFA origins and the angle of the DFA offspring, a two-wire technique should be applied for treatment of these lesions. Using two 0.018 wires, this can be easily done via a 6-french sheath. Different approaches are possible: In patients with a low plaque burden in the DFA ostium and absence of a significant stenosis, it is sufficient to place a safety wire in the DFA during balloon dilatation of the SFA ostium. In patients with coincident stenosis of the SFA and DFA ostium, a kissing balloon technique should be applied with simultaneous inflation of overlapping balloons in the SFA and DFA. Using this technique, one has to be careful not to oversize the balloons in the CFA since the diameter of the two balloons add up and may lead to severe injury or even rupture of the CFA. In patients where simultaneous inflation of two balloons in the SFA and DFA seems not feasible due to a small diameter of the CFA, sequential balloon inflations have to be performed. Bifurcation stent techniques as used in the coronary arteries (crush stenting, mini-crush, reverse crush, etc.) should not be used for the femoral bifurcation since these techniques require the use of balloon-expanding stents, which should not be used in this location.

9.6   Revascularisation

- Balloon dilatation remains the standard for revascularisation of CFA, DFA, and SFA lesions. We first attempt balloon angioplasty in almost all patients. The balloon to artery ratio for balloon dilatation in these segments should be 1:1. Only in heavily calcified CFA lesions, undersized balloon dilatation might be necessary to avoid the risk of arterial rupture. Ideally, the length of the balloon should be adapted to the length of the lesion. Today, very long balloons (up to 200 mm) enable comfortable treatment also of very long lesions. We keep the balloon inflated between 1 and 2 min. The angiographic results seem better after long balloon inflations, and even long dissections can be sealed by prolonged balloon inflation. However, admittedly, there are no scientific data proving that prolonged balloon dilatation improves midterm outcomes after angioplasty.
- Stent Implantation. Self-expanding nitinol stents are the standard implants for the entire femoral segment. These stents are flexible, and the newest generation may withstand the mechanical stress in the femoral arteries. Although nitinol stents have less radial force than balloon-expanding stents, most lesions can be adequately handled, but predilatation and lesion preparation are frequently necessary. Indications for nitinol stenting are residual stenosis after balloon dilatation, flow-limiting dissection, and elastic recoil. Nitinol stents have also been proven superior to balloon angioplasty in longer and complex lesions and therefore frequently are used in patients with lesions above 5–10 cm in length. Today, stents with a length of up to 200 mm are available, thus overlapping of multiple stents can be reduced even in very long lesions. We recommend

pre-dilatation and post-dilatation for all nitinol stent implantations to guarantee an adequate vessel wall alignment of the stents. The stent-to-artery ratio should be 1:1–1.2:1. Severe oversizing should be avoided since this increases the risk for restenosis

- Alternative to self-expanding stents, balloon-expanding stents can be used in very short and very rigid lesions. These devices should be used in a 1:1 stent-to artery ratio. These stents have an optimal radial force, but bear the risk of stent compression or stent crush through outside forces, particularly in the CFA. Therefore, most interventionists are reluctant in implanting balloon-expanding stents in the femoral segment.

- Stent Grafts. The implantation of stent grafts was originally indicated for the treatment of aneurysmatic disease or complications like perforation and bleeding. Recently, stent grafts are also used for long and complex SFA lesions. Usually, self-expanding stent grafts should be used for the SFA only, and stent graft should be used in the CFA and DFA only for emergency indications. Stent graft implantation requires relatively large introducer sheaths (8–9 french) and adequate vessel preparation (predilatation) as well as post-dilatation. The major disadvantage of stent graft implantation is the occlusion of all collateral vessels in the covered segment. Occlusion of stent grafts therefore may lead to a worsening of the initial clinical situation.

- Alternative revascularisation techniques include cutting balloon angioplasty, atherectomy using different devices (rotational atherectomy, Silver-Hawk atherectomy), laser-angioplasty, or cryoplasty. All these methods are technically feasible, improve the immediate outcome, and have niche indications, but have not been proven effective in long-term randomized trials. Most important indications for these devices are extremely calcified lesions to reduce the plaque burden and prepare the lesion for stent implantation.

- Aspiration and Thrombolysis. Patients with huge thrombus load (e.g., due to embolic disease, acute stent thrombosis, or acute graft thrombosis) should undergo aspiration thrombectomy and thrombolysis. We perform purely mechanical aspiration using a 6-french soft-tiped guiding catheter. Alternatively, several mechanical aspiration systems (Rotarex, Angiojet) are available. For thrombolysis, rt-PA or Urokinase can be used. Both substances should be used in conjunction with full-dose unfractioned heparin. We apply Urokinase (100.000 Units per hours locally). The dosage of rt-PA is a bolus of up to 20 mg followed by a continuous infusion of

1–4 mg per hour. We recommend to use a perfusion catheter system for local thrombolysis where the thrombolytic system is injected directly to the lesion. Local thrombolysis requires regular monitoring of coagulation parameters including apTT, thrombocyte count, and fibrinogen in 4-h intervals during thrombolysis.

9.7 Access Site Management

We prefer to use arterial closure devices in 80–90% of the patients, unless a 4-french sheath has been implanted. In these cases, manual compression is applied. Prerequisites for the use of an arterial closure device are puncture of the CFA, absence of a significant stenosis at the puncture site, absence of any major side-branch (DFA) at the puncture site and a diameter of the CFA of at least 5 mm. The use of arterial closure devices in other locations than the CFA has been reported (DFA, SFA, popliteal artery, brachial artery), but our experience in these locations is not convincing with relatively high rates of complications.

10 Post-Procedure Management and Follow-up Protocol

After the removal of the sheath a compression bandage is applied. After the use of an arterial closure device patients are mobilized at 4 h. Similarly, after use of a 4-french sheath bed rest is recommended only for 4 h. Patients who underwent manual compression after a 6-french or larger intervention without use of an arterial closure device have to keep bed-rest overnight with a compression bandage.

Continuous hemodynamic monitoring is not done routinely after femoral interventions, unless the patient has any symptoms or complaints. Patients are usually discharged 1 day after the intervention. Before discharge, the access site and the treated segment are investigated by duplex ultrasound to exclude puncture-site complications and to document the result of revascularisation. Furthermore, all patients undergo ABI measurements and oscillography.

Patients are invited for follow-up investigations including clinical evaluation, ABI, and oscillography every 3 months postintervention for the first year.

11 Complications and Management

Complications occur in 5–10% of femoral interventions. Fortunately, most complications are relatively harmless and can be handled easily during the intervention. Nevertheless, one has to be prepared for the following events:

• Access site complications. These are the most frequent incidents including bleeding (retroperitoneal), pseudoaneurysms, dissections, thrombotic occlusions, infections, and hematoma. These complications may occur directly in the cath-lab, or hours after the intervention or even after discharge. Adequate puncture technique and access site management are crucial to avoid these complications. Today, many minimal invasive therapies exist to handle access-site complications, e.g., pseudoaneurysms can be treated by ultrasound guided compression therapy, percutaneous thrombin injection, coil embolisation, or overstenting using stent grafts (Fig. 25.6).

• Perforation and Rupture. Fortunately, this complication very rarely occurs in the femoral segment, unless balloons are grossly oversized or stiff wires are handled without care. The first action after a rupture and massive bleeding is to inflate an occlusion balloon at low pressure above or across the lesion. Depending on the extent of bleeding, heparin should be reversed by administration of protamine (which is hardly ever necessary in femoral interventions). Furthermore, the bleeding site can be compressed from outside. If the bleeding continues, the segment should be sealed using a stent graft. If bleeding occurs from a side branch or if no wire can be crossed by the ruptured segment, the bleeding artery can be sealed by coil embolization.

• Dissection. This is a frequent finding after balloon angioplasty at the dilated segment and requires prolonged balloon dilatation or stent implantation. Of course, dissection may also occur at the puncture site or as a complication in any other vascular segment, where a wire has been placed without care.

• Embolization occurs in 2–5% of femoral interventions. Usually, emboli can be aspirated using a 6-french aspiration catheter. Very rarely local thrombolysis is required either as a bolus or followed by continuous infusion. Alternatively, balloon angioplasty or stent implantation may help to solve the problem.

• Restenosis. This is the most frequent long-term complication after femoral interventions (Fig. 25.7), and in this context, the femoral artery remains the Achilles heel of the interventionist.

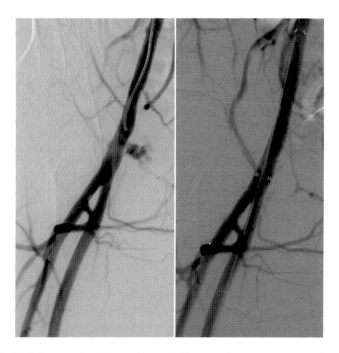

Fig. 25.6 Overstenting of a massive arterial leakage after percutaneous angiography in a patient unfit for surgery

- Stent Fractures. First-generation nitinol stents showed fracture rates of up to 50%. These fractures were associated with restenosis and even bleeding complications due to pseudoaneurysm formation. Fractures have to be treated by repeat stent implantation or use of a stent graft. New stent designs make fractures a rare complication.

12 Outcomes: Open Versus Endovascular Treatment

- Technical Success Rates. Immediate technical success rates of endovascular treatment of CFA, DFA, and SFA stenosis are close to 100% and similar to open surgery. Chronic total occlusions, particularly of the SFA, are treated with an above 90% technical

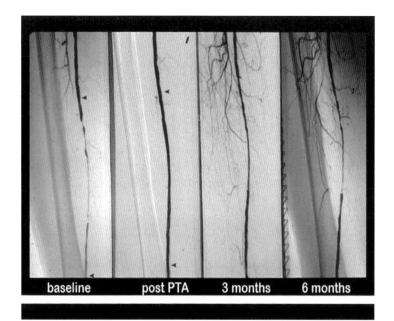

Fig. 25.7 Occurrence of restenosis after long segment balloon angioplasty of the superficial femoral artery

success rate in experienced centers. Stenting guarantees an excellent immediate result even in very long lesions (Fig. 25.8). However, surgery has an almost 100% success rate in these indications, independent of the length of the lesion.

- Complications. Major complications after endovascular procedures in the femoral area occur in less than 1% to maximum 5%, and minor complications are reported in 3–15% of endovascular procedures. Open surgical procedures have a major complication and death rate of 3–8% and a minor complication rate of 8–30%.
- Restenosis Rates. Restenosis rates depend on the segment treated. Good data are available only for the SFA: After balloon angioplasty, restenosis rate mainly depend on the length of the treated segment. In short lesions (below 5 cm), 12 and 24 months restenosis rates are 30% and 40%, in lesions longer than 5 cm restenosis rates increase to 60% and higher at 1 year. After nitinol stent implantation, restenosis rates seem to be less dependent on lesion

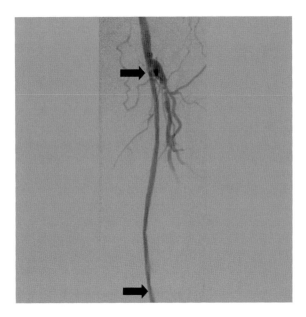

Fig. 25.8 Long segment stent implantation for the treatment of a chronic total occlusion

length. Depending on the implanted stent type, the 12 and 24 months restenosis rates are 15–30% and 25–45%, respectively. Stent grafts show restenosis/reocclusion rates of about 15–20% at 12 months and 20–25% at 24 months, respectively. In comparison, vein graft surgery offers the best long-term results for SFA treatment: patency rates at 1, 3, and 5 years are around 90%, 75% and 60%, respectively. Prosthetic bypass grafts show higher failure rates with more than 50% reocclusions at 5 years.

13   Table/Flowchart on the Role of Endovascular Treatment

An overview on the role of endovascular treatment of patients with femoral artery disease is given in Fig. 25.9. This refers to patients with chronic limb ischemia. In patients with acute critical limb ischemia, the treatment algorithm depends on the clinical stage: patients

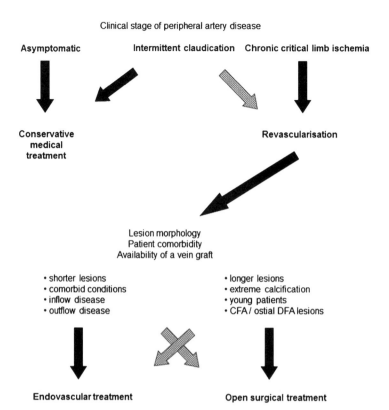

Fig. 25.9 Flow chart summarizing the role of endovascular treatment of the femoral artery In patients with acute onset of symptoms of leg ischemia, athero-embolic, or cardioembolic disease has to be considered as a differential diagnosis. Most frequently, emboli arise from atrial fibrillation, and alternatively, aortic aneurismal disease or aortic plaques may cause distal embolisation. However, acute onset of disease may also occur in patients with atherothrombotic disease due to rapid progression of atherosclerotic disease in the femoral artery. Regarding treatment, the differential diagnosis of embolic and atheroslerotic disease is crucial to enable the optimal revascularisation strategy and guarantee an optimal prophylaxis against recurrent events. Briefly, in patients with embolic obstruction, removal of the thrombus by embolectomy (open surgical or endovascular) is the treatment of choice, and alternatively in patients with incomplete ischemia, thrombolysis can be considered. In contrast, in patients with atherosclerotic disease, endarterectomy or bypass surgery as well as balloon angioplasty or stent implantation are the classical treatment options. Regarding pharmacotherapy, patients with (cardio-)embolic disease typically will undergo oral anticoagulation with vitamin K antagonists, whereas patients with atherosclerotic disease usually will receive treatment with an antiplatelet drugs like aspirin or clopidogrel

with acute complete ischemia (pain, pallor, pulselessness, paresthesia, plegia, prostration) and immediate danger of the leg, emergent open vascular surgery is the treatment of choice. Patients with acute, but incomplete ischemia (absence of paresthesia, plegia, and prostration) are urgently treated by either an endovascular or open surgical approach depending on the same factors as in patients with chronic critical limb ischemia.

References

1. Norgren L, Hiatt WR, Dormandy JA, Nehler MR, Harris KA, Fowkes FG. TASC II Working Group. Inter-Society Consensus for the Management of Peripheral Arterial Disease (TASC II). J Vasc Surg. 2007;45(Suppl S): S5–67.
2. Schillinger M, Sabeti S, Loewe C, Dick P, Amighi J, Mlekusch W, Schlager O, Cejna M, Lammer J, Minar E. Balloon angioplasty versus implantation of nitinol stents in the superficial femoral artery. N Engl J Med. 2006;354(18):1879–88.
3. Krankenberg H, Schlüter M, Steinkamp HJ, Bürgelin K, Scheinert D, Schulte KL, Minar E, Peeters P, Bosiers M, Tepe G, Reimers B, Mahler F, Tübler T, Zeller T. Nitinol stent implantation versus percutaneous transluminal angioplasty in superficial femoral artery lesions up to 10 cm in length: the femoral artery stenting trial (FAST). Circulation. 2007;116(3):285–92.
4. Pereira CE, Albers M, Romiti M, Brochado-Neto FC, Pereira CA. Meta-analysis of femoropopliteal bypass grafts for lower extremity arterial insufficiency. J Vasc Surg. 2006;44(3):510–7.

Chapter 26
Superficial Femoral and Popliteal Artery Disease

Marc Bosiers and Koen Deloose

1 Anatomy

The common femoral artery (CFA) originates from the external iliac artery at the inguinal ligament. At about 4 cm distal to the inguinal ligament, the CFA splits into the deep femoral artery (DFA), also called the profunda, and the superficial femoral artery (SFA). The DFA origin is located on the lateral side of the CFA and runs on to the medial side of the femur. The two main arteries branching off the DFA are the lateral and the medial femoral circumflex arteries. The first, which originates in the proximal portion of the DFA and ends in the genicular branches at the level of the knee, is often an important collateral route in case of SFA occlusions. The medial femoral circumflex artery provides blood to the proximal adductor compartment.

The CFA changes into the SFA at the level of the branching of the DFA. From this point the SFA runs distally towards the adductor

M. Bosiers, M.D. (✉)
Department of Vascular Surgery, A.Z. St. Blasius Hospital,
Dendermonde, Belgium
e-mail: Marc.bosiers@telenet.be

K. Deloose, M.D.
Department of Vascular Surgery, A.Z. St. Blasius Hospital,
Dendermonde, 9200, Belgium

A. Kumar and K. Ouriel (eds.), *Handbook of Endovascular Interventions*,   349
DOI 10.1007/978-1-4614-5013-9_26,
© Springer Science+Business Media New York 2013

hiatus (Canal of Hunter), which is located about 5 cm above the knee, where it becomes the popliteal artery. The start of the popliteal artery is often referred to as P1. The popliteal artery crosses the patella (at P2) and ends at the origin of the anterior tibial artery (P3). Around the knee, a natural collateral vasculature is formed by the superior, middle and inferior genicular arteries that branch from the popliteal artery in pairs. The distal popliteal artery ends below the knee what is sometimes wrongly called the "trifurcation". In reality, it consists of two separate bifurcations, where the anterior and posterior tibial arteries branch off.

Variations that can sometimes be seen:

- The medial or lateral femoral circumflex arteries originate from the CFA instead of the DFA in roughly 20% of people.
- In 0.4% of cases, popliteal artery ends in a trifucation, as the origin of the anterior and posterior arteries coincides.

2 Disease Definition

- Stenosis or occlusion due to atherosclerosis
- Aneurysm
- Pseudo-aneurysm

3 Disease Distribution

Stenotic lesions in the superficial femoral artery often have a diffuse aspect. Some lesions may result from thrombosis due to local plaque formation at the level of the Canal of Hunter. Occurrence of femoro-popliteal artery aneurysms is associated with the presence of an aortic aneurysm in approximately 50% of the patients. Whereas lesions in the deep femoral artery are more common in patients presenting with diabetes, this particular association does not exist for SFA lesions.

4 Diagnosis: Clinical

Indication for Treatment: Symptomatic Disease

Clinical categories of limb ischaemia. Rutherford-Becker classification

(a) Class 0 : asymptomatic—normal treadmill; normal stress test
(b) Class 1 : mild claudication—the patient can complete the tread-mill test; after exercise an ankle pressure of more than 50 mm Hg is measured, which is at least 25 mm Hg lower than the brachial pressure
(c) Class 2: moderate claudication—the patient scores worse than Class 1, but better than Class 3
(d) Class 3: severe claudication—the patient cannot complete the treadmill test; after exercise an ankle pressure of less than 50 mm Hg is measured
(e) Class 4: ankle pressure measured at rest is below 40 mm Hg, peak velocity ratio at the ankle or metatarsal is flat or barely pulsatile; the toe pressure lies below 30 mm Hg
(f) Class 5: minor tissue loss (i.e., non-healing ulcer, focal gangrene with diffuse pedal edema)—the ankle pressure at rest is below 60 mm Hg, peak velocity ratio at the ankle or metatarsal is flat or barely pulsatile; the toe pressure lies below 40 mm Hg
(g) Class 6 : major tissue loss—the ankle pressure at rest is below 60 mm Hg, peak velocity ratio at the ankle or metatarsal is flat or barely pulsatile; the toe pressure lies below 40 mm Hg

5 Diagnostic imaging: CFDU/CTA/MRI/Diagnostic Angiography

5.1 Color-Flow Doppler Ultrasound

Colour-Flow Doppler Ultrasound (CFDU) is a commonly used screening method. It owns its popularity as a means of post-op surveillance because it is readily available, cheap and carries a low risk. However, caution is advised when interpreting CFDU measurements as it is operator dependent.

5.2   Computed tomography Angiography (CTA)

Computed tomography angiography (CTA) is a non-invasive study, which combines the luminal information of digital subtraction angiography images with the cross-sectional view information of axial computed tomography angiography. CTA images visualise the vessel wall, extraluminal processes and anatomic relationships with adjacent structures. The most important disadvantages of CTA are: the high contrast load needed to visualize the vasculature, and the fact that it is a relatively investigator-dependent technique. Overestimation of degree of stenosis on computed tomography angiopgraphy images is possible due to "blooming artefacts". Also, heavily calcified eccentric plaques preclude a correct reading. Furthermore, the arterial lumen can be covered up by ring-like calcifications in the vessel wall.

5.3   Magnetic resonance angiography (MRA)

Magnetic resonance angiography (MRA) is another non-invasive imaging modality. It uses flow-induced signal variations to render blood vessels and to obtain quantitative blood flow information concerning velocity and direction and allows the creation of 3D reconstructions. Two types exist: (1)unenhanced magnetic resonance angiography, which relies only on flow effects and therefore only depicts the movement of blood, and (2) contrast-enhanced magnetic resonance angiography, which uses a contrast agent to visualise the vessel lumen. Unenhanced MRA shows extravascular tissue, allowing the correlation of blood flow abnormalities with associated soft tissue pathologies. Yet, because it is based on complex flow phenomena and is sensitive to flow and movement, it is prone to lead to artefacts in the imaging generated. Enhanced MRA does not require any exposure to ionising radiation or nephrotoxic iodinated contrast media and offers image quality comparable to on-table angiography, but is sensitive to movement and, because the vascular enhancement is a transient and dynamic process, timing of the acquisition is key.

5.4   Digital subtraction angiography (DSA)

Digital subtraction angiography (DSA) is an invasive technique that has long been the only means to visualise the arterial tree. Typically, the common femoral artery is punctured to gain access to the arterial system, which is followed by the introduction of an angiographic catheter and the injection of iodinated contrast medium. Digital subtraction angiography is capable of providing dynamic images, information that cannot be obtained with standard computed tomography angiography and magnetic resonance angiography techniques.

6   Management: Treatment Choice: TASC II 2007 Lesion Classification

(h) Type A – Endovascular treatment is the treatment of choice

  1. Single stenosis of maximum 10 cm length
  2. Single occlusion of maximum 5 cm length

(i) Type B – Endovascular treatment is the preferred treatment, after verification of the patient's co-morbidities

  1. Multiple stenoses or occlusions, each maximum 5 cm long
  2. Single stenosis or occlusion of maximum 15 cm, not involving the infra-geniculate popliteal artery
  3. Single or multiple lesions in the absence of continuous tibial arteries to improve inflow for a distal bypass
  4. Heavily calcified occlusion of maximum 5 cm long
  5. Single popliteal stenosis

(j) Type C – Surgery is the preferred treatment, in good-risk patients

  1. Multiple stenoses or occlusions, with a cumulative length of more than 15 cm, with or without heavy calcification
  2. Recurrent stenoses or occlusions that need treatment after two endovascular interventions

(k) Type D – Surgery is the treatment of choice

  1. Chronic total occlusions of the common or superficial femoral artery of more than 20 cm, involving the popliteal artery
  2. Chronic total occlusion of the popliteal artery and the proximal infra-geniculate arteries

6.1 List of Open Operative Choices

Venous bypasses are always preferred over prosthetic grafts. Results with in situ and reversed are equal, and use of any of these two techniques depends on the preference of the operator. Toe, forefoot or wound amputation is normally delayed for 6–10 days after bypass surgery, after reperfusion assessment. Next to bypass surgery, profundaplasty plays an important role in surgical treatment of femoropopliteal treatment, as the deep femoral artery is the most important collateral route for a blockage of the superficial femoral artery. This is often performed in combination with treatment of the common femoral artery.

1. Longer length infra-inguinal bypass (in decreasing order of preference).

   (a) Autologous vein – first choice whenever possible

      1. Ipsilateral greater saphenous vein
      2. Contra-lateral greater saphenous vein
      3. Spliced vein

   (b) PTFE
   (c) Human umbilical vein
   (d) Radial artery
   (e) Cryopreserved vein

2. Shorter length infra-inguinal bypass (10–15 cm)

   (a) Eversion endarterectomy of the superficial femoral artery, with anastomosis to the available vein segment
   (b) Arm vein
   (c) Lesser saphenous vein
   (d) PTFE (above-knee bypass)
   (e) Dacron (above-knee bypass)

3. Amputation

   (a) Toe
   (b) Forefoot
   (c) Wound

4. Profundaplasty

7 Intervention: Techniques and Pitfalls

All patients receiving endovascular therapy should receive aspirin and clopidogrel (75 mg per day) for four days prior to procedure. During the procedure intravenous heparin administration is necessary to maintain an activated clotting time between 250 and 300.

7.1 Contra-lateral Procedure

1. Access is made by puncturing the common femoral artery at the contra-lateral side using the Seldinger technique.
2. A short (11 cm) 6 F straight sheath is installed at the puncture site.
3. Bifurcation crossing is performed with a 0.035″ hydrophilic guidewire of 260 cm, which is advanced into the aorta with a crossover catheter of choice of 65 or 100 cm (e.g., RIM, Simmons 1, Simmons 2, Universal Flush, Berenstein).
4. Crossover catheter is placed in the common femoral artery on the lesion side and over a stiffer guidewire (e.g., Bent Terumo, Amplatz,…)
5. A long 4F-6F sheath (e.g., Destination) is installed in the common femoral artery
6. Intraluminal lesion passage is done by advancing the hydrophilic guidewire and crossover catheter into the superficial femoral artery (SFA) of the contralateral limb. Subintimal lesion passage can be attempted if intraluminal passage with the guidewire does not work.
7. Intraluminal lesion passage is performed with the catheter (of choice) over the guidewire
8. Lesion treatment is done by means of

    (a) Thrombolysis
    (b) PTA
    (c) Stent placement

        1. Flexible self-expanding nitinol
        2. Long self-expanding nitinol
        3. Drug-eluting self-expanding nitinol

9. A completion angiography is performed. If the result is insufficient after PTA (residual stenosis ≥30% or flow-limiting dissection), a prolonged balloon dilation can be performed. When the result remain unsatisfying, stent placement is done.

7.2   Ipsilateral Procedure

(a) Access is made by puncturing the common femoral artery at the ipsilateral side using the Seldinger technique. The entrance into the Common Femoral Artery should be in the upper half of the femoral head. If not the wire shall invariably go into the profunda femoris/deep femoral artery. In this event it is almost invariably better to remove the needle and hold pressure for a few minutes. Subsequently a reattempt at a higher level should be done.

(b) The remaining steps are the same as for contra-lateral access with the exception that crossover does not have to be achieved.

8   Complications and Management

8.1   Embolisation

Distal embolisation during infra-inguinal endovascular treatment is more likely to occur in patients with (near-)occlusions, when calcification is present, in long and diffuse lesion settings, or when there is an intravascular filling defect. Each maneuver with balloons, stents, guidewires and catheters can potentially trigger embolic debris to loosen from the vessel wall. Yet, the incidence of athero-embolisation can be minimised by good patient selection, prevention with pharmacological treatment, the use of long low-profile flexible devices, and expert operator techniques. Scraping of the arterial wall should be avoided in all circumstances. Therefore, catheter progression or removal should always be performed over the guidewire. Although protection devices have been advocated by some in order to prevent distal embolisation, it remains debatable whether this solution is necessary and cost-effective.

Next to systemic anti-coagulation, several treatments for embolisation at the femoro-popliteal tract exist. Immediate removal of thrombus with the aid of a balloon embolectomy catheter is performed, with which several passes are made until no more debris can be extracted. Also, backbleeding through guiding catheters, after guidewire removal, enables to remove debris. Endovascular techniques to treat embolisation offer certain potential benefits compared to surgery. With catheter-directed thrombolysis the micro-circulation, which cannot be reached by means of catheters, can be addressed. Moreover, it reveals the underlying stenoses or occlusions, which can afterwards be easily treated with endovascular therapy. Also, percutaneous aspiration thrombectomy is a minimally invasive method to safely remove debris in the femoro-popliteal tract, without the risk of bleeding associated with lytic therapy and delayed reperfusion.

8.2 Dissection

It is not uncommon to generate a flow-limiting dissection by dilation of a culprit lesion. Whenever this occurs, prolonged balloon dilation (at least one minute) should be attempted first in order to solve the problem. If the dissection then still persists stent placement is indicated.

8.3 Re-stenosis

Occurence of re-stenosis after PTA is not uncommon but is easily treatable by means of endovascular re-intervention. On the other hand, in-stent re-stenosis remains the Achilles' Heel of femoropopliteal endovascular treatment. Unfortunately, very little evidence is available as to what is the best way to treat it. Recent thrombus can be treated with thrombolysis, but often requires additional procedures. Although several devices, such as atherectomy systems or specifically designed balloon types, have been proposed as a solution for longer-term in-stent re-stenosis, they did not yield satisfactory results. Sub-analysis of the Zilver PTX trial showed acceptable outcome, for stent-in-stent placement of drug-eluting stents, with a freedom of target lesion revascularisation of 78% after 12 months.

Also, subgroup analysis of the Thunder trial hinted that drug-coated balloons might be a promising tool to treat in-stent re-stenosis, but further investigation is definitely warranted.

8.4   Perforation, Rupture, Pseudoaneurysm

Possible causes of ruptures or perforations are injuring the arterial wall during the passage of guidewires or catheters, or ulceration due to stent struts "scraping" against the arterial wall resulting in a local or systemic infection. Often a pseudoaneurysm develops. The transition between the superficial femoral artery and the popliteal artery or at the bifurcation of the tibiofibular trunk is most prone to be perforated. Usually these are self-limiting, however, in case of a sustained perforation or rupture placement of a covered stent or stent-graft is indicated in order to seal off the injured segment of the artery. In severe cases, an emergency surgical bypass is indicated.

9   Outcomes (Table 26.1)

For TASC A&B femoropopliteal lesions, several controlled randomised trials (CRT) have been published, evaluating percutaneous transluminal angioplasty (PTA) versus nitinol stenting. These CRTs show no benefit for stenting over PTA in TASC A lesions. However, stent implantation yields better results than PTA for treating TASC B lesions, approximating a 12-month primary patency rate of 70%, together with low stent fracture rates. For TASC C&D femoropopliteal lesions, no data from CRT's have currently been published.

10   Flowchart Summerizing the Role of Endovascular Treatment

Figures 26.1 and 26.2

Table 26.1 Outcomes of endovascular treatment of femoro-popliteal lesions

Study	N	Lesion length	Primary patency after 1 year	Stent fracture after 1 year
FAST (Bard)				
PTA	121	4.5 cm	61%	N/A
Luminexx stent	123	4.5 cm	68%	N/A
RESILIENT (Edwards)				
PTA	69	6.4 cm	38%	N/A
LifeStent	137	7.1 cm	80%	3%
ASTRON (Biotronik)				
PTA	39	8.4 cm	39%	N/A
Astron stent	34	8.4 cm	66%	-
ABSOLUTE VIENNA (Abbott)				
PTA	53	12.7 cm	37% (31% @2 year)	N/A
Absolute stent	51	13.2 cm	63% (54% @2 year)	2% (2% @2 year)
Zilver PTX randomised (Cook)		No data available yet		
Bare Zilver stent	240			
Zilver PTX stent	240			
Zilver PTX registry (Cook)				
Total population	718	9.9 cm	89% (725/818)[a]	1.6% (n = 1,413)
Lesions <15 cm (TASC A&B)	540	6.1 cm	92% (574/627)[a]	0.9% (n = 816)
Lesions ≥15 cm (TASC C&D)	178	22.9 cm	79%(143/182)[a]	2.6% (n = 584)
In-stent re-stenosis	110	12.6 cm	78% (93/120)[a]	1.1% (n = 267)

[a]Freedom from target lesion revascularisation

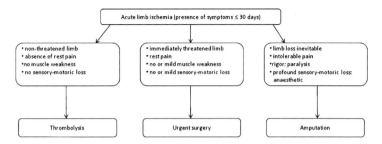

Fig. 26.1 Acute limb ischaemia

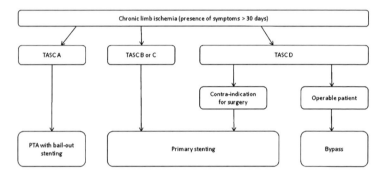

Fig. 26.2 Chronic limb ischaemia

References

1. Norgren L, Hiatt WR, Dormandy JA, Nehler MR, Harris KA, Fowkes FG, et al. Inter-Society Consensus for the Management of Peripheral Arterial Disease (TASC II). J Vasc Surg. 2007;45:S5–67.
2. Hirsch AT, Haskal ZJ, Hertzer NR, Bakal CW, Creager MA, Halperin JL, et al. ACC/AHA 2005 guidelines for the management of patients with peripheral arterial disease (lower extermity, renal, mesenteric, and abdominal aortic): executive summary a collaborative report from the American Association for Vascular Surgery/Society for Vascular Surgery, Society for Cardiovascular Angiography and Interverntions, Society for Vascular Medicine and Biology, Society of Interventional Raidology, and the ACC/AHA Task Force on Practice Guidelines (Writing Committee to Develop Guidelines for the Management of Patients With Peripheral Arterial Disease) endorsed by the American Association of Cardiovascular and Pulmonary Rehabilitation; National Heart, Lung, and Blood Institute; Society for Vascular Nursing; TransAtlantic Inter-Society Consensus; and Vascular Disease Foundation. J Am Coll Cardiol. 2006;47:1239–312.

3. Bosiers M, Deloose K, Verbist J, Peeters P. Present and future of endovascular SFA treatment: stents, stent-grafts, drug coated balloons and drug coated stents. J Cardiovasc Surg (Torino). 2008;49(2):159–65.
4. Lyden SP, Shimshak TM. Contemporary endovascular treatment for disease of the superficial femoral and popliteal arteries: an integrated device-based strategy. J Endovasc Ther. 2006;13 Suppl 2:41–51.

Chapter 27
Infrapopliteal Occlusive Disease

Michael Glasby and Amman Bolia

1 Anatomy

The superficial femoral artery becomes popliteal artery, as it enters the adductor hiatus. It lies deep to the vein (for this reason, there is a risk of arterio-venous fistula formation complicating a popliteal puncture). The artery divides into the anterior tibial (AT) artery and tibio-peroneal trunk (TPT). The TPT divides into the posterior tibial (PT) artery and peroneal artery. The AT becomes the dorsalis pedis at the foot which anastomoses with the plantar arch and then gives off branches contributing to the supply of the toes. The PT artery after giving off the circumflex fibula artery descends the leg medially and passes behind the medial malleolus. It divides into the medial and lateral plantar arteries. The peroneal artery descends in the posterior compartment giving off muscular branches It terminates at the ankle and anastomoses with the distal anterior tibial artery.

Angiosomes concept (Taylor 1982): Understanding which territory is supplied by which vessel can guide therapy and predict the outcome of the intervention. Generally, the AT and DP supply the

M. Glasby, M.D.
X-ray Department, Derby Royal Infirmary, Derby, UK

A. Bolia, M.D. (✉)
Department of Imaging and Interventions, Leicester Royal Infirmary
NHS Infirmary Square, Leicester, Weicestershire, LE15WW, UK
e-mail: abolia@hotmail.com

A. Kumar and K. Ouriel (eds.), *Handbook of Endovascular Interventions*,   363
DOI 10.1007/978-1-4614-5013-9_27,
© Springer Science+Business Media New York 2013

anterior leg and dorsum of the foot. The peroneal artery supplies the heel and lateral ankle and the PT supplies the heel, plantar surface of foot and medial ankle. However, with multiple occlusions and subsequent collateralisation, these territories may become less distinct.

1.1 Anatomic Variations

Many variants exist. Most important is the relationship of the popliteal artery with the muscles/tendons of the popliteal fossa which may lead to popliteal entrapment syndrome, the treatment for which is open surgery.

Other variants of the origins of the crural vessels, such as high take off of the AT artery or conjoint origins, commonly exist.

2 Disease Definition

Below-the-knee occlusive disease can have a multitude of etiologies.

Atherosclerosis This is the most commom cause of below-the-knee occlusive disease. Risk factors as elsewhere (increasing age, smoking, diabetes, hyperlipidaemia, family history, hyperhomocysteinemia, chronic renal insufficiency).

Popliteal aneurysm Popliteal aneurysm can occlude or release emboli that can occlude the run-off vessels distally. 50 % of these are found bilaterally.

Trauma Blunt or penetrating trauma can result in vascular injury that can result in occlusion or dissection.

Thrombosis (hypercoagulable syndromes)

Blue toe syndrome (cholesterol emboli from proximal atherosclerosis)

Fibromuscular dysplasia

Peripheral emboli (ususally cardiac in origin)

Popliteal entrapment Suspect in young patients with popliteal occlusion/claudication.

Vasculitis such as Takayasu's

Thromboangiitis obliterans (Buerger's disease)

Rare causes such as popliteal artery adventitial cyst and *Pseudoxanthoma elasticum*

3 Disease Distribution

Peripheral vascular disease is usually a result of systemic atherosclerosis and therefore cerbrovascular, coronary and renovascular disease often coexist. For this reason, patients with critical limb ischaemia have a 20 % mortality in the first year of presentation. Due to their co-morbidities, endovascular treatment is an invaluable option for treatment of critical limb ischaemia.

Rarer causes such as vasculitis and popliteal entrapment syndrome are seen in a much younger population.

4 Classification/Disease Patterns

The Inter-Society Consensus for the management of peripheral arterial disease (TASC II) addresses the classification for occlusive disease. However while there is a diagnostic-treatment algorithm for aorto-iliac and femoro-popliteal disease, no such classification has been suggested for the infra-popliteal segment. There are however some treatment recommendations made by this group and are discussed below.

5 Differential Diagnosis

1. Neuropathic pain

   (a) Diabetes
   (b) Nerve root/spinal compression
   (c) Peripheral non-diabetic sensory neuropathy

2. Ulcerating conditions

   (a) Venous insufficiency
   (b) Infections

3. Buerger's disease
4. Night cramps

6   Diagnosis: Clinical and Laboratory

Clinical: Calf claudication is typically not an indication to do a below-knee intervention. However, foot claudication or signs/symptoms of critical limb ischaemia such as rest pain, ulceration or gangrene are.

Once diagnosed clinically there are several non-invasive tests available for further work-up of the extent and severity of the stenosis/occlusion of the below-knee vessels.

Hand-held doppler ultrasound: The doppler probe, typically a 8-MHz probe, is placed over the dorsalis pedis and posterior tibial arteries at the ankle to give a subjective assessment of flow through the vessel. Here the phasicity—monophasic versus biphasic, is more important than the strength of the signal.

ABPI (ankle brachial pressure index) (also known as ABI—ankle brachial index) less than 0.90 is diagnostic of perpiperal vascular disease. An ABI less than 0.4 is reflective of severe peripheral vascular disease. Exersise stress testing ABI and active pedal plantar flexion are tests used for patients with isolated iliac disease who have palpable pulses at baseline, but with the classic symptoms of claudication.

False-negative results may occur in calcified, non-compressible vessels (particularly in long-standing diabetes and renal failure). The ABI may be >1.40 in these patients, and the Doppler signal at the ankle cannot be obliterated even at cuff pressures of 300 mm Hg. Other test should be considered in these patients.

Toe pressures and the toe-brachial index (TBI): Useful in patients with non-compressible calcified tibial vessels. A normal TBI should be >0.70. TBI cannot be carried out if there is ulceration or tissue loss in the first two toes.

Segmental plethysmography or pulse volume recordings: Using brachial, thigh, calf and ankle cuffs, a plethysmograph measures limb volume and produces a pulse volume recording (PVR). The amplitude of the tracing reflects the volume changes in the limb during arterial pulsitility.

Laboratory Tests: Complete blood count along with biochemistry and coagulation screening are baseline tests to perform on any patient for angiography. Homocysteine levels or other inflammatory markers such as C-reactive protein (CRP), erythrocyte sedimentation rate (ESR), and hypercoagulable work-up are other tests, if there is clinical suspicion of non-atherosclerotic cause.

7 Diagnostic Imaging: USG/CT/MRI/Diagnostic Angiography

Ultrasound is the first modality to use to diagnose peripheral vascular disease.

Colour flow doppler showing flowing blood displayed as colour is the first non-invasive test to be done. This is superimposed on the B-mode image, allowing simultaneous visualization of anatomy and flow dynamics

Duplex ultrasound: Colour doppler and spectral doppler (which shows a graphical representation of flow velocities) are displayed simultanously. This allows the visualization and calculation of flow wave form and velocites, respectively. The degree of stenosis and anatomical location can then be accurately assessed. Doppler waveforms progress from a normal triphasic pattern to a biphasic and, ultimately, monophasic appearance in those patients with significant peripheral arterial disease.

Ultrasound of the infrapopliteal vessels is technically challenging and therefore operator dependent. It is also limited by patient factors (obesity, heavy calcification, presence of wounds/dressings).

Computed tomography (CT angiography): This modality is now being increasingly used with the increasingly faster multidetector scanners with high spacial resolution. Accuracy of stenosis quantification can be limited by heavy calcification as well as the smaller calibre of the vessels. There is a risk of contrast induced nephropathy/allergy as well.

Magnetic resonance angiography: Most commonly, IV contrast enhanced sequences are used. Sequences that increase the temporal resolution such as TRICKS (time-resolved contrast kinetics) can be helpful in the peripheral vessels. There is a risk of gadolinium-induced NSF (nephrogenic systemic sclerosis) in patients with renal insufficiency. Non-IV sequences are available (time of flight, phase contrast) but are of limited value in the crural vessels. Imaging of infrapopliteal vessels can be spoilt by contamination with venous signal.

Digital subtraction angiography: This remains the gold standard for imaging of the below-the-knee vessels. However, it is invasive and carries a small risk of complications such as access site bleeding, but has the advantage that one can proceed immediately to treatment in the same setting.

8   Management

The management is determined by the severity of the ischaemia.

Patients with claudication are first managed by medical optimization using risk factor modification such as smoking cessation, strict glycemic control, management of hypertension and cholesterol. Equally important is to develop an exercise regimen.

If conservative measures are unsuccesful and claudication becomes worse and lifestyle limiting consider therapeutic intervention with revascularisation.

Critical limb ischaemia: While wound care with topical dressing is important, in the absence of revascularization procedures, healing is unlikely to happen. This should be endovascular in the first instance. Whilst the systemic morbidity and mortality with an Endovascular approach is low, it is important to bear in mind Endovascular intervention doesnot preclude a subsequent open Bypass operation.

Acute ischemia: Treatment options include the following:

(a) Systemic anticoagulation
(b) Surgical embolectomy/bypass
(c) Endovascular treatment. Catheter-directed pharmacological thrombolysis causes gradual clot lysis and will reveal any underlying stenosis needing angioplasty. Contraindications are similar to that of systemic thrombolysis. Systemic thrombolysis has no role in acute limb ischaemia. Percutaneous aspiration thrombectomy using a large bore catheter and a syringe to aspirate the thrombus/embolus is another method of clot removal—but useful mainly when there is limited burden of clot. Effectiveness will be limited if there is large volume thrombus. Mechanical thrombectomy devices are available and are useful in larger thrombus loads. Rheolytic devices such as the AngioJet Ultra Thrombectomy System (Medrad, USA) use pulsatile high-velocity stream of saline to fragment the thrombus which is then immediately aspirated.

9 List of Open Operative Options

1. Bypass surgery. Typically femoro-popliteal (below knee) for popliteal occlusion or femoro-distal/popliteal-distal bypass (to the run-off vessels) using vein graft or synthetic graft. The patency of femoro-distal bypass is related to the quality of the outflow vessel rather than the level chosen for the anastomosis. The long-term patency of vein grafts is significantly superior to that of synthetic grafts for the infra-geniculate segment.
2. Surgical embolectomy. If the occlusion is acute from fresh thrombus-in-situ or from embolus, surgical embolectomy is operative procedure of choice.
3. Endarterectomy. Uncommonly performed
4. Sympathectomy. Pain control
5. Debridement. Remove infected/necrotic material to aid healing of remaining viable tissues. This is often followed by VAC application.
6. Amputation. If all other treatments fail an amputation is recommended. This is helpful both for pain control as well as to start the rehabilitation for ambulation with an artificial limb as soon as possible.

10 Intervention: Techniques and Pitfalls

10.1 Technique

1. Puncture: Usually an antegrade ipsilateral common femoral puncture. One has to ensure that the entry into the common femoral artery is in the upper one-third so that the wire may go down the superficial femoral artery (SFA). Contra-lateral retrograde common femoral can also be performed but has less favourable pushabiltiy and torque control of the catheters. Longer catheters and guidewires are needed for a contra-lateral "up & over" approach. Ultrasound-guided antegrade popliteal puncture is used in cases where the SFA is occluded and unable to be endovascularly recanalized. Lastly, the subintimal arterial flossing with antegrade-retrograde intervention (SAFARI) can be used for difficult cases which are not possible in a purely antegrade manner.

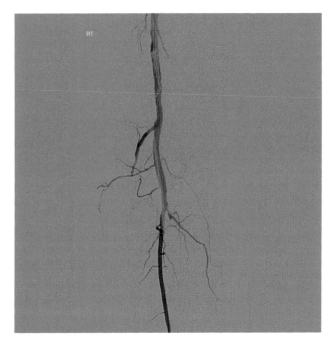

Fig. 27.1 Occluded anterior tibial artery

2. Modified seldinger technique: Single wall puncture. Guidwire inserted down the needle and all catheter exchanges are over a guidewire.

3. Endoluminal angioplasty: The occlusion is crossed with a guidewire within the true lumen of the vessel, and angioplasty is carried out. This method is best used in vessels with a lot of calcification. The wire to be used varies from a 0.014″ to a 0.035″ wire, depending upon the operator's preference. We typically use a 0.035″ system (Figs. 27.1–27.4). There are a host of balloons present for use at this level, both over the wire as well as monorail. In addition, there are newer drug eluting balloons, the data for which is still evolving.

4. Subintimal angioplasty: A hydrophilic angle-tipped guidewire is made to form a loop by its natural tendency to do so when the tip catches on a plaque or when it encounters the occlusion. The guidewire is then used to create a dissection between the intima and the media. The wire/catheter combination is advanced within

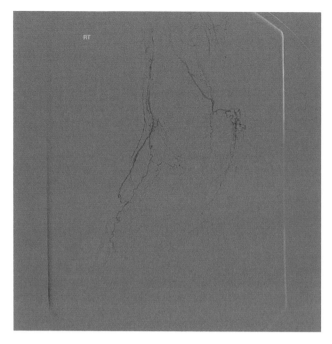

Fig. 27.2 Reconstituted anterior tibial artery at ankle

this plane to bypass the occlusion. The guidewire will naturally tend to break back into the true lumen when it again encounters normal vessel. The newly created false lumen is then angioplastied or stented.

5. Stenting: Stents have a limited role in the popliteal artery because the flexion of the knee causes metal fatigue and subsequent stent fracture. Some newer stents are more flexible and are licenced for use in the popliteal artery. The small calibre of the crural vessels makes them susceptible to re-occlusion with thrombus or intimal hyperplasia. The use of stents here remains unproven.

6. Mechanical atherectomy: Mechanical atherectomy devices are available such as the Turbohawk (eV3, Plymouth, MN, USA), which physically removes the artheroma in order to replicate the effect of a surgical endarterectomy. These devices may play a role in recurrent lesions refactory to repreated conventional angioplasty or to treat instent stenosis.

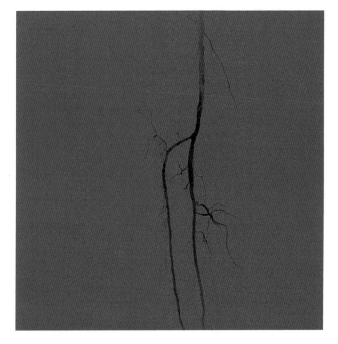

Fig. 27.3 Recanalized anterior tibial artery—proximal

10.2 Pitfalls

Fresh thrombus: A short history or recent sudden deterioration of symptoms should raise suspicion of fresh thrombotic occlusion. This is a critical thing to look for in the preintervention ultrasound. Missing this finding places one at risk of catastrophic embolization with angioplasty. The guidewire will pass through the occlusion very easily. Careful injection of a small volume of contrast produces a characteristic appearance. A suction embolectomy can be attempted, if however unsuccessful angioplasty should be delayed by at least 3 months.

Vasospasm: Very common in small distal vessels. Vasodilators such as GTN (50–250 mcg) or tolazoline (5 mg) can be used, being injected intra-arterially for direct delivery.

Elastic recoil: The vessel fails to remain open despite administering vasodilators and performing repeated prolonged angioplasty. Self-expanding stents are the only method of treating this; however, they

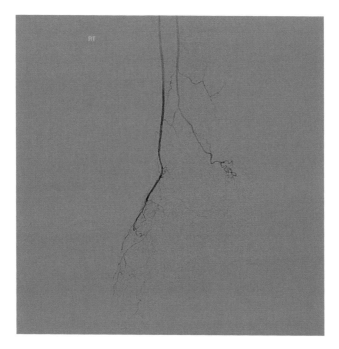

Fig. 27.4 Recanalized anterior tibial artery—distal

have their long-term patency problems as discussed earlier. The subintimal channel is likely to thrombose acutely.

Re-entry failure: When performing subintimal angioplasty, re-entry into the true lumen can sometimes be problematic, particularly in heavily calcified vessels. Various devices are availavle to aid re-entry such as the Outback catheter (Cordis, Bridgewater, NJ, USA) or IVUS-guided Cross Point catheter (Medtronic, Santa Rosa, California, USA).

10.3   Post-procedure Mangement and Follow-up Protocol

Local department protocols apply.

If a closure device is used, the Instructions for use of that particular device are used including the recommended duration of bed rest.

Typically 6–8 h bed rest is recommended, depending upon the sheath size and if a closure device is not used.

Regular observations of HR, BP, O2 saturations, groin/puncture site for bleeding, foot perfusion.

These patients are usually on dual anti-platelet medications as a result of their co-morbidities, but in the event that they are not, they are started on aspirin and clopidogrel. These are continued for a duration of one month, after which aspirin alone is maintained for life.

11   Complications and Managment

11.1   Haemorrhage

(a) Wire perforation. Crural vessels are more fragile and are therefore at greater risk of perforation. These are almost always self-limiting. They are treated by creating a new subintimal dissection to bypass the perforation, balloon tamponade, external compression or stent graft. Consider coil embolization of the subintimal tract if persistent (this does not prevent a repeat attempt at a later date).

(b) Vessel rupture. Can occur during balloon inflation. Alert for persistent pain after balloon deflation. Treat with balloon tamponade/external compression ± stent-graft insertion.

(c) Groin haematoma. If this occurs around the catheter entry site during the procedure consider exchanging for a larger sheath. If occurs post-procedure control haemorrhage with manual compression. Surgical closure is occasionally necessary.

(d) False aneurysm. If small, <1 cm, they may resolve spontaneously and initially only need a follow-up ultrasound to see progression/resolution. Othewise use ultrasound-guided compression or ultrasound guided thrombin injection. If the aneurysm has a wide neck or previous treatment has failed, consider balloon occlusion with thrombin injection or stent-graft. If the patient is unstable or minimally invasive measures have not/unlikely to work, surgical repair is indicated.

(e) Embolus. Percutaneous aspiration thombo-embolectomy (PAT) using a 5–8 F catheter passed up to the embolus and a 50-ml syringe is attached to apply suction. The embolus is aspirated into the catheter and withdrawn under continuous suction with the syringe (pitfall: the thrombus may become lodged into the sheath which will then need to be cleared).

"Push and park". If the embolus is large for example saddle embolus in the popliteal bifurcation, and cannot be aspirated it can be pushed distally to allow flow into other vessels. This method relys on there being at least one other patent run-off vessels to maintain perfusion to the foot.

Surgical embolectomy or bypass surgery. If endovascular methods fail and the perfusion of the limb is compromised, surgery is indicated.

12   Outcome: Open Versus Endovascular

Infra-popliteal disease is a problematic group by any treatment modality. For subintimal angioplasty, a high initial technical success (78–86 %) can be acheived. Reported long-term patency is variable but limb salvage rates (81–94 %) can be expected.

Very few randomised controlled trials comparing endovascular therapy with surgery or best medical therapy have been carried out. Bypass versus angioplasty in severe ischaemia of the leg has been studied (BASIL trial). BASIL concluded that angioplasty first stratergy has a broadly similar outcome to surgery first in terms of amputation free survival but surgery is more expensive in the short term. However, in patients who survive for greater than 2 years surgery appears to provide an advantage. This trial did not look specifically at infra-popliteal disease.There have been no randomised control trials to date that have compared specifically infra-popliteal angioplasty with femoral-distal bypass grafting and best medical therapy.

A systematic review of subintimal angioplasty in peripheral vascular disease has been carried out (ref-). Primary patency in crural vessels is lower than femoro-popliteal angioplasty (46–53 %) but high limb salvage rates are achievable (87–94 %). Patients with CLI and a crural lesion demonstrate a survival after 1 year of from 65 to 78 %, in contrast to a survival of between 86 and 100 % after 1 year for patients with mixed disease and a femoral lesion.

References

1. Bolia A, Sayers RD, Thompson MM, Bell PR. Subintimal and intraluminal recanalisation of occluded crural arteries by percutaneous balloon angioplasty. Eur J Vasc Surg. 1994;8(2):214–9.
2. Ingle H, Nasim A, Bolia A, Fishwick G, Naylor R, Bell PR, Thompson MM. Subintimal angioplasty of isolated infragenicular vessels in lower limb ischemia: long-term results. J Endovasc Ther. 2002;9(4):411–6.
3. Adam DJ, Beard JD, Cleveland T, Bell J, Bradbury AW, Forbes JF, Fowkes FG, Gillepsie I, Ruckley CV, Raab G, Storkey H. Bypass versus angioplasty in severe ischaemia of the leg (BASIL): multicentre, randomised controlled trial, BASIL trial participants. Lancet. 2005;366(9501):1925–34.
4. Met R, Van Lienden KP, Mark JW, Koelemay SB, Legemate DA, Reekers JA. Subintimal angioplasty for peripheral arterial occlusive disease: a systematic review. Cardiovasc Intervent Radiol. 2008;31(4):687–97.

Chapter 28
Caval and Iliac Vein Disease

Olaf Kaufman, Haraldur Bjarnason, and Peter Gloviczki

1 Anatomy

The *external iliac vein* (EIV) begins at the inguinal ligament and ends anterior to the sacroiliac joint where it joins the internal iliac vein (IIV) to form the common iliac vein (CIV). The IIV is a short vein, formed by its extra- and intrapelvic tributaries. The CIV*s* join at the right side of the fifth lumbar vertebra to form the IVC. In contrast to the right CIV, which ascends vertically to the IVC, <u>the left CIV</u> takes an almost transverse course and underlies the <u>right common iliac artery</u>, which may compress it against the lumbar spine (May-Thurner syndrome). The IVC takes a cephalic course at the right anterior aspect of the spine, and it passes through the liver and then through the diaphragm at the level of the 10th thoracic vertebra and joins the right atrium at the T9 level.

O. Kaufman, M.D., Ph.D. • H. Bjarnason, M.D.
Divisions of Vascular and Interventional Radiology, Gonda Vascular Center,
Mayo Clinic, 200 First Street SW, Rochester, MN 55905, USA

P. Gloviczki, M.D. (✉)
Vascular and Endovascular Surgery, Gonda Vascular Center,
Mayo Clinic, Rochester, MN, USA
e-mail: gloviczki.peter@mayo.edu

A. Kumar and K. Ouriel (eds.), *Handbook of Endovascular Interventions*,   377
DOI 10.1007/978-1-4614-5013-9_28,
© Springer Science+Business Media New York 2013

Tributaries of the IVC are the lumbar veins, the right gonadal (spermatic, ovarian) vein, the renal veins, the right suprarenal, the right inferior phrenic, and the hepatic veins. The left gonadal and suprarenal veins join the left renal vein. In case of IVC obstruction, anastomoses between the veins of the chest and abdominal wall (thoraco-epigastric, internal thoracic, and epigastric veins), the lumbar-azygos connections, and the vertebral plexuses are the important collaterals.

Embryologically, the iliocaval segment develops from multiple veins. The bilateral posterior cardinal veins form the iliac veins. Most of the left-sided embryologic veins regress resulting in a right-sided IVC. The right supracardinal vein develops into the infrarenal IVC. At the level of the kidneys, the IVC is formed from the right sub-supracardinal anastomosis and above that from the right subcardinal vein . The hepatic segment is formed directly by hepatic sinusoids.

Variations

Prevalence of

1. Duplicated infrarenal IVC secondary to persistence of left supracardinal vein: 2%
2. Left-sided IVC (drains into left renal vein) with absent right IVC: 0.5%
3. Absence of hepatic IVC, with the infrarenal IVC joining the azygos/hemiazygos system and draining into the superior vena cava (SVC): <0.5%

2   Disease Definition

(a)   Acute iliofemoral venous thrombosis (Chapter 29)
(b)   Chronic venous obstructions

  1. Benign

    • Nonthrombotic

      – Primary iliac vein compression/obstruction (May-Thurner syndrome)

        (a)   Anatomical compression
        (b)   Congenital malformation (synechia)

    – Compression or obstruction by retroperitoneal fibrosis, benign tumor, aortic or iliac aneurysms, abscess, cyst, pregnancy, previous trauma, radiation, or surgery

- Thrombotic:
    - Chronic spontaneous deep vein thrombosis (with or without May-Thurner syndrome)
    - Iatrogenic thrombosis – IVC filters, central venous access (femoral or translumbar), pacemaker leads, etc.

2. Malignant
    - Primary venous leiomyosarcoma
    - Secondary caval tumors
        - Renal cell carcinoma
        - Hepatic or adrenal tumors, metastases
        - Germ cell tumors – seminomas and teratomas

(c) Valvular incompetence (Pelvic congestion syndrome, pelvic, vulvar or scrotal varicosity)
(d) Venous aneurysms
(e) Congenital malformations (venous or arteriovenous)

3   Disease Distribution

(a) 275,000 new cases of venous thromboembolism/year in the USA
(b) 5% of the adult Western population has chronic venous insufficiency with skin changes or ulcers
(c) 33–67% of patients with iliac or iliocaval outflow obstruction have postthrombotic syndrome
(d) Chronic ilio-caval thrombosis has 75% female predominance with ~2/3 occurring on the left side.

4   Classification and Outcome Assessment

(a) The Clinical, Etiologic, Anatomic, and Pathophysiologic (CEAP) classification provides a system to stratify and communicate the multiple variations in clinical presentation of venous disease in a standardized manner.

1. Most patients present with stage C3 (swelling) or C4 (skin changes) disease
2. Symptoms at presentation usually include swelling (>90%) and with exercise (venous claudication, >75%).
3. IVC occlusions/hypoplasia/agenesis with patent iliac veins and good collaterals maybe asymptomatic for many years

(b) Venous Clinical Severity Score (VCSS) is designed to measure changes in severity (signs and symptoms) of chronic venous disease and define clinical outcome of a treatment over time.

5   Clinical and Laboratory Exam

(a) Should exclude malignancy and establish any underlying thrombophilia
(b) Thrombophilia workup is performed on patients without causes of external compression, acute thrombosis in young patients, or thrombosis without obvious cause
(c) Venous plethysmography is helpful to evaluate the functional status of the venous system as a follow-up study after intervention, but otherwise is of questionable clinical use.

6   Diagnostic Imaging

Duplex scanning (DS), Computer tomographic angiography/venography (CTA/CTV), Magnetic resonance imaging (MRI), Magnetic resonance angiography/venography(MRA,MRV), and diagnostic venography with direct venous pressure measurements

(a) Duplex scanning

1. Duplex scanning with ultrasound may be used to interrogate flow in the pelvic vessels and vena cava

   • Limited by patient body habitus
   • May reveal collateral vessel formation
   • Provides flow rates to help evaluate stenoses and flow dynamic

- Excellent to establish the nature of infrainguinal (in-flow) venous occlusion or valvular incompetence
- Useful to monitor stent or by-pass patency

2. Intravascular ultrasound (IVUS)

  - Helps to delineate
    - External compression
    - Congenital developmental abnormalities

      (a) Intravascular webs
        - Degree of narrowing

          - May assist with accurate placement of vascular stents and angioplasty

3. Trans-vaginal ultrasound

  - Useful to establish pelvic varicosity or malformation

(b) Noninvasive imaging with MRI /MRA/MRV, CTA/CTV

1. May reveal underlying lesions causing external compression
2. CTA/CTV is useful to delineate occluded caval and iliac vein disease and give clues to chronicity

   - Extensive collaterals and calcification suggest long-standing disease
   - Reconstruction in multiple planes allows planning of interventions
   - Dehydration and variation in hydration status can cause vein narrowing and therefore misinterpretation

3. MRI /MRV has similar attributes as CT, and it is useful in patients with tumors, vascular malformations, pelvic congestion syndrome, IVC absence, or congenital variants

   - 3D reconstructions
   - Direction and speed of flow may be calculated using appropriate protocols

(c) Venography

  - Ascending venography

    - Technique

(a) Angiocatheter placed in a dorsal foot vein for contrast injection
(b) The procedure is performed on a tilt table with the head end elevated in order to delay flow of contrast to the upper body and allow more time to evaluate the anatomy of the deep and superficial venous systems
(c) Tourniquets may be helpful to decrease superficial flow for more directed diagnosis of the deep veins

   – Direct visualization of stenoses/obstruction and collateral vessels. Among other things it may assist in localization of perforators, thrombosis, and embryologic abnormalities.
   – Great saphenous vein may be evaluated
   – Limitations

(a) Contrast may be diluted upon reaching iliac veins precluding good examination of the iliac veins and the IVC
(b) Ascending venography is not a functional study, but collaterals may indicate hemodynamically significant obstructions

   • Iliocavography

     – Frequently required with femoral vein puncture to evaluate the iliocaval, renal, and gonadal veins. Can be used with direct venous pressure measurements

   • Descending venography

     – Injection into the ipsilateral common femoral vein (CFV) either from contralateral CFV, internal jugular vein, or less favorably from the ipsilateral CFV
     – Performed on a tilt table with the head elevated to provide gravitational effect and with the patient performing valsalva maneuver. Limitations: Good for proximal incompetence but may not detect isolated peripheral incompetence
     – Retrograde injection into the ovarian or IIV vein establishes the diagnosis of ovarian or IIV reflux and confirms pelvic venous congestion. Venographic criteria for pelvic congestion syndrome include

(a) An ovarian vein diameter ≥ 6 mm
(b) Contrast retention > 20 s
(c) Congestion of the pelvic venous plexus and/or opacification of the ipsilateral (or contralateral) internal iliac vein and/or
(d) Filling of vulvo-vaginal and thigh varicosities.

7 Management Paradigm and Indications

(a) Treatment is based on symptoms not responding to compression therapy and lifestyle modification

1. Indications

   - Leg or thigh pain, venous claudication, and swelling
   - Chronic, nonhealing ulcers
   - Severe lipodermatosclerosis
   - Varicosities
   - Pelvic pain, dyspareunia, feeling of fullness and congestion, dysuria, perineal varicosity
   - Presence of large venous aneurysm, history of pulmonary embolism, surgically fit patient

(b) Operative procedures

1. Open surgical bypass

   - Palma procedure (femoro–femoral saphanous vein bypass, PTFE bypass
   - Femoroiliac , femorocaval bypass
   - IVC replacement or patch after tumor excision (PTFE, spiral saphenous vein, or femoral vein graft)

2. Excision ovarian vein (with or without left renal vein transposition for associated left renal venous congestion (Nutcracker syndrome)

3. Reconstruction for IVC or iliac venous aneurysm (aneurysmorrhaphy or graft replacement)

8 Endovascular Interventions: Technique and Pitfalls

(a) Angioplasty and stent placement

1. Approach

   - Access jugular and/or ipsilateral femoral/common femoral veins using US guidance

Table 28.1 Vessel/stent size

Vessel	Size (mm)
IVC	20–22
Common iliac veins	14–16
External iliac veins	12–16
Common femoral veins	10–14

- Use long introducer sheaths from right internal jugular vein (IJV)IJ to avoid looping catheters in RA and causing arrhythmias

- If iliac vein occlusion is bilateral, usually attempt to traverse the side anticipated to be the most challenging first
- Suggest hydrophilic (glide) wires followed by glide catheters. Attempt to "float" them through recanalized thrombus rather that "drill" through chronic thrombus

  - Spinning guide wire rapidly while slowly advancing helps "float" wire through

- Measure pressure gradient after obstructive lesion passed
- To enhance access, it is possible to snare wire distally and create through and through access for better tension control and stiffness
- If lesion is bilateral repeat above process for contralateral side making sure to stay in same plane
- Angioplasty initially with 4–8 mm low-profile balloon allows easier passage of larger balloons

2. Stent placement (Table 28.1)

- Stent placement in IVC can be performed from either jugular or femoral approach with deployment just above bifurcation and proceeding cephalad
- Usually start with 20–22 mm diameter Wallstents in IVC
- May place Gianturco (20 mm by 50 mm) stents inside the Wallstents for further support
- Avoid covering the renal veins unless they are chronically thrombosed in which case retroperitoneal collaterals have already taken over
- Iliac and CFV can be dilated to 14 mm (12 mm) smaller women with common iliac to 16 mm

- Self-expanding stents of identical size are almost always placed
- Iliac vein stents may be placed either from femoral or jugular vein approach with approximately 0.5 cm to 1 cm of overlap. While various opinions exist, we place stents such that they barely extend into IVC if the IVC is patent
- If bilateral iliac stents are placed, place kissing stents at bifurcation simultaneously and into the proximal CIVs
- Continue deployment in a caudal direction until you reach portion of veins that will provide sufficient inflow
- Crossing the inguinal ligament has not caused problems, it is much more important to establish adequate inflow.

3. Most venous recanalizations may be performed with conscious sedation; however, for IVC recanalizations propofol, anesthesia is helpful and general anesthesia may be required
4. Single prophylactic antibiotic dose may be given, but stent infections have not been reported
5. During the procedure, intravenous heparin is administered to maintain an activated clotting time between 250 and 300 seconds

(b) Embolization of ovarian veins, IIVs, or pelvic malformations

1. Start the procedure similar to diagnostic venography, establishing access through the groins or IJV.
2. Embolization depends on the size of the veins and the presence or the absence of malformation and a–v shunting; usually a combination of coils, plugs, or alcohol sclerotherapy can be used.

9 Postprocedure Management and Follow-up Protocol After Stenting

(a) Low Molecular Weight Heparin (LMWH) started immediately after the procedure until therapeutic INR achieved—(INR 2.5–3.5)
(b) Anticoagulation for at least 2 months, longer depending on hypercoagulability work-up, inflow and other contributing factors
(c) No literature to support aspirin or clopidogrel but we tend to give 75 mg of clopidogrel for 6 weeks following stent placement

(d) Clinical follow-up with the USA of treated area at 3 months, 6 months, 12 months, and annually or less frequently from then on as needed
(e) Compression stockings, 30–40 mm Hg knee high in most cases for life

10 Complications and Management

(a) Occlusion—less than 5% of stents occlude
(b) Bleeding complications during dilation of chronically thrombosed veins is very rare. However, bleeding and other problems have been encountered in radiated areas and following recent surgery around the treated veins
(c) Lower back pain is common following the procedure but generally subsides in 2–3 weeks
(d) Restenosis/Thrombosis −1.5% (<30 days)

  1. Primary patency of IVC stents 49–100%
  2. Almost all stents develop instent restenosis

(e) AV fistulas have been placed in selected cases to keep stented areas open but this is not widely practiced
(f) Stent compression, especially at the left common femoral vein level, is encountered. Nitinol stents may not have enough radial force
(g) Stent migration is rare and is usually caused by under sizing or the stents are caught on balloons during the procedure
(h) Access site complications – hematoma

11 Outcomes

(a) Raju et al. presented that 82% iliac vein stenting were patent at 2 years with healing of 66% venous ulcers
(b) Delis et al. showed that 83% of venous wounds healed within 8.4 months of iliac vein stenting with the reduction of one CEAP clinical class on average

(c) Neglen et al. demonstrated that 23% of ilio-caval stents had no in-stent restenosis at 42 months, 61% had greater than 20% diameter stenosis, and only 15% had $\geq$50% stenosis. Also median pain score and degree of swelling decreased significantly post-stent placement

(d) Transcatheter embolotherapy improves symptoms of pelvic venous congestion in 50–80% of the patients. Chang showed it was better than alternative therapies, including open surgery.

References

1. Neglen P, Hollis KC, Olivier J, Raju S. Stenting of the venous outflow in chronic venous disease: long-term stent-related outcome, clinical, and hemo-dynamic result. J Vasc Surg. 2007;46(5):979–90.
2. Delis KT, Bjarnason H, Wennberg PW, Rooke TW, Gloviczki P. Successful iliac vein and inferior vena cava stenting ameliorates venous claudication and improves venous outflow, calf muscle pump function, and clinical status in post-thrombotic syndrome. Ann Surg. 2007;245(1):130–9.
3. Jost CJ, Gloviczki P, Cherry Jr KJ, et al. Surgical reconstruction of iliofemoral veins and the inferior vena cava for nonmalignant occlusive disease. J Vasc Surg. 2001;33(2):320–7.
4. Raju S, Neglen P. Percutaneous recanalization of total occlusions of the iliac vein. J Vasc Surg. 2009;50(2):360–8.
5. Chung MH, Huh CY. Comparison of treatments for pelvic congestion syndrome. Tohoku J Exp Med. 2003;201(3):131–8.

Chapter 29
Deep Venous Thrombosis: Upper and Lower Extremity

Anthony J. Comerota and Subhash Thakur

1 Anatomy

1.1 Lower Extremity

Three sets of paired venae comitantes paralleling the course of three named arteries begin in the distal calf. The paired veins join in the mid calf. The anterior tibial vein drains the anterior compartment, the posterior tibial vein drains the posterior compartment, and the peroneal vein drains the lateral compartment of the leg. They join to form the popliteal vein in the popliteal fossa.

Distally, the popliteal vein proceeds medially to the artery, and in proximal portion, it is lateral to the artery. In the distal thigh in the abductor canal, the popliteal vein becomes the femoral vein. The

---

A.J. Comerota, M.D., F.A.C.S., F.A.C.C. (✉)
Jobst Vascular Institute, The Toledo Hospital, 2109 Hughes Dr Suite 400, Toledo, OH 43606, USA

Department of Surgery, University Of Michigan, 1500 E. Medical Center, Ann Arbor, MI 48109, USA
e-mail: marilyn.gravett@promedica.org

S. Thakur, M.D.
Jobst Vascular Institute, The Toledo Hospital, 2109 Hughes Dr Suite 400, Toledo, OH 43606, USA

A. Kumar and K. Ouriel (eds.), *Handbook of Endovascular Interventions*,   389
DOI 10.1007/978-1-4614-5013-9_29,
© Springer Science+Business Media New York 2013

deep femoral vein drains the soft tissues of the thigh and is the major collateral venous drainage when the femoral vein is occluded. The deep femoral vein joins the femoral vein laterally in the proximal femoral triangle to form the common femoral vein. At the inguinal ligament, the common femoral vein becomes the external iliac vein. The external iliac vein joins the internal iliac vein in the pelvis and becomes the common iliac vein, which drains into the vena cava.

There are hundreds of deep venous valves, the majority of which are located in the distal veins, with progressively fewer in the larger proximal veins. Venous sinuses are located in the soleal muscles, which drain into the posterior tibial vein. The gastrocnemius veins, an interlacing valved venous network in the gastrocnemius muscle, drain into the popliteal vein.

1.2   Upper Extremity

The deep veins of the upper extremity are, like the lower extremity, paired with arteries in the arm. The basilic vein ascends up the inner side of the arm, pierces the deep fascia at mid-arm, and, after joining the venae comites of the brachial artery, forms the axillary vein. At the outer border of the first rib, the axillary vein becomes the subclavian.

2   Disease Definition

Acute deep venous thrombosis (DVT) is defined as acute thrombosis occurring in the deep veins of the upper or lower extremity. It is generally the consequence of coagulation thrombosis as opposed to a platelet-fibrin thrombus, which initiates arterial thrombosis.

Thrombosis in the venous circulation results from a combination of stasis, endothelial damage, and hypercoagulabilities. Risk factors include age, malignancy, surgery, trauma, immobilization, oral contraceptives, hormone replacement therapy, pregnancy and the puerperium, obesity, neurologic disease, cardiac disease, and antiphosphilopid antibodies. Genetic causes include deficiencies of antithrombin, proteins C and S, factor V Leiden, prothrombin

20210A, hyperhomocysteinemia, dysfibrinogenemia, dysplasmino-genemia, reduced heparin cofactor II activity, elevated levels of clotting factors such as factors XI, IX, VIII, VIII, X, and II, and plasminogen activator inhibitor-1.

Primary axillary and subclavian vein thrombosis often result from obstruction of the subclavian vein in the thoracic outlet (inlet), which has been termed the Paget Schroetter syndrome, often presenting in healthy, muscular, physically active individuals. Secondary axillary and subclavian DVT result from indwelling catheters or pacemaker wires. Other less common causes include mediastinal tumors.

3   Disease Distribution

It has been recently estimated that in the USA, there are more than 900,000 cases of venous thromboembolism per year. Put in this per-spective, it exceeds the annual incidence of heart disease and stroke. Acute DVT leads to pulmonary embolism and the postthrombotic syndrome (PTS). There are over 300,000 venous thromboembolic related deaths each year in the USA. Ninety-five percentage of DVT occurs in the lower extremity and approximately 5% in the upper extremity. The incidence of the postthrombotic syndrome (PTS) is high. A recent prospective analysis of patients treated with anticoagu-lation alone for acute DVT demonstrated that 43% had PTS at two years' follow-up. Predictors of severe PTS include extensive DVT, iliofemoral DVT, high body mass index, and older age.

4   Diagnosis: Clinical and Laboratory

The diagnosis of DVT must be confirmed by an objective laboratory test, as the clinical diagnosis of acute DVT is erroneous in 50%. When symptoms are present, they include a dull ache or pain in the calf or leg or edema. With extensive DVT involving the proximal iliofemoral or axillosubclavian veins, symptoms may include significant swelling, pain, cyanosis, and dilated superficial veins. Iliofemoral DVT may present as phlegmasia alba dolens (swollen, white, painful leg) or phlegmasia cerulean dolens (swollen, blue, painful leg). The severity of symptoms at presentation generally is related to the degree of venous obstruction.

D-dimer (a breakdown fragment of complexed fibrin) is helpful when negative since a negative test essentially excludes DVT when associated with low clinical suspicion. Elevated D-dimer levels are often not helpful (due to numerous reasons for false positives), other than to raise concern that thrombosis may be present.

5   Diagnostic Imaging: USG/CT/MRI/Diagnostic Angiogram

1. *Venous duplex* is the most commonly used diagnostic test for acute DVT. It includes B-mode imaging with and without probe compression and assessing Doppler velocity patterns. The most common diagnostic parameter is noncompressibility of the involved vein. It carries sensitivity and specificity rates of greater than 95% for proximal DVT. It is painless, requires no contrast, is safe in pregnancy, and can be repeated as indicated.

2. *Computed tomography (CT) and magnetic resonance (MR) venography* are helpful to evaluate thrombosis of the iliac veins and inferior and superior vena cavas. CT scans of the chest, abdomen, and pelvis in patients with proximal DVT have demonstrated asymptomatic pulmonary emboli in 40–60% of patients. Importantly, a high incidence of associated underlying pathology has been identified, especially in patients with idiopathic iliofemoral DVT.

3. *Phlebography* has been largely replaced by noninvasive studies; however, it continues to have a role when the diagnosis remains in doubt after other tests have been performed. Phlebograms are always performed when catheter-based techniques are used to eliminate thrombus. It is always important to evaluate the vena cava to identify its degree of involvement whenever mechanical or pharmacomechanical intervention is planned. Phlebography also helps to identify the left common iliac vein compression due to right common iliac artery or other intraluminal pathology requiring correction. In axillary subclavian DVT, phlebography should be performed with the arm in hyperextended position to assess extrinsic compression of subclavian vein at the thoracic outlet as it crosses the first rib.

6 Management

The primary treatment of venous thromboembolism is systemic anticoagulation. Anticoagulation can be considered prophylactic, as it helps to prevent thrombus extension and embolization, but does little to resolve thrombus. Anticoagulant agents interrupt (slow) thrombus formation to reduce thrombus propagation, embolic complications, and reduce the risk of recurrence. However, they do not clear thrombus from the deep venous system.

1. *Anticoagulation*

   Early and continuously therapeutic anticoagulation is important. Patients treated with unfractionated heparin (UFH) who become subtherapeutic early in their care face a 15-fold risk of recurrence. Low-molecular-weight heparin (LMWH) has improved bioavailability compared to UFH and does not require monitoring.

   The majority of patients with acute DVT can be managed with systemic anticoagulation alone. Heparin should be started and continued for at least 5 days during which oral anticoagulation with vitamin K antagonist (warfarin) is instituted. A target international normalized ratio (INR) of 2.0–3.0 for 2 consecutive days is recommended before stopping heparin.

   (a) *Heparin (UFH)*

       The initial dose of UFH is weight-based at 80 units/kg bolus followed by 18 units/kg/h as a continuous infusion. It is monitored by measuring the APTT which should be therapeutic, defined as >1.5× control value. Alternatively, a sustained high dose (i.e., 2,000 μ/h) can be given to patients at low risk of bleeding.

   (b) *Low-molecular-weight heparin*

       LMWH is now the preferred initial treatment for acute DVT. It is administered subcutaneously and does not require monitoring. Its use is not recommended in patients with severe renal dysfunction (CrCl ≤30). Pregnant patients are preferably treated with LMWH (enoxaparin 1 mg/kg every 12 h or 1.5 mg/kg daily).

   (c) *Direct thrombin inhibitors* (indicated for heparin-induced thrombocytopenia (HIT))

Table 29.1 Recommended duration of anticoagulation

Patients	Modifier	Recommendation	Grade
1st episode DVT Calf Proximal	Transient (reversible) risk factor	3 months VKA	1A
1st episode DVT	Idiopathic	At least 6–12 months **and** consider indefinite	1A 2A
VTE patients	Rx'ed with VKAs	INR 2.0–3.0 *Against* high intensity	1A 1A
1st episode DVT	Cancer	LMWH × 3–6 months **and** anticoagulation indefinitely (or until cancer resolved)	1A 1C
1st episode DVT	Antiphospholipid Ab **or** ≥2 other thrombophilic conditions	Indefinite anticoagulation	2A
Recurrent DVT		Indefinite anticoagulation	2A
VTE patients	Indefinite anticoagulation	Reassess risk/benefit at routine intervals	1C

- *Hirudin* is cleared by kidneys so must be used with caution in patients with compromised renal function. Initial dose is a bolus of 0.4 mg/kg over 15–20 s followed by 0.15 mg/kg/h.
- *Argatroban* is metabolized in the liver so must be used with caution in patients with compromised hepatic function. Initial dose is 2 mcg/kg/min as continuous IV infusion. The APTT should be maintained at 1.5–3 times the baseline.

(d) *Vitamin K antagonists (warfarin)* should be started after parenteral anticoagulation to avoid paradoxical transient hypercoagulability resulting from reduction of proteins C and S (which are vitamin K dependent). The goal of treatment is an INR of 2.0–3.0.

Proper duration of anticoagulation as recommended by the 2008 ACCP guidelines are shown in Table 29.1.

2. *Compression therapy and ambulation*

At the time of diagnosis and initiation of anticoagulation, the involved leg(s) should be wrapped snugly from the toes to the thigh and the patient encouraged to ambulate. This significantly reduces early morbidity, improves thrombus resolution, and reduces postthrombotic morbidity. Elastic compression stockings with a gradient of 30–40 mmHg should be prescribed long term, to be worn from the time the patient awakens in the morning until going to bed at night. This reduces the risk of postthrombotic morbidity by 50%.

3. *Inferior vena cava filters*

(a) *Absolute indications*

- Contraindication to anticoagulation
- Documented failure of anticoagulation
- Complications of anticoagulation

(b) *Relative indications*

- Large free floating thrombus in vena cava (especially prior to intervention)
- Massive PE
- Patients undergoing pulmonary embolectomy
- Recurrent PE in the presence of filter
- Patients undergoing thrombolysis for iliofemoral DVT
- DVT with limited cardiopulmonary reserve

(c) *Prophylactic indications*

- Absence of DVT or PE in a patient with high risk of PE (i.e., pelvic fracture)

4. *Strategy of thrombus removal*
Removal of thrombus from the deep venous system is an appropriate goal of treatment, especially in patients with extensive DVT. Successful thrombus removal eliminates venous obstruction and increases the likelihood of maintaining valvular function.

(a) *Thrombolytic therapy*
Systemic thrombolysis is generally inadequate because very little of the infused plasminogen activator penetrates the clot to activate fibrin-bound plasminogen. The delivery of a thrombolytic agent directly into the venous clot allows efficient activation of fibrin-bound plasminogen with small doses of plasminogen activator. Clinical success rates have been encouragingly high using pharmacomechanical techniques during catheter-based intervention.

Patients with acute axillosubclavian vein thrombosis are well served with catheter-directed or pharmacomechanical thrombolysis. Following lysis, an underlying stenosis is often found, usually in the subclavian vein as it passes between the first rib and clavicle. This is best treated by excision of the first rib followed by balloon venoplasty and stenting, if necessary. Stenting of the subclavian vein as it crosses the first rib should be avoided prior to first rib resection, as the stent will be crushed, resulting in reocclusion and a potentially worse outcome.

(b) *Venous thrombectomy*

Contemporary venous thrombectomy is an effective technique designed to remove clot from the entire lower extremity venous system. An associated small arteriovenous fistula (AVF) and a small distal catheter through which heparin is infused to achieve systemic anticoagulation are techniques which help to reduce rethrombosis.

A large multicenter randomized trial in patients with iliofemoral DVT comparing venous thrombectomy, AVF, and anticoagulation versus anticoagulation alone showed significantly better patency, lower venous pressure, less edema, and fewer postthrombotic symptoms at 6 months, 5 years, and 10 years.

7 Open Operative Procedures

1. Venous thrombectomy for acute DVT
2. First rib resection for thoracic outlet decompression in selected cases of axillary and subclavian DVT where subclavian vein compression is documented as it crosses the first rib. It is beyond the scope of this chapter to review the operative techniques for 1st rib resection. However, we believe that the transaxillary approach achieves complete decompression of the thoracic outlet with the best cosmetic result.

8 Interventional Goals: A Strategy of Thrombus Removal

- Prevent pulmonary embolism
- Restore venous patency and unobstructed venous drainage from the involved extremity
- Preserve valve function
- Reduce or eliminate postthrombotic morbidity

9 Interventions

1. *Technique of catheter-directed thrombolysis*

   (a) Under ultrasound guidance, the popliteal vein is cannulated and an appropriately sized sheath is placed.

   (b) An ascending phlebogram is performed to define the extent of thrombosis. It is important to visualize the vena cava to assess whether thrombus extends into the inferior vena cava (IVC) and whether it is occlusive or nonocclusive.

   (c) A hydrophilic guidewire and catheter is advanced through the clot and into the IVC.

   (d) A pharmacomechanical thrombectomy catheter, the Trellis-8 catheter (Covidien, Mansfield, MA), is advanced through the sheath and through the thrombosed veins. The cephalad balloon is positioned above the thrombus. Both balloons are inflated and 2–5 mg of recombinant tissue plasminogen activator (rt-PA) injected into the infusion port. The catheter is activated and spins at 1500 rpm. After 15–20 min, the plasminogen activator solution is aspirated, the balloons deflated, and contrast injected to evaluate treatment results. If residual thrombus persists, treatment can be repeated. If thrombus is cleared, the catheter is repositioned to treat additional thrombus. If persistent thrombus exists following use of the Trellis catheter, catheter-directed thrombolysis with drip infusion or through an EKOS LySus® catheter system (EKOS Corp., Bothell, WA) is performed. Low-dose, high-volume infusion is preferred (1 mg rt-PA in 50–100 cc per hour). Phlebograms are repeated at routine intervals (approximately 12 h) to assess progress and need for catheter repositioning.

(e) Following clearance of the thrombus, the venous system is assessed for an underlying lesion. Frequently, on the left side, an underlying stenosis of the common iliac vein is identified (May-Thurner syndrome) and corrected with venoplasty and stenting (14–16 mm Wall stent). Any lesion must be corrected to reduce the risk of rethrombosis.

(f) Therapeutic anticoagulation is mandatory to prevent rethrombosis.

(g) External pneumatic compression is applied to improve venous return, while the patient is in bed (during and after treatment).

2. *Venous Thrombectomy*

(a) An incision is made in the inguinal area, and control of the common femoral vein, femoral vein, saphenofemoral junction, and profunda femoris vein(s) is obtained.

(b) A longitudinal femoral venotomy is performed, the leg is elevated, and extrusion of infrainguinal clot is attempted.

(c) If infrainguinal (femoropopliteal) thrombus persists, exposure of the posterior tibial vein in the lower leg is performed to complete the infrainguinal thrombectomy with balloon catheter and hydraulic techniques.

(d) Following balloon catheter thrombectomy and flushing residual thrombus from the leg with a heparin-saline solution, 200 cc of saline with 10 mg of rt-PA is infused into the infrainguinal venous system after clamping the femoral vein below the venotomy.

(e) A #8–10 Fogarty venous thrombectomy catheter is used for the iliofemoral thrombectomy, which is performed under fluoroscopic guidance. Contrast is used to inflate the balloon.

(f) Iliac vein compression, or other lesions, should be treated with balloon angioplasty and stenting (14–16 mm stent with high radial strength) to ensure unobstructed venous drainage into the vena cava.

(g) The venotomy is then closed with 6-0 Prolene.

(h) The proximal PTV is cannulated with a small pediatric feeding tube, which is brought into the wound through a separate stab wound and secured with a looped 2-0 Prolene suture.

(i) The catheter is used for postoperative anticoagulation with UFH, ensuring maximal heparin concentration where it was needed most—in the previously thrombosed veins.

(j) Construction of a small arteriovenous fistula is performed to increase venous blood flow velocity to assist in maintaining patency. A side branch of the proximal great saphenous vein or the great saphenous vein itself is anastomosed to the proximal SFA.

(k) If unobstructed ipsilateral drainage into the vena cava cannot be established, a cross pubic bypass with a 10-mm externally supported PTFE graft combined with an arteriovenous fistula is constructed.

(l) Therapeutic anticoagulation is required to prevent rethrombosis.

(m) External pneumatic compression is applied during the postoperative period to improve venous return.

10   Complications and Management

1. *Bleeding* is the most common complication of anticoagulation. In patients treated for venous thromboembolism, major bleeding occurs in up to 7%. To decrease the risk of bleeding over the long term with warfarin compounds, dose adjustment and monitoring by an anticoagulation clinic are advised. Some patients are best served by self-monitoring and dose adjustment.

2. *Heparin-induced thrombocytopenia (HIT)*

   (a) HIT occurs in 3–5% of patient treated with heparin.

   (b) Platelet counts should be monitored in all patients receiving heparin. A drop in platelet count by 50% from baseline or a count below 100,000 should raise suspicion of HIT

   (c) If this occurs, heparin administration is immediately stopped and blood tests for HIT sent. Treatment with direct thrombin inhibitors is begun.

   • *Hirudin* is cleared by the kidneys; therefore, it must be used with caution in patients with compromised renal function. The initial dose is a bolus of 0.4 mg/kg over

15–20 s followed by a continuous infusion of 0.15 mg/kg/h.

- *Argatroban* is metabolized in the liver; therefore, it must be used with caution in patients with compromised hepatic function. Initial dose is 2 mg/kg/min as a continuous IV infusion. During infusion, the APTT should be maintained at 1.5–3 times the baseline.

(d) Confirm the diagnosis of HIT using:

- Enzyme-linked immunosorbent assay (ELISA). It is highly sensitive but does not have good specificity.
- Serotonin release assay (SRA). It is poorly sensitive but highly specific.

(e) Warfarin should be started only when the platelet count has returned to baseline or recovered substantially.

11 Outcomes

Following catheter-directed thrombolysis, patency is restored in 80–90% of patients. The degree of thrombus resolution is directly correlated to the postthrombotic morbidity. The more complete the thrombus removal, the better the patient's outcome. Many patients will retain valve function if complete thrombus removal is achieved. Bleeding complications occur in 5–10% of patients; however, since lower doses of t-PA are being used, reports published in the last 6 years generally report major bleeding complications in less than 5% of patients. Fortunately, fatal PE, intracranial bleed, and death due to thrombolysis are rare.

Adding mechanical techniques to catheter-directed thrombolysis improves outcomes, shortens treatment times, and reduces the dose of plasminogen activator used.

Eighty percentage of the patients treated for acute axillosubclavian venous thrombosis can expect a good or an excellent outcome.

12   Flowchart

RECOMMENDATIONS FOR THE DIAGNOSIS AND TREATMENT OF ACUTE DEEP VEIN THROMBOSIS

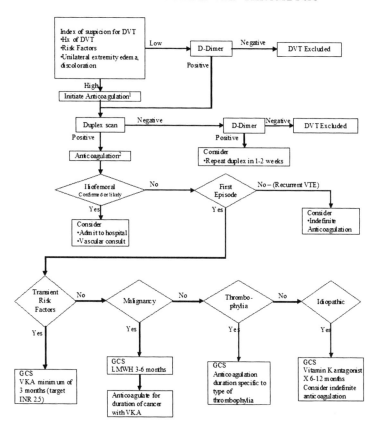

GCS = graduated compression stockings
VKA = Vitamin K antagonist (Warfarin)

Management of Iliofemoral DVT

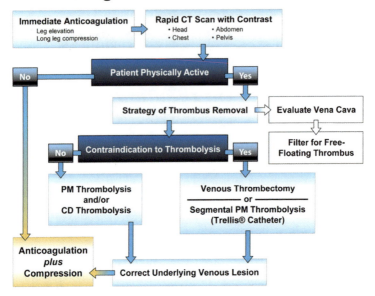

References

1. Comerota AJ, Gale SS. Technique of contemporary iliofemoral and infrainguinal venous thrombectomy. J Vasc Surg. 2006;43(1):185–91.
2. Kearon C, Kahn SR, Agnelli G, Goldhaber SZ, Raskob G, Comerota AJ. Antithrombotic therapy for venous thromboembolic disease: ACCP evidence-based clinical practice guidelines (8th ed). Chest. 2008;133(6):454S–545S.
3. Kahn SR, Shrier I, Julian JA, Ducruet T, Arsenault L, Miron MJ, et al. Determinants and time course of the postthrombotic syndrome after acute deep venous thrombosis. Ann Intern Med. 2008;149(10):698–707.
4. Comerota AJ, Gravett MH. Iliofemoral venous thrombosis. J Vasc Surg. 2007;46(5):1065–76.
5. Warkentin TE, Greinacher A, Koster A, Lincoff AM. Treatment and prevention of heparin-induced thrombocytopenia: American College of Chest Physicians Evidence-Based Clinical Practice Guidelines (8th Edition). Chest. 2008;133(6 Suppl):340S–80S.

Chapter 30
Pulmonary Embolism and SVC Syndrome

Huiting Chen and Peter H. Lin

1 Pulmonary Embolism

1.1 Disease Definition

Pulmonary embolism (PE) is a potentially fatal condition caused by embolic occlusion of the pulmonary artery or one of its branches due to thrombotic material that has traveled through the bloodstream from elsewhere in the body. The majority of emboli are thrombi from the deep veins of the legs; less likely causes can be fat, air or amniotic fluid emboli. PE is a highly lethal condition that affects more than 600,000 patients annually in the United States and is responsible for 150,000 to 200,000 deaths every year.

H. Chen, M.D.
Department of Surgery, University of Michigan Health System,
Ann Arbor, MI, USA

P.H. Lin, M.D. (✉)
Baylor College of Medicine, HVAMC (112), 2002 Holcombe Blvd,
Houston, TX 77030, USA
e-mail: plin@bcm.tmc.edu

A. Kumar and K. Ouriel (eds.), *Handbook of Endovascular Interventions*, 403
DOI 10.1007/978-1-4614-5013-9_30,
© Springer Science+Business Media New York 2013

1.2 Disease Distribution

Pulmonary embolism is the third most cause of cardiovascular death. The average annual incidence of venous thromboembolism (VTE) in the United States is 1 per 1000, with about 250,000 incident cases occurring annually. The actual incidence of PE is likely higher since autopsy studies show that an additional similar number of patients are diagnosed with PE during autopsy. This has led to an estimated incidence 650,000 to 900,000 fatal and nonfatal VTE events in the US per year. The incidence of venous thromboembolism has not changed significantly in the past four decades.

1.3 Classification

PE can be classified based on the onset of the condition into either acute or chronic PE. Additional classification within acute PE can be divided into massive or submassive based on the severity of symptoms.

1. Acute PE: The etiology in acute PE is sudden obstruction of pulmonary vessels which results in immediate symptoms and signs

   (a) *Acute massive PE*: This condition involves significant hemodynamic compromise circulatory collapse due in part to cardiogenic shock. Presence of hemodynamic instability further supports the diagnosis of acute massive PE, which is defined as systolic arterial pressure <90 mm Hg or a drop in systolic arterial pressure of at least 40 mm Hg for at least 15 min. Because this condition accounts for the majority of PE-related fatality, the diagnosis and treatment strategies in the remainder of this chapter are focused on acute massive PE.

   (b) *Acute submassive PE*: This is characterized by acute PE with signs of right ventricular dysfunction or right heart failure. Since right heart failure is a frequent cause of sudden fatality in patients with PE, the presence of right ventricular dysfunction is indicative of poor prognosis if prompt treatment is not initiated.

2. Chronic PE: The etiology of chronic PE is a progression of an acute PE leading to pulmonary hypertension that results in slowly progressive dyspnea over the course of months or years.

1.4   Diagnosis

Patients with PE present with nonspecific individual symptoms; clinical suspicion of PE should be based on the presentation as a whole with a thorough evaluation of risk factors. Signs and symptoms include acute onset of dyspnea, pleuritic chest pain, tachypnea, tachycardia, jugular venous distention, and accentuated pulmonic component of the second heart sound. Acute massive PE results in acute RV failure indicated by increased jugular venous pressure, a right-sided S3, and a parasternal lift. Approximately half of patients will show signs or symptoms of lower extremity DVT, including edema, tenderness, erythema, or a palpable cord in the thigh or calf. Less than 10% of patients present with circulatory collapse brought on by a massive PE. Routine labs usually yield nonspecific results such as leukocytosis and an increased erythrocyte sedimentation rate (ESR). D-dimer is a degradation of cross-linked fibrin, and a level of >500 ng/ml is typically abnormal. Depending on the type of assay used, d-dimer sensitivity may reach approximate 95% and specificity may reach over 60%.

1.5   Diagnostic Imaging

Patients with acute massive PE present with high-risk signs of shock or hypotension. In this life-threatening situation, patients may forego nonspecific tests such as electrocardiogram and chest radiograph and proceed directly to CT if it is immediately available.

Echocardiography: Abnormal findings of an acute massive PE include indirect signs of acute pulmonary hypertension and right ventricular overload such as increased RV size, decreased RV function, and tricuspid regurgitation.

Nuclear scintigraphic ventilation-perfusion V/Q scanning of the lung: V/Q scanning should be considered whenever the diagnosis of PE is suspected and no alternative diagnosis can be proved. A normal V/Q scan virtually excludes PE. However, V/Q scan should not be used alone to confirm or exclude the diagnosis of PE. A repeat V/Q scan is indicated before stopping anticoagulation in a patient with irreversible risk factors for DVT and PE because recurrent symptoms are common and a reference "posttreatment" V/Q scan can serve as a new baseline for comparison, often sparing the patient the need for a future angiogram.

Multidetector computed tomographic angiography (MDCTA): High-resolution MDCTA has become the first line of diagnostic imaging modality in patients suspected of having PE. This has been shown to have sensitivity and specificity similar to that of contrast pulmonary angiography, and, in recent years, has become accepted both as the preferred primary diagnostic modality and as the criterion standard for making or excluding the diagnosis of pulmonary embolism. It is noteworthy that MDCTA is more likely to miss lesions in a patient with pleuritic chest pain due to multiple small emboli that have lodged in distal vessels, but these lesions also may be difficult to detect using conventional angiography.

Magnetic resonance angiography (MRA): MRA is potentially limited by respiratory and cardiac motion artifact, magnetic susceptibility effects from the adjacent air-containing lung, and complicated blood flow patterns. Technological advances show promise for increased MRA use in the future.

Pulmonary angiography: This is a catheter-based imaging study in which a diagnostic catheter is placed in the pulmonary artery for angiographic evaluation. It was once considered the gold standard in the diagnosis of acute PE before the introduction of MDCTA. A negative pulmonary angiographic exam excludes clinically relevant PE. However, in the setting of hemodynamic instability, pulmonary angiography can confirm the presence of PE and permits the initiation of catheter-directed pulmonary artery thrombolysis.

1.6 Management

Acute massive PE is an emergency with a mortality rate of approximately 30% without treatment. Indications for treatment: acute massive PE with cardiogenic shock and/or persistent arterial hypotension with no absolute contraindications such as ischemic stroke in preceding 6 months or hemorrhagic stroke. Catheter-directed thrombolysis has been shown to be efficacious in patients with acute massive and PE with rapid symptomatic improvement and stabilization of hemodynamic condition.

1.7 Open Operative Treatment

Traditional open surgical treatment for acute massive PE is open thromboembolectomy of the pulmonary artery via mediastinotomy. Initiation of circulatory arrest with cardiopulmonary bypass is necessary to perform this procedure. Because of the underlying hemodynamic instability in these patients, operative mortality of this formidable surgical approach remains as high as 30%.

1.8 Intervention

Consider catheter-directed thrombolysis in patients with acute massive PE. Systemic anticoagulation with intravenous heparin (50–100 units/kg of heparin bolus followed by a constant infusion of 15–25 units/kg/h) should be given for patients with symptomatic PE. For patients with acute massive PE who are undergoing catheter-directed thrombolysis, an activated clotting time between 250 and 300 should be maintained to achieve adequate anticoagulation.

Technical steps for catheter-directed thrombolysis for acute massive PE:

1. Obtain femoral vein access using a micropuncture needle and catheter and place a 6 F introducer sheath. Bilateral femoral access should be obtained for bilateral catheter-directed thromobolysis in patients with bilateral PE.
2. Place a 260-cm 0.035″ Bentson guidewire guided by a MONT-1 pulmonary angiographic catheter to traverse across the right atrium and right ventricle to enter the main pulmonary artery. Pulmonary angiogram is performed using power injector to identify the location of the pulmonary arterial thrombus. Selective right and left pulmonary artery angiogram should be performed to further delineate the thrombus extent in the pulmonary arterial circulation.

3. Exchange the pigtail catheter with a multi-infusing thrombolytic catheter so the infusion portion of the catheter is embedded within the pulmonary arterial thrombus. Consider placing bilateral pulmonary thrombolytic catheters if PE is identified in bilateral pulmonary arteries, which may require bilateral femoral venous access with introducer sheath placement.

4. Infusion of thrombolytic agent using tissue plasminogen activator can be performed via the catheter-directed thrombolytic catheter at an infusion rate of 1 mg/h. heparin is commonly used during thrombolysis which is delivered at 500 μ/h via the femoral sheath to reduce pericatheter thrombosis. Alternatively, heparin can also be given systematically via peripheral intravenous route to achieve full systemic anticoagulation with an aPTT at 1.5–2 times the control value.

5. In all patients receiving thrombolysis and heparin, serial blood monitoring including the aPTT, platelet counts, fibrinogen, and fibrin degradation products should be checked on a continuing basis every 8–12 h. Heparin is contraindicated in the presence of anti-heparin antibodies due to dangerous thrombocytopenia can develop. Although not routinely ordered, an assay for the antibody is available.

6. For PE catheter-directed thrombolysis, interval pulmonary angiography should be performed 12–48 h after initiation of catheter-based interventions to determine the need to continue or stop thrombolysis. Criteria for stopping thrombolytic therapy are based on the following conditions:

   (a) No change in clot burden after 24 h
   (b) Resolution of clinical symptoms despite the presence of residual clot or
   (c) A decrease in the mean pulmonary arterial pressure of at least 50%

1.9 Complications and Management

Bleeding is the most common complication following thrombolytic therapy. Often bleeding occurs at sites of invasive procedures such as pulmonary angiography or arterial puncture. Noncomplicated bleeding from vascular puncture sites should be controlled with manual compression followed by a pressure dressing. Patients with significant or refractory bleeding may be transfused ten units of cryoprecipitate and two units of fresh frozen plasma. Additionally, protamine sulfate may be administered to reverse the effect of any heparin that remains in the patient's plasma.

1.10 Outcomes

Endovascular treatment of acute massive pulmonary embolism by catheter-directed thrombolysis has shown complete thrombus removal in up to 100% of cases. Recently, a novel treatment strategy using ultrasound-accelerated thrombolytic therapy has shown efficacious outcome in patients with both acute massive and acute submassive PE. Specifically, ultrasound-accelerated thrombolysis decreases the amount of thrombolytic agents and infusion time, which lowers the incidence of hemorrhagic complications. Postprocedural hemorrhage is low as 0% in ultrasound-accelerated thrombolysis compared to approximately 21% in catheter-directed thrombolysis. Retrievable IVC filters may be placed and subsequent retrieved within a year without complication. With either method of thrombolysis, patients compliant on long-term oral anticoagulation therapy with warfarin may achieve 0% recurrence of PE.

References

1. Lin PH, Annambhotla S, Bechara CF, et al. Comparison of percutaneous ultrasound-accelerated thrombolysis versus catheter-directed thrombolysis in patients with acute massive pulmonsty embolism. Vascular 2009; S137–S147.
2. Goldhaber SZ, Visani L, De Rosa M. Acute pulmonary embolism: clinical outcomes in the International Cooperative Pulmonary Embolism Registry (ICOPER). Lancet 1999; 353:1386–9.
3. Kuo WT, van den Bosch MA, Hoffmann LV, et al. Catheter-directed embolectomy. fragmentation, and thrombolysis for the treatment of massive pulmonary embolism after failure of systemic thromolysis. Chest 2008; 134:250–4.
4. Chamsuddin A, Nazzal L, Kang B, et al. Catheter-directed thrombolysis with the Endowave system in the treatment of acute massive pulmonary embolism: a retrospective multicenter case series. J Vasc Interv Radiol 2008;19:372–6.
5. Spies C, Khandelwal A, Smith TH, et al. Percutaneous mechanical thrombectomy for massive pulmonary embolism using a conservative treatment strategy. J Interv Cardiol 2008;21:566–71.

2 Superior Vena Cava Syndrome

2.1 Anatomy

The superior vena cava (SVC) is the primary vessel that receives venous drainage of the head, neck, upper extremities and upper torso. The SVC begins where the right and left brachiocephalic join at the lower edge of the right first costal cartilage and terminates where it joins the right atrium at the lower edge of the right third costal cartilage. The brachiocephalic veins form on each side at the junction of the internal jugular and the subclavian veins. The left brachiocephalic vein crosses midline and joins with the right brachiocephalic vein to form the SVC. Compression of the SVC from malignancy is usually due to extrinsic masses in the middle or anterior mediastinum, right paratracheal or precarinal lymph nodes or tumors originating from the right lobe bronchus. As these masses increase in size and compress the SVC, there is increased resistance to venous blood flow and eventual development of collaterals to relieve the obstruction.

2.2 Disease Definition

Superior vena cava syndrome (SVCS) is the obstruction of flow through the superior vena cava from the upper torso to the right atrium. Etiologies are secondary to:

1. Stenosis of the brachiocephalic veins or SVC
2. Occlusions of the brachiocephalic veins or SVC

2.3 Disease Distribution

SVCS is predominantly associated with malignancy involving the thoracic cavity. Approximately 2–4% of patients with carcinoma of the lung will develop SVCS during their disease course. Lymphoma and lung cancer account for over 90% of malignant causes of SVCS.

Presently in the United States, more than 90% of patients with SVCS have an associated malignancy as the cause. This is in sharp contrast with historical causes of SVCS in the 1940s when nonmalignant infectious etiologies such as syphilis and tuberculosis were the primary causative factors. The incidence of these infectious etiologies has declined significantly since then due to improvement of antibiotic therapy. There are other nonmalignant causes of SVCS which include thrombosis from central venous instrumentation including central venous catheter, pacemaker, or defibrillator placement. In developing countries, nonmalignant infectious causes represent a significant contributor in the pathogenesis of SVCS.

2.4 Classification or Disease Pattern

Based on the etiology of vascular obstruction, SVCS may be classified based on the following disease pattern:

1. Intravascular thrombus from neoplastic invasion of the vessel wall—This frequently results in complete obstruction of the SVC due to both intravascular thrombus and extrinsic compression. Incomplete SVC obstruction may occur which is typically caused by extrinsic compression without thrombus formation.
2. Extrinsic pressure exerted by tumor mass or lymphadenopathy— This is the most common etiology as neoplasms account for approximately 80% of all SVCS. The most common malignancies that cause SVCS are bronchogenic carcinomas (75–80% of neoplasms causing SVCS) with the majority of which being small cell carcinomas of the lung. Non-Hodgkin lymphomas account for 10–15% of the cases. Significant mediastinal lymphadenopathy may also exert a mass effect.
3. Stenosis by intravascular devices (Fig. 30.1)—Central venous devices such as pacemakers, defibrillators, central venous infusion ports, or chronic hemodialysis catheters may lead to central venous endothelial irritation resulting in intraluminal fibrosis. With an ever-growing aging population, this etiology is on the rise.
4. Mediastinal fibrosis due to infectious processes or radiation— Nonmalignant etiologies include infectious processes such as tuberculosis and radiation-induced mediastinal fibrosis.

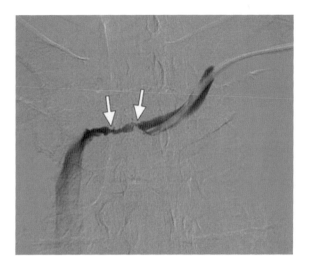

Fig. 30.1 SVC stenosis

2.5 *Diagnosis*

Patients with SVCS present with signs of venous occlusion of the head, neck, upper thorax, and arms. Dyspnea is common as edema impinges on the larynx and pharynx. Additional sighs include face and neck swelling, cough, dysphagia, plethora, distended veins in upper thorax, neck and arms, and upper limb edema. Cerebral edema may also result, leading to mental status changes, headache and lightheadedness.

Symptoms present gradually with progressing intensity as neoplasms increase in size and invasiveness, resulting in increasing obstruction. Though the overall course is that of worsening symptoms, patients may experience intermittent improvement of symptoms as venous collaterals develop. Histological diagnoses are not necessary to diagnose SVCS, although they can be valuable in distinguishing malignant from benign etiologies. A tissue diagnosis may be necessary for patients who present with SVCS without a prior diagnosis of a neoplasm. In such cases, minimally invasive techniques such as sputum cytology and biopsy of enlarged peripheral lymph nodes are preferred. More invasive techniques such as bronchoscopy, VATS, thoracotomy, and mediastinoscopy may be necessary to diagnose subtypes of lymphoma. Suspected non-Hodgkin lymphoma and small cell lung cancers can be diagnosed and staged with bone marrow biopsies.

2.6 Diagnostic Imaging

Chest radiograph: Most patients with SVCS have an abnormal chest radiograph reflecting the underlying neoplastic etiology. The most common findings on chest X-ray are mediastinal widening followed by pleural effusion.

Contrast-enhanced computed tomography angiography (CTA): CTA of the chest and neck with particular focus on the venous structure represent the <u>most useful study for SVCS</u> as it is able to define the underlying cause of venous obstruction, identify the extent of occlusion, and evaluate any collateral venous drainage pathways. Identification of venous collaterals is a sound indicator for SVCS (specificity 96%, sensitivity 92%).

Magnetic resonance venography (MRV): This is an alternative imaging modality to CT scan for patients who cannot receive contrast administration due to allergy or suffer from CT scanning-associated claustrophobia.

Diagnostic Venography: This imaging modality requires catheter placement from either femoral or upper extremity venous system to identify underlying SVC pathology. It offers the advantage of concomitant endovascular intervention such as venous stenting at the time of diagnostic imaging. Venography of the upper limbs bilaterally is the gold standard for identifying SVC obstruction and delineating the extent of thrombus formation. However, unlike CT scans, conventional venography is unable to identify the cause of the SVC obstruction unless thrombosis is the exclusive etiology.

2.7 Management

Symptomatic SVCS should be approached as a clinical emergency. Immediate therapy includes head elevation and steroid administration to reduce edema and compressive symptoms.

Indications for treatment:

1. Symptomatic disease

   (a) Chronic or recurrent SVC nonmalignant obstruction: consider operative or endovascular interventions
   (b) Acute severe malignant SVCS: chemoradiation therapy to achieve initial tumor response followed by operative or endovascular therapy.

2. Asymptomatic disease: is not an indication for treatment.

2.8   Open Operative Choices

For malignant tumor, consider surgical treatment with tumor resection via mediastinotomy and SVC bypass. Prosthetic bypass conduit with Dacron or expanded polytetrafluoroethylene (ePTFE) graft can be used for SVC bypass. Autogenous bypass conduit with jugular vein or femoral vein interposition graft can also be used. Due to potential vein graft diameter mismatch, large caliber prosthetic graft is more commonly used compared to autogenous vein graft conduit. However to reduce the size mismatch, spiral vein grafts are used.

2.9   Endovascular Interventions

Consider catheter-based interventions with SVC balloon angioplasty and stenting as the first-line treatment strategy for nonmalignant SVCS due to its less invasive nature and rapid patient recovery. Systemic anticoagulation with intravenous heparin (50–100 units/kg of heparin bolus followed by a constant infusion of 15–25 units/kg/h) should be given for patients with symptomatic SVC thrombosis. For patients who are not on systemic anticoagulation, an intraprocedural IV bolus of heparin (100 U/kg) should be administered prior to endovascular intervention with either balloon dilation or stenting placement. During the procedure, an activated clotting time between 250 and 300 should be maintained to achieve adequate anticoagulation.

Technical steps for SVCS balloon angioplasty and stenting:

1. Establish femoral venous access with an 8 F introducer sheath.
2. Place a 260-cm 0.35″ Bentson guidewire guided by an angled catheter in the SVC.
3. Cathether exchange to place a diagnostic pigtail catheter in the SVC. Perform venography using a power injector to visualize lesions involving the SVC and/or brachiocephalic veins.
4. Whenever possible, use a floppy 260 cm 0.035″ hydrophilic guidewire to traverse across the SVC lesion. If the lesion involves a long segment of SVC, ipsilateral brachiocephalic vein, or SVC occlusion, a guidewire exchange may be performed so a stiff 0.035″ Amplatz or a Lunderquist wire for improved tractability for angioplasty balloon catheter or stent catheter delivery. In the event of venous occlusion involving bilateral brachiocephalic veins, establish bilateral upper extremity venous access via either a brachial or basilica vein approach to facilitate the catheterization of the central vein occlusion.
5. Balloon angioplasty is routinely performed to first dilate the SVC or brachiocephalic vein stenosis with either 10 mm diameter balloon angioplasty catheter.
6. For long lesions encompassing the SVC and brachiocephalic vein where a curved segment of central vein is involved, consider using a 12 mm or 14 mm diameter self-expanding stents with either Wallstent or nitinol-based stent. For focal lesions involving either the SVC or brachiocephalic vein alone, consider using a balloon-expandable stent. When a self-expandable stent is used, poststenting balloon dilatation should be performed.
7. Deploy additional placement if a single stent is insufficient to cover the entire lesion length. Ensure at least 10 mm of the stent is bridged beyond the lesion segment.
8. If the segment of SVC adjacent to the stricture is greater than 16 mm in diameter, perform a bilateral brachiocephalic kissing stent technique using either 12 mm or 14 mm diameter self-expandable stents via either the bilateral femoral vein or a bilateral upper extremity approach. In the kissing stent technique, position the proximal self-expandable stent in the proximal SVC, whereas the distal stent is extended to the respective brachiocephalic vein. Simultaneously perform bilateral poststenting kissing billion dilatation across the lesion.

9. Perform a completion venography to document the treatment result
10. Remove the introducer sheaths and guidewires and apply manual pressure compression to achieve hemostasis.

2.10   Postprocedure Management

Following stent placement, patients should receive systemic antico-agulation with heparin for 3–6 days. During this time, initiate oral anticoagulation with warfarin to maintain an international normalized ratio between 2.0 and 3.0. Long-term anticoagulation may be achieved with low-dose warfarin: 1 mg daily. If there is a contraindi-cation to such therapy, an alternative is a three-month course of dual antiplatelet therapy with clopidogrel and aspirin. This is how our group manages postprocedural medication.

2.11   Complications and Management

Early procedural related complications as well as late treatment failure can occur following SVC stenting procedures.

1. Early complications:

   (a) Pulmonary embolism (PE)—due to catheter manipulation during balloon angioplasty or stent placement in thrombosed SVC or brachiocephalic vein. Initial treatment includes antico-agulation. In severe cases PE with hemodynamic compromise, consider catheter-directed thrombolysis of the pulmonary artery.

   (b) Stent migration—due to placement of undersized stent. Appropriate stent sizing with approximate 15–20% stent over-size compared to normal adjacent lesion-free SVC segment will avoid the possibility of stent undersize and migration. If a stent is severely undersized and migrated to the heart, con-sider stent retrieval using a snare cathether from a femoral vein approach.

(c) Perforation or rupture of the SVC—a rare complication commonly due to oversized balloon angioplasty. If contrast extravasation is detected suggesting SVC rupture, reinserted a smaller balloon angioplasty catheter and inflate the angioplasty catheter for 10 min to achieve SVC tamponade and vessel wall hemostasis.

2. Late complications—Stent occlusion due to thrombotic occlusion or intimal hyperplasia is a known late treatment complication. Reintervention with catheter-directed thrombolysis or thrombectomy may be considered in the event of acute stent thrombosis. Balloon angioplasty with additional stent placement may be considered if late stent occlusion is due to recurrent of SVC compression or intimal hyperplasia.

2.12 Outcomes

Percutaneous stenting of SVCS has shown up to 100% technical success and up to 96% symptomatic improvement of both malignant and benign etiologies. Periprocedural complications may be as low as 0%. A single stent was used in 68% of patients, whereas 32% of patients required multiple (2–3 kissing) stents. Primary patency in patients with malignant and benign causes of SVCS were 64% and 76% respectively, 1 year postintervention. Twenty five percent of patients with benign SVCS underwent reintervention due to symptom recurrence. Of these, half were successfully treated with balloon dilatation and half were treated with repeat stent placement. Overall symptom-free survival from all causes of SVCS ranged from 1 to 34 months (mean 14.8 months).

References

1. Barshes NR, Annambhotla S, Sayed H, et al. Percutaneous stenting of superior vena cava syndrome: treatment outcome in patients with benign and malignant etiology. 2007; 15(5): 314–321.
2. Yim CD, Sane SS, Bjarnason H. Superior vena cava stenting. Radiol Clinic North Am 2000; 38: 409–24.

3. Gregorio Ariza MA, Gamboa P, Gimeno MJ, et al. Percutaneous treatment of superior vena cava syndrome using metallic stents. Eur Radiol 2003; 853–62.
4. Garcia MR, Bertoni H, Pallota G, et al. Use of self-expanding vascular endo-prostheses in superior vena cava syndrome. Eur J Cardiothorac Surg 2003; 24:208–11.
5. Uberoi R. Quality assurance guidelines for superior vena cava stenting in malignant disease. Cardiovasc Intervent Radiol 2006; 29:319–22.

Chapter 31
Varicose Veins: Comprehensive Management

Eric Mowatt-Larssen, Manj Gohel, Cynthia Shortell, and Alun Davies

1   I. Anatomy

1. The venous system of the lower extremity consists of three interconnected systems: the deep system, the superficial system, and the perforating veins.

   (a) **Deep veins** run deep to the superficial fascia and drain the extremity muscular compartments from distal to proximal. Most venous blood draining from the lower extremity leaves via the common femoral vein.

   (b) **Superficial veins** run superficial to the superficial fascia and drain the skin from distal to proximal and from superficial to deep. **Saphenous veins** are surrounded by the saphenous fascia, easily identifiable on transverse ultrasound as the "saphenous

E. Mowatt-Larssen, M.D.
Department of Surgery, Duke University Health System, Durham, NC, USA

M. Gohel, M.D. • A. Davies, M.D. (✉)
Charing Cross Hospital, Fulham Palace Rd., London, UK
e-mail: a.h.davies@imperial.ac.uk

C. Shortell, M.D. (✉)
Department of Surgery, Duke University, DUMC 3538, Durham, NC 27710, USA
e-mail: Short018@mc.duke.edu

A. Kumar and K. Ouriel (eds.), *Handbook of Endovascular Interventions*,   419
DOI 10.1007/978-1-4614-5013-9_31,
© Springer Science+Business Media New York 2013

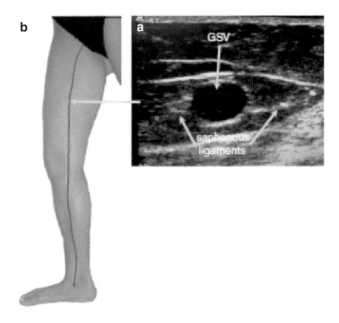

Fig. 31.1 The saphenous eye of the great saphenous vein. Transverse B mode ultrasound image of GSV (**a**). Probe position on the thigh (**b**)

eye" (Fig. 31.1). **Tributary veins** route blood from the skin to the saphenous veins.

(c) The **great saphenous vein** (GSV) starts in the medial foot, ascends in the leg in the saphenous sheath anterior to the medial malleolus, and runs along the medial border of the tibia. It passes medial to the knee and then runs medial to the femoral vein. At the groin, it drains into the common femoral vein at the saphenofemoral junction (SFJ).

(d) Multiple **perforator veins** perforate the superficial fascia and route blood from superficial to deep veins.

2. Some individuals have accessory saphenous veins, which can also run in sheaths with ultrasound saphenous eyes. The **anterior accessory saphenous vein** (AASV), often present, runs lateral to the GSV. The AASV can be distinguished from the GSV by the alignment sign, or its position superficial to the femoral vein and artery on transverse ultrasound.

3. The SFJ has a constant terminal valve located 1–2 mm distal to the SFJ on the GSV, and usually another preterminal valve 2 cm

distally along the GSV, marking the limit of the SFJ. Proximal veins draining the abdominal wall and pudendum terminate at the SFJ. Additionally, distal veins, such as the AASV or posterior accessory saphenous vein, often drain at or near the SFJ.

4. The **small saphenous vein** (SSV) begins in the lateral foot, ascends in the leg posterior to the lateral malleolus, then runs in the midline posterior calf between the two heads of the gastrocnemius to the popliteal fossa. The SSV, like all saphenous veins, runs in a sheath with the ultrasound saphenous sign. It terminates most often at the SPJ, draining into the popliteal vein superior to the popliteal crease. The SSV often continues as a thigh extension draining into deep veins more proximally, or can also continue as the Giacomini vein, draining into the GSV.

2   Disease Definition

Patients have **chronic venous disease** when they have either symptoms (pain or swelling) or physical signs (varicose veins, telangiectasias, dermatologic complications) attributable to abnormal venous flow or venous reflux.

(a) **Varicose veins** are blue dilated subcutaneous veins usually over 3 mm diameter, and they most often bulge outside the skin surface.

(b) **Reticular varicosities** are blue dilated subdermal veins usually less than 3 mm in diameter.

(c) **Telangiectasias**, also called spider veins, are red or purple dilated intradermal venules usually less the 1 mm in diameter.

(d) **Chronic venous insufficiency** is diagnosed when a patient has either edema or dermatologic complications from chronic venous disease.

(e) Dermatologic complications of venous reflux: An **ulcer** is a full thickness skin defect. **Lipodermatosclerosis** is a localized fibrosis of the skin and subcutaneous tissues. **Atrophie blanche** is a localized area of white, atrophic skin areas surrounded by dilated capillaries. **Venous pigmentation** is brown and due to extravasated blood. **Venous eczema** is red and can weep, blister, or scale. **Corona phlebectactica** is a fan-shaped pattern of small intradermal veins.

3   Disease Distribution

Chronic venous disease signs, such as telangiectasias, varicose veins, and venous ulcers, are common but notoriously underdiagnosed. Telangiectasias have over 80% prevalence, while varicose veins have around 25% prevalence. More severe vein disease is thankfully less common, but around 1% of the population has an active or healed venous ulcer.

A first-degree family history of varicose veins in a parent is the greatest risk factor for the development of chronic venous disease, with a corrected odds ratio of over 2. Other risk factors are increased age, female sex, pregnancy, high body mass index, taller height, and prolonged standing.

4   Disease Classification

(a) Chronic venous disease is classified using the **CEAP system**, based on clinical manifestations (C), etiology (E), anatomic disease distribution (A), and pathophysiology (P). The "C" from CEAP is most often used in venous studies and in clinical practice.

(b) C6 patients have an active venous ulcer.

(c) C5 patients have a healed venous ulcer.

(d) C4 patients have dermatologic complications from venous disease other than ulcer, as discussed in IId.

(e) C3 patients have venous edema.

(f) C2 patients have varicose veins.

(g) C1 patients have telangiectasias and/or reticular varicosities.

(h) C0 patients have no visible signs of venous disease. These patients can still have pain or swelling from venous reflux.

5   Diagnosis: Clinical

(a) **Pain** is the most common symptom. Patients often describe their pain as aching, heaviness, fatigue, soreness, or burning. Location is typically at varicose vein sites, or along the path of the GSV (medial ankle, calf, and/or thigh) or SSV (posterior or distal lateral calf), but can also consist of generalized leg pain. It usually

worsens with prolonged standing and improves with extremity elevation.
(b) **Swelling** is also common. Venous edema usually begins around the medial malleolus, although it can spread proximally throughout the extremity. It typically worsens with prolonged standing and improves with extremity elevation.
(c) Telangiectasias, varicose veins, swelling, and skin changes are the common signs.

6 Diagnostic Imaging

Duplex ultrasound is the key to diagnosis and management of chronic venous disease. This test rules out deep venous thrombosis as a cause of patient symptoms. It also defines the anatomy and extent of venous reflux critical in determining patient management. It is important to note that most ultrasound studies performed on the lower extremity evaluate only the presence or the absence of thrombus and do not investigate the patient's valvular function. Therefore, a "negative" venous ultrasound usually does not rule out the possibility of valvular insufficiency unless it is performed in a vascular lab that specializes in venous disorders. In phlebological ultrasound, superficial, deep, and perforator systems are examined for reflux and obstruction. Superficial venous examination is performed along the course of all saphenous veins and their junctions, as well as any other refluxing tributary veins. The source of reflux for all superficial varices should be determined.

Venous reflux is defined as blood flow in the reverse direction to physiologic flow (for example, towards the floor in a standing patient). Pathologic reflux lasts for more than 0.5 s. Reflux can be elicited by several methods including calf squeeze, muscle squeeze, vein cluster manual compression, Valsalva maneuver, active foot dorsiflexion and relaxation, or pneumatic calf cuff deflation. The most common finding in patients with varicose veins is reflux within the GSV.

Occasionally, patients may need **magnetic resonance venography**, if ultrasound is insufficient to fully evaluate the relevant pathology. Patients with unusual skin or duplex ultrasound findings may have a vascular malformation. Iliac vein compression can present with severe pain and swelling which can be posttraumatic or congenital

(May-Thurner Syndrome, in which the left iliac vein is compressed by the right iliac artery). Patients can have pelvic congestion syndrome, with pelvic pain and varicosities due to pelvic vein reflux. This can be confirmed by venography.

7 Management

Table 31.1 lists the indications for treatment of superficial venous reflux. The main contraindication for superficial venous ablation is superficial or deep venous obstruction.

Compression therapy is used for patients with any level of venous reflux. Compression improves venous hemodynamics, improves quality of life for patients with chronic venous disease, reduces edema and skin discoloration, and improves the venous ulcer-healing rate. The main contraindication to compression use is peripheral arterial disease, especially with ankle-brachial index less than 0.5. Commercially available compression stockings are most often used. Inelastic compression, such as Unna boots and multilayer compression dressings are also used in patients with active ulcers.

Refluxing veins are corrected in the following order: great saphenous, small saphenous, other superficial veins, perforator vein(s), deep vein(s). The main contraindication to reflux treatment is venous obstruction. Indications for perforator vein ablation are controversial, but it is generally accepted that correction of perforator reflux is indicated for patients with class C5–C6 disease. In addition, perforator reflux should be reevaluated by duplex ultrasound following successful superficial ablation because they often normalize afterward, especially if the patient has no deep venous reflux. Deep venous reflux treatments carry a higher risk, have more variable success rates, and are usually treated only for patients with particularly severe symptoms, and only at specialized centers.

Table 31.1 Indications for superficial venous treatment	General appearance
	Significant pain attributable to venous disease
	Significant edema attributable to venous disease
	Skin changes attributable to venous disease
	Leg ulcer attributable to venous disease
	History of superficial thrombophlebitis
	History of bleeding varicose veins

8   Open Operative Choices

(a) The classic surgical procedure for GSV reflux is ligation of the GSV at the SFJ and saphenous trunk **stripping**. Often the below-knee GSV is preserved due to a significant risk of saphenous nerve injury. This surgical procedure has become less common, as the risks for recurrent varicosities after treatment due to neovascularization have become clear. SSV surgery is also possible, but is plagued by highly variable anatomy, high varicosity recurrence rates, and injuries to the popliteal vein, popliteal nerve, and sural nerve.

(b) **Ambulatory phlebectomy** (AP) can be used for remaining visible and palpable tributary or localized varicosities after superficial axial vein ablation. In this method, the patient's varicosities are marked preoperatively in the standing position. The patient is placed supine and tumescent anesthesia is administered. One to 3 mm incisions are made vertical to the varicosity, which is hooked and then grasped by a hemostat or a Size 3 Oesch hook. Gentle traction is then applied to tease the vein out of the wound. The vein is divided and the ends extracted by a combination of rotation, traction, and massage. At the completion of the procedure, a compression dressing is applied and the patient is ambulated. Complications are rare but include blister formation, transient pigmentation, and telangiectatic matting, with superficial thrombophlebitis, hematoma, and dysesthesias less common.

(c) **Transilluminated, powered phlebectomy** using the TriVex system (Smith & Nephew, North Ryde NSW, Australia) can be used in place of AP, especially in patients with extensive varicose veins, since this technique requires in less operating time and fewer patient incisions. The procedure has similar patient satisfaction and complication rates as AP. In the current technique, the patient's varicosities are marked preoperatively in the standing position. The patient is positioned supine, and first-stage tumescence is applied. The tumescent fluid hydrodissects the veins, allows for better vein visualization, and allows better light diffusion from the transilluminator. The varicosities are resected using the powered resector under active transillumination. After initial resection, second-stage tumescence is applied by placing the illuminator/irrigator into the resection channels, and residual blood is irrigated out and the treated veins are tamponaded shut.

Additional wound drainage sites are made using a 2–3 mm dermal punch or #11 blade to decrease the hematoma risk. Clear effluent should be obtained. In third-stage tumescence, an 18-gauge spinal needle is placed into the subcuticular plane and a peau d'orange effect is obtained on the skin. Wounds are left to drain, reducing hematoma risk. The patient is then wrapped with a compression dressing and ambulated. Compression and regular ambulation should be continued for 2–3 weeks.

(d) **Subfascial endoscopic perforator vein surgery** (SEPS) is indicated for patients with CEAP Class 4–6 disease and persistent incompetence after superficial venous correction. During the procedure, an endoscope under carbon dioxide insufflation is used to identify abnormal perforator veins, which are then occluded and divided by harmonic scalpel, electrocautery, or clipped and cut with scissors. First, the subfascial space is explored, then paratibial fasciotomy is performed to access posterior tibial perforators. SEPS is likely superior to open surgery because of lower wound complication rates, but wound infection, deep venous thrombosis, ulcer recurrence, and paresthesias have been reported. Actual SEPS results have been variable with regard to ulcer healing.

9   Intervention: Technique and Pitfalls

9.1   *Endovenous laser ablation of the GSV*

(a) This procedure can be used, with specific differences depending on the target vein, for both saphenous and tributary veins, as long as the vein is long and straight enough to be cannulated. Ablation of the GSV is the most common scenario. Ultrasound is used throughout to verify correct anatomical placement.

(b) Patients are advised that the GSV is successfully ablated around 94% of the time at three-year follow-up. They can expect mild pain and bruising after the procedure for 3–4 weeks. The main risk of the procedure is deep venous thrombosis. With current techniques, that risk is around 1%.

(c) The patient is placed supine and in 10–20° of reverse Trendelenburg. This step helps enlarge the vein somewhat and make an easier target.

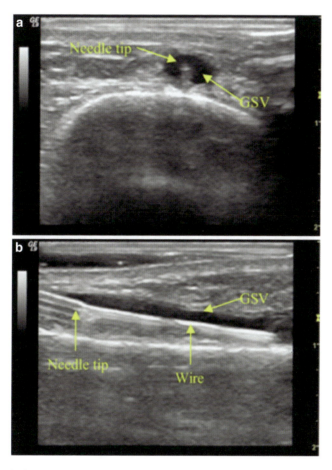

Fig. 31.2 Venous access. Cross-sectional (**a**) and longitudinal (**b**) view

(d) The course of the target vein is marked using ultrasound.

(e) The patient is cleaned and prepped.

(f) The target vein is accessed using a micropuncture system and ultrasound (Fig. 31.2). The patient can now be placed in 10–20° of Trendelenburg position to help compress the vein.

(g) The guide wire is placed through the micropuncture catheter and advanced to the SFJ, verified by ultrasound.

(h) The catheter is advanced over guide wire, with the tip placed 2 cm from the SFJ, verified by ultrasound (Fig. 31.3).

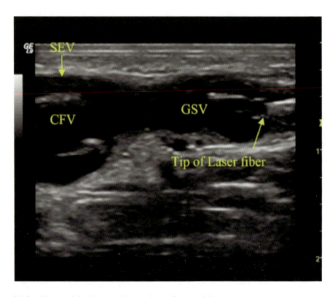

Fig. 31.3 Tip positioning at the saphenofemoral junction

(i) The laser fiber is advanced through the catheter, with the tip placed 2 cm from the saphenofemoral junction, verified by ultrasound. Placement at this spot allows good efficacy while minimizing risk of deep venous thrombosis.

(j) Tumescent anesthesia is placed around the target vein with a 1-cm circumferential halo placed around the catheter and laser fiber, verified by ultrasound, along the entire course of the segment of GSV treated (Fig. 31.4). The GSV should also be at least 1 cm below the skin to prevent skin burns. A total of 5–10 mL per cm of treated vein is typically needed. Tumescent anesthesia provides analgesia, compresses the vein, and acts as a heat sink protecting structures adjacent structures to the treated vein. To prepare the tumescent anesthetic solution, mix 50 ml 1% lidocaine in 500 ml cold normal saline to create a 0.01% lidocaine solution.

(k) Laser safety goggles are applied to the patient and all healthcare providers.

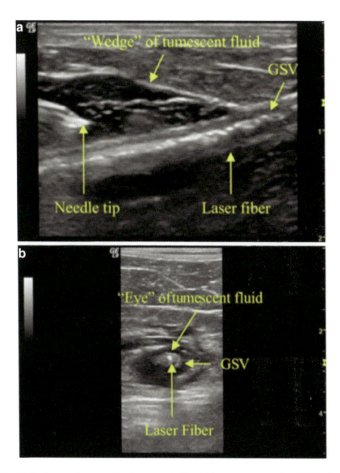

Fig. 31.4 Tumescent anesthesia. Longitudinal (**a**) and cross-sectional (**b**) views

(l) Laser fiber energy is delivered in continuous wave at 70–80 Joules per cm of vein. A setting of 13 watts continuous wave with pullback speed of 6 s per cm is most commonly used. The laser is turned to standby before removal of the catheter and laser fiber from the skin.

(m) Ultrasound verifies GSV ablation and lack of deep venous thrombosis during and immediately after the procedure.

(n) A compression dressing is applied to the needle entry site.

(o) The patient is ambulated for a minimum of 20 min.

9.2 Radiofrequency Ablation (RFA) of the GSV

(a) This procedure can be used, with specific differences depending on the target vein, for saphenous and tributary veins, as long as the vein is long and straight enough to be cannulated. The GSV ablation is the most common scenario. Ultrasound is used throughout to verify correct anatomical placement.

(b) Patients are advised that the GSV successfully ablated 97% of the time with the new Closure Fast catheter at 1-year follow-up. Patients can expect mild pain and bruising after the procedure for 3–4 weeks. The main risk of the procedure is deep venous thrombosis. With current techniques, that risk is around 1%.

(c) The patient is placed supine and in 10–20° of reverse Trendelenburg. This step helps enlarge the vein somewhat and make an easier target.

(d) The course of the target vein is marked using ultrasound.

(e) The patient is cleaned and prepped.

(f) The target vein is accessed using a micropuncture system and ultrasound (Fig. 31.2). The patient can now be placed in 10–20° of Trendelenburg position to help compress the vein.

(g) The radiofrequency catheter is advanced over guide wire, with the tip placed 2 cm from the SFJ, verified by ultrasound (Fig. 31.3). Placement at this spot allows good efficacy while minimizing risk of deep venous thrombosis.

(h) If the laser or RFA catheter does not advance easily, straightening of the leg or extrinsic thigh compression may facilitate advancement of the catheter. Some RFA systems (such as the VNUS® ClosureFAST™) have a channel for a 0.014″ wire, which may help to traverse tortuous segments of the vein.

(i) Tumescent anesthesia is placed around the target vein with a 1 cm circumferential halo placed around the catheter and laser fiber, verified by ultrasound, along the entire course of the segment of GSV treated (Fig. 31.4). The GSV should also be at least 1 cm below the skin to prevent skin burns. A total of 5–10 mL per cm of treated vein is typically needed.

(j) Radiofrequency energy is delivered at 120°C for 20–60 s per each 7 cm segment. Typically, 40 s is delivered at the SFJ, and 20 s at each distal segment, but a longer duration can be used for large diameter or aneurismal segments. This translates to using two 20 s RF cycles at the SFJ and one RF cycle for the remainder of the GSV.

(k) Ultrasound verifies GSV ablation and lack of deep venous thrombosis during and immediately after the procedure.

(l) A compression dressing is applied to the needle entry site.

(m) The patient is ambulated for a minimum of 20 min.

9.3 Differences Between EVLA and RFA

(a) Endovenous laser procedures must be performed in an approved setting and require specific safety measures including eye protection and staff training.

(b) The size of sheath or type of venous access catheter may vary depending on the type and manufacturer of EVLA and RFA used.

(c) Laser catheters should be used with the slow withdrawal or pulsed ablation techniques (depending on the specific laser device used)

(d) Lase wavelengths ranging from 810 nm to 1,470 nm are available, and laser catheters may be bare fiber (forward firing) or radial.

(e) With numerous EVLA and RFA devices currently available, the choice of ablation catheter will depend on the personal expertise and preference of the operator

9.4 Potential Pitfalls and Technical Tips

(a) Small or friable veins may be difficult to cannulate, and multiple needle punctures may result in venous spasm. Challenging cannulation may be facilitated by the use of a tourniquet or microvascular access needle. Despite these measures, open venous cutdown may be necessary and can be performed using local anesthesia.

(b) If the laser or RFA catheter does not advance easily, straightening of the leg or extrinsic thigh compression may facilitate advancement of the catheter. Some RFA systems (VNUS^R Closure FAST^TM) have a channel for an 0.014" wire, which may help to traverse tortuous segments of the vein.

(c) Always verify the position of the tip of the catheter before venous ablation. Changes in the position of the patient (particularly flexion or extension of the knee) and infiltration of tumescent anesthesia may cause the catheter to move.

(d) Ensure that the ablation catheters is clearly visualized at all stages of the procedure. The catheter may pass preferentially into the deep venous system via a perforating vein.

9.5 Sclerotherapy

Position the leg at 30° elevation. Use gentle probe massage and ankle dorsiflexion to advance the foam up the vein to be treated.

(a) Sclerotherapy techniques can be used to treat almost any abnormal surface vein. Sodium tetradecyl sulfate is FDA approved as a liquid sclerosant. Ultrasound guidance should be used when the target vein is not visible on the skin surface, or when the target vein is near a deep vein in order that the echogenic sclerofoam can visualized and kept out of the deep vein (Fig. 31.5).

(b) Foam sclerotherapy is more effective than liquid sclerotherapy, but also generally has more side effects. Foam sclerotherapy is used for varicose veins, while liquid sclerotherapy is the first choice for reticular varicosities or telangiectasias.

(c) Foam is generated by the Tessari method, mixing two syringes: one of liquid sclerosant (polidocanol: 0.5–3%) or sodium tetradecyl sulfate: 1–3%), and the other of air, attached by a three-way stopcock, back and forth over 20 times (Fig. 31.4). The usual volume ratio is liquid to air of 4:1. The resulting solution is effective for around 45–60 s.

(d) The main risk of sclerotherapy is also deep venous thrombosis, occurring at a rate below 1% for most veins. Neurological complications, including rare strokes, have also been reported.

(e) Higher concentrations of sclerosant are usually more effective than lower concentrations but carry a higher risk of complications and side effects. Larger veins need higher sclerosant concentrations. Table 31.2 is a general guide to sclerosant concentration.

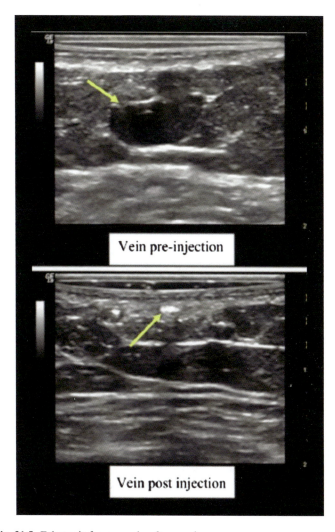

Fig. 31.5 Echogenic foam seen by ultrasound

If initial therapy is ineffective, the concentration should be doubled.

(f) Foam volumes per injected site should be limited per Table 31.2. Total volume of sclerofoam injected per day should not exceed 10 mL.

Table 31.2 Sclerotherapy guidelines

Vein type	Starting concentration of STS sclerofoam (%)	Maximum volume per injection site (mL)
Great saphenous vein	3.0	6.0
Small saphenous vein	1.0	4.0
Tributary vein	1.0	6.0
Perforator vein	1.0	4.0
Varicosity diameter 7–10 mm	0.50–1.0	2.0
Varicosity diameter 3–6 mm	0.25–0.50	2.0
Reticular varicosity	0.25 liquid (not foam)	1.0
Telangiectasia	0.25 liquid (not foam)	0.5

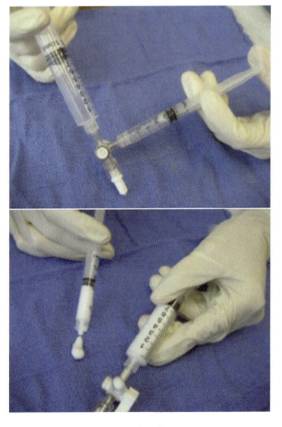

Fig. 31.6 Tessari method to generate sclerofoam

(g) *Ultrasound-guided foam sclerotherapy* (UGFS): The area is cleaned and prepped. The target vein is accessed by needle and syringe with saline under ultrasound visualization, and syringe shows a good blood return. The patient is placed in 10–20° of Trendelenburg position. Sclerofoam is generated using the Tessari method described above in 10 cc (Fig. 31.6). Any nearby superficial-deep venous junctions are compressed. The sclerofoam is placed in the target vein under ultrasound visualization, ensuring no passage into deep veins (Fig. 31.5). The sclerofoam can also be "massaged" by hand into more proximal refluxing varicosities. The patient is left in Trendelenburg position for 15 min to allow the foam to turn into liquid, and thus reduce the risk of deep venous thrombosis or stroke. A light compression bandage is placed at the treated area, and the patient is ambulated.

(h) Technique for **sclerotherapy** of localized abnormal veins: The area is cleaned and prepped. When the target vein is visible on the skin surface and not near a deep vein, a butterfly can be placed into the target vein. Correct placement is verified by blood return. The sclerofoam generated per the Tessari method described in Sect. 31.10c above is injected. The treated vein should blanch when the sclerofoam replaces blood. The patient is placed in Trendelenburg when possible as long as venous access is still possible. The patient should wait at least 15 minutes after any sclerofoam delivery to allow the sclerofoam to turn into liquid. The injected sites are then compressed, and the patient is ambulated.

10 Perforator Venous Techniques

(a) *Radiofrequency ablation* (RFA): Specially designed catheters can be used to access the perforator vein under ultrasound guidance. The catheter should be placed be at least 5 mm away from the deep vein and 10 mm below the skin surface. Tumescent anesthesia is delivered around the perforator vein and heat is delivered, typically for 85°C for 4–8 min.

(b) *Endovenous laser ablation* (EVLA): Specially designed laser fibers can be used to access the perforator vein directly under ultrasound guidance. The catheter should be placed at least

10 mm away from the deep vein and below the skin. Tumescent anesthesia is delivered around the perforator vein, and heat is delivered similar to GSV treatment. There is no published experience with EVLA of incompetent perforator veins with follow-up over one month.

(c) *Ultrasound-guided foam sclerotherapy* (UGFS): Foam is injected into a neighboring vein, not directly into the abnormal perforator vein directly, in order to avoid having the foam pass into the nearby deep vein. Ultrasound guidance is particularly important both to avoid inadvertently cannulating the nearby perforator artery and to ensure foam does not pass into deep veins. Injection volume should be less than 2–4 mL.

11 Postoperative Management

(a) Following vein treatment, the patient uses **compression** stockings to allow a scar to form in the treated vein for successful ablation. Compression stockings also help prevent deep venous thrombosis. A reasonable compression protocol is continuous compression for one week (except showering), followed by daily compression when not lying down for the second week. Alternatively, one can use wool and elastic compression bandaging for 48–72 h, replaced with thigh length Class II compression stockings (30–40 mm Hg) for 2 weeks. Early and regular **ambulation** following endovenous procedures is also important to prevent deep venous thrombosis. Ibuprofen is used to reduce the inflammatory response and provide analgesia.

(b) **Ultrasound** is usually performed 1–3 days after endovenous procedures to ensure there is no endovenous heat-induced thrombus (EHIT). It is not clear whether a heat-induced thrombus carries a similar risk to embolize as de novo thrombus, but most experts believe the clinical sequelae of this event are minimal. Nevertheless, any EHIT needs to be watched closely with regular ultrasound every 2–3 days. The patient should be counseled to follow up to an emergency department should they develop symptoms of pulmonary embolism, such as shortness of breath, chest pain, or syncope. When to use anticoagulation is controversial, but most physicians anticoagulate patients in whom EHIT extends over 50% of the diameter of the common femoral vein and discontinue once thrombus resolution is seen on ultrasound (usually between 7 and 14 days). Initial anticoagulation with enoxaparin and conversion to warfarin is the typical regimen used, if indicated.

(c) There are evolving data that the longer the physician waits to perform **adjunctive procedures**, the less frequently they need to be done. After saphenous treatment, for example, it is common to wait 1–3 months to treat nonsaphenous symptomatic veins.

(d) Patients with chronic venous disease are prone to **recurrence**. A significant number of these patients may have currently unpreventable recurrence due to genetic predisposition. Patients with recurrent symptoms or signs of chronic venous disease should have full duplex ultrasound performed typically done at about 12 months. Reflux may recur in treated veins, or it may have developed in previously normal veins. Patients treated with surgery can have neovascularization, or growth of new venous channels between ligated and even surgically removed veins.

12   Complications and Management

1. <u>Bruising and hematoma:</u> May occur particularly at phlebectomy sites or along the length of the vein ablated using laser or radiofrequency. This is usually mild and self-limiting, but may be reduced by good intraoperative hemostasis following phlebectomy and compliance with postoperative compression.

2. <u>Deep vein thrombosis:</u> A highly important, but rare complication occurring in <1% of venous procedures. May be prevented by careful catheter positioning before ablation and appropriate thromboprophylaxis.

3. <u>Skin burn:</u> May occur if the laser or radiofrequency catheter is too superficial during ablation. Take care to ensure that the catheter is >1 cm from the skin surface during ablation. If thermal skin damage does occur, treat with flamazine dressings and analgesia. Secondary ulceration may require multilayer compression bandaging.

4. <u>Recurrence</u>: Recurrence may occur early or late and may be due to recanalization (or failure of ablation) of treated veins, or de novo reflux in new veins. In all cases of recurrent varicose veins, perform a duplex scan and plan further treatment accordingly. To avoid failed ablation, ensure that adequate energy levels are delivered to the vein during ablation (e.g., >60 J/cm for EVLA).

5. <u>Parasthesia and neuralgia</u>: Usually self-limiting and mild, but may be a troublesome side effect for some patients. Ensure that superficial nerves are avoided during hook phlebectomy.

6. <u>Skin matting and staining</u>: Can occur following UGFS and may be avoided by aspiration of thrombus in sclerosed veins.

13   Outcomes: Open Versus RFA Versus EVLA

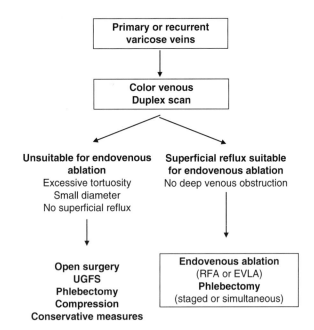

Technical success rates at 1 year exceed 80% with all modalities. Neovascularization at the SFJ is seen in up to 20% of patients following GSV stripping, whereas this is uncommon after RFA or EVLA. UGFS can achieve high rates of vein occlusion, although additional treatments are more likely to be necessary than with other modalities. A recent meta-analysis reported 1-year technical success rates of 81% after UGFS, 88% following RFA, and 93% after endovenous laser ablation. However, with the latest segmental RFA catheters and radial 1,470 nm laser fibers, 1-year occlusion rates approaching 100% have been reported.

14 Flow Chart Summarizing Role of Endovenous Treatment

References

1. Bergan JJ, Schmid-Schonbein GW, Coleridge Smith PD, Nicolaides AN, Boisseau MR, Eklof B. Mechanisms of disease: chronic venous disease. N Engl J Med. 2006;355:488–98.
2. van den Bos R, Arends L, Kochaert M, Neumann M, Nijsten T. Endovenous therapies of lower extremity varicosities: a meta-analysis. J Vasc Surg. 2009;49:230–9.
3. Min RJ, Khilnani N, Zimmet SE. Endovenous laser treatment of saphenous vein reflux: long-term results. J Vasc Interv Radiol. 2003;14:991–6.
4. Merchant RF, Pichot O, Closure Study Group. Long-term outcomes of endovenous radiofrequency obliteration of saphenous reflux as a treatment for superficial venous insufficiency. J Vasc Surg. 2005;42:502–9.
5. Breu FX, Guggenbichler S, Wollmann JC. 2nd European Consensus Meeting on Foam Sclerotherapy 2006. Vasa. 2008;S/71:3–29.
6. Gohel MS, Davies AH. Radiofrequency ablation for uncomplicated varicose veins. Phlebology. 2009;24 Suppl 1:42–9.

Chapter 32
Arteriovenous Grafts: Stenosis, Thrombosis and Aneurysms

Robyn A. Macsata, Allison C. Nauta, and Anton N. Sidawy

1 Anatomy

1.1 Arterial (Fig. 32.1)

The arterial supply of the upper extremity begins at the aortic arch; the right subclavian artery originates from the innominate (brachio-cephalic) artery, while the left subclavian artery originates directly from the aortic arch. After crossing the first rib, the subclavian becomes the axillary artery; after crossing the lower border of the teres major, it becomes the brachial artery. In the antecubital fossa, the brachial artery bifurcates into the radial and ulnar arteries. The radial artery courses laterally in the forearm and then posterior at the wrist to the anatomical snuffbox where it forms the major branches of the deep palmar arch and communicates with the deep branches of the ulnar artery. The ulnar artery courses medially in the forearm to the

R.A. Macsata, M.D., F.A.C.S.
Department of Surgery, Veterans Affairs Medical Center, Washington, DC, USA

A.C. Nauta, M.D.
Georgetown University School of Medicine, Washington, DC, USA

A.N. Sidawy, M.D., M.P.H.(✉)
Georgetown University Medical Center, 50 Irving St., NW (2A155),
Washington, DC 20422, USA
e-mail: ansidawy@aol.com

A. Kumar and K. Ouriel (eds.), *Handbook of Endovascular Interventions*,   441
DOI 10.1007/978-1-4614-5013-9_32,
© Springer Science+Business Media New York 2013

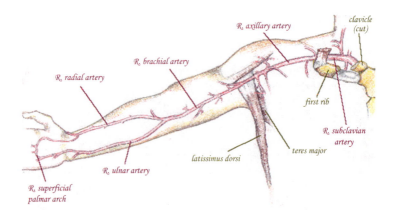

Fig. 32.1 Arterial anatomy of the upper extremity

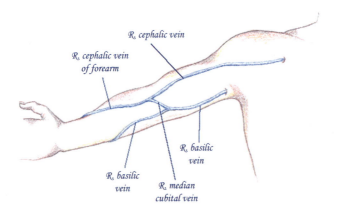

Fig. 32.2 Superficial venous anatomy of the upper extremity

wrist, where it forms the major branches of the superficial palmar arch and communicates with the superficial branches of the radial artery.

1.2 Venous (Fig. 32.2)

Superficial

The superficial venous system consists of the cephalic vein, which runs laterally from the wrist to its insertion into the axillary vein, and

the basilic vein, which runs posterior and medial throughout the forearm crossing anterior to the antecubital fossa to its insertion into the axillary vein.
Deep

The deep venous system usually is paired and courses parallel to the arteries; it consists of the superficial and deep palmar arch, which form to produce the radial and ulnar veins, which combine to produce the brachial followed by the axillary and subclavian vein. The main variation from arterial anatomy is proximal; both the right and left subclavian vein combine with their respective internal jugular veins, to form both a right and left innominate (brachiocephalic) vein; the right and left innominate vein combine to form the superior vena cava.

2   Disease Definition

The National Kidney Foundation-Dialysis Outcomes Initiative (NKF-KDOQI) recommends that patients be referred to a vascular access surgeon for permanent dialysis access when their creatinine clearance is less than 25 mL/min.

3   Disease Distribution

In 2005, data from the U.S. Renal Data System (USRDS) showed more than 106,000 new patients began therapy for end-stage renal disease (ESRD) while the prevalent dialysis population reached 341,000. Total Medicare costs for ESRD patients neared $20 billion; this accounts for 6% of the total Medicare spending in 2005.

4   Classification of Treatment Modalities

4.1   Dialysis Catheters

Short-term dialysis catheters are double lumen noncuffed nontunneled catheters that are placed at beside without fluoroscopic guidance; these catheters are placed in patients needing acute dialysis access and are used for less than 3 weeks duration. *Long-term dialysis catheters* are double lumen cuffed tunneled catheters that are placed with fluoroscopic guidance; these catheters are placed in patients needing long-term dialysis access usually while awaiting permanent arteriovenous (AV) access and are intended to be used over weeks to month's duration. Both short- or long-term dialysis catheters may be placed in the internal jugular, subclavian, or femoral veins; for highest flow and lowest complications, the right internal jugular approach with the catheter tip just above the atrial-caval junction is preferred. To decrease the risk of central venous stenosis and subsequent venous hypertension, the subclavian approach is avoided if at all possible.

4.2   Autogenous Arteriovenous (AV) Access

Autogenous AV access, previously referred to as an AV fistula, is formed with a direct anastomosis between an artery and a superficial vein; after the AV access matures, the venous outflow tract is used for cannulation during dialysis sessions. A direct configuration is used when the venous outflow tract is already superficial and easily accessible, as seen with the cephalic vein; a transposed configuration is used when the venous outflow tract is deep or not easily accessible, as seen with the basilic vein; a translocated configuration is used when the venous outflow tract is relocated entirely, as seen with the greater saphenous vein.

Autogenous AV access has consistently been shown to have excellent patency rates when compared to prosthetic AV access as well as fewer complications related to infection, pseudoaneurysms, and seromas; therefore, autogenous AV access is always preferred to prosthetic AV access. With these benefits, the drawbacks of autogenous AV access, including longer maturation times and failure of maturation, are felt to be acceptable.

4.3   Prosthetic Arteriovenous (AV) Access

Prosthetic AV access, previously referred to as an AV graft, is formed with prosthetic material placed between an artery and a superficial or deep vein; after the AV access matures, the prosthetic material is used for cannulation during dialysis sessions. A straight configuration is used when the artery is located distal to the venous outflow tract, as seen with the brachial artery and axillary vein; a loop configuration is used when the artery is located adjacent to the venous outflow tract, as seen with the brachial artery and antecubital vein.

5   Preoperative Evaluation

5.1   History and Physical Examination

A thorough patient history is taken documenting patient's dominant extremity, recent history of peripheral and central venous lines including pacemakers and defibrillators, any history of trauma or previous surgeries to the extremity, and all previous AV access procedures. On physical examination, a full pulse examination of the bilateral brachial, radial, and ulnar arteries including modified Allen's test is performed. The superficial venous system is evaluated with and without a pressure tourniquet in place, examining for distensibility and interruptions; to evaluate the deep venous system, any prominent venous collaterals or extremity edema is noted.

5.1.1   Modified Allen's Test

The patient is instructed to clench his/her fist. Then using one's fingers, apply occlusive pressure to the ulnar and radial arteries of the patient at the wrist. This maneuver will obstruct the blood flow to the hand and should lead to a blanching of the hand. If this does not happen then one has not completely occluded the arteries with the fingers. Once complete occlusion has been achieved, release the pressure on the ulnar artery. This should lead to a flushing of the hand within 5–15 s.

5.1.2   Results

Positive Modified Allen's test: Normal flushing of the hand.
Negative Modified Allen's test: Failure of normal flushing within the
  expected time. This is reflective of the lack of adequate circulation

by the ulnar artery alone and thus the radial artery should *not* be accessed.

The overall utility of the Allen's test is questionable

5.2   Arterial Assessment

If any abnormality is noted on the clinical arterial examination, the patient is further evaluated with segmental pressures and arterial duplex. If any pressure gradient is noted between the bilateral upper extremities or arterial diameter is less than 2.5 mm, the patient is further evaluated with an arteriogram; any inflow abnormalities are treated with angioplasty and/or stent placement or open surgical methods.

5.3   Venous Assessment

If any abnormality is noted on the superficial venous exam, the patient is further evaluated with superficial venous duplex; only veins with diameter greater than 2.5 mm that are noted to be distensible and continuous are used for autogenous AV access. If any abnormality is noted on the central venous exam, the patient is further evaluated with deep venous duplex followed by venogram if more information is needed; any venous outflow abnormalities are treated with angioplasty and/or stent placement or open surgical methods.

6   Operative Choices

Table 32.1 lists the various types of autogenous and prosthetic AV accesses available in the upper and lower extremities and body wall. When planning AV access, a few general principles apply.

1. Upper extremity access sites are used first, with the nondominant arm given preference over the dominant arm.
2. AV accesses are placed as far distally in the extremity as possible.

Table 32.1 Arteriovenous access configuration

Upper Extremity

Forearm

1. Autogenous
   (a) Autogenous posterior radial branch-cephalic wrist direct access (Snuff-box Fistula)
   (b) Autogenous radial-cephalic wrist direct access (Brescia-Cimino-Appel Fistula)
   (c) Autogenous radial-cephalic forearm transposition
   (d) Autogenous brachial (or proximal radial)-cephalic forearm looped transposition
   (e) Autogenous radial-basilic forearm transposition
   (f) Autogenous ulnar-basilic forearm transposition
   (g) Autogenous brachial (or proximal radial)-basilic forearm looped transposition
   (h) Autogenous radial-antecubital forearm indirect greater saphenous vein translocation
   (i) Autogenous brachial (or proximal radial)-antecubital forearm indirect looped greater saphenous vein translocation
   (j) Autogenous radial-antecubital forearm indirect femoral vein translocation
   (k) Autogenous brachial (or proximal radial)-antecubital forearm indirect looped femoral vein translocation
2. Prosthetic
   (a) Prosthetic radial-antecubital forearm straight access
   (b) Prosthetic brachial (or proximal radial)-antecubital forearm looped access

Upper Arm

1. Autogenous
   (a) Autogenous brachial (or proximal radial)-cephalic upper arm direct access
   (b) Autogenous brachial (or proximal radial)-cephalic upper arm transposition
   (c) Autogenous brachial (or proximal radial)-basilic upper arm transposition
   (d) Autogenous brachial (or proximal radial)-brachial vein upper arm transposition
   (e) Autogenous brachial (or proximal radial)-axillary (or brachial) upper arm indirect greater saphenous vein translocation
   (f) Autogenous brachial (or proximal radial)-axillary (or brachial) upper arm indirect femoral vein translocation

Lower Extremity

1. Autogenous
   (a) Autogenous femoral-greater saphenous lower extremity (straight or looped) transposition

(continued)

Table 32.1 (continued)

   (b) Autogenous tibial (anterior or posterior)-greater saphenous lower
        extremity direct access
   (c) Autogenous femoral–femoral (vein) lower extremity (straight or looped)
        transposition
2. Prosthetic
   (a) Prosthetic femoral-femoral (vein) lower extremity looped access
Body Wall
1. Prosthetic
   (a) Prosthetic axillary-axillary (vein) chest (straight or looped) access
   (b) Prosthetic axillary-internal jugular chest looped access
   (c) Prosthetic axillary-femoral (vein) body wall access

(Adapted from Sidawy AN et al. Recommended standards for reports dealing
with arteriovenous hemodialysis accesses. *JVS.* 2002;35:603-610)

3. Autogenous AV access is always preferred to prosthetic AV
   access.
4. Autogenous AV access configurations order of preference is direct
   anastomosis, venous transpositions, followed by venous
   translocations.

7   Surveillance

Postoperatively, the AV access is followed by clinical examination
until maturation; from the time of access placement, autogenous AV
access should be mature and ready for cannulation by 12 weeks and
prosthetic AV access should be mature and ready for cannulation by
as early as 2 weeks. After initial maturation, the AV access is monitored routinely while on dialysis, with physical examination and
monthly determinations of access flow. If any access is noted to be
failing, it is further examined with duplex followed by fistulogram if
more information is needed. Thrombosed accesses are diagnosed by
clinical exam; this may be confirmed by duplex.

8 Management Paradigm (Fig. 32.3)

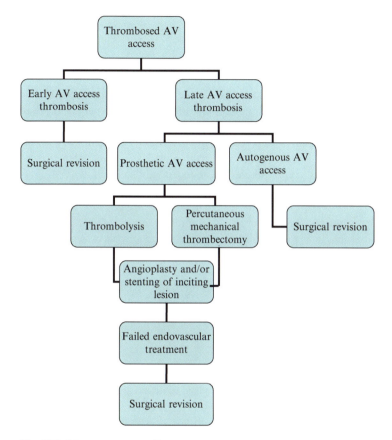

Fig. 32.3 Management paragdigm

8.1 Failed/Thrombosed Access

8.1.1 Early AV Access Failure

Early access thrombosis occurs within 30 days of surgery and is due to a technical failure; it is most commonly associated with inadequate venous outflow, which may be secondary to inadequate caliber of the outflow vein or central venous stenosis. Other less common causes include poor arterial inflow and anastomotic stenosis. Endovascular or open surgical means of thrombolysis or thrombectomy rarely work; surgical revision is required.

8.1.2   Late AV Access Failure

Late access thrombosis usually occurs 1–2 years after access placement and is most commonly due to intimal hyperplasia. In an autogenous access, this occurs anywhere in the outflow tract; in a prosthetic access, this occurs at the graft venous anastomosis. A second common cause of late access thrombosis is central venous stenosis due to intimal hyperplasia associated with central lines.

Endovascular or open surgical means of thrombolysis or thrombectomy rarely work with an autogenous AV access; surgical revision is required. Endovascular thrombolysis or thrombectomies are attempted in prosthetic AV access if thrombosis has occurred within 14 days of presentation; both techniques are followed by a fistulogram and repair of the inciting venous stenosis with angioplasty and/or stent placement to prevent recurrent thrombosis. If endovascular means fail, open surgical thrombectomy and revision is required.

8.2   Failing Access

Similar to failed access, failing accesses are due to either intimal hyperplasia in the venous outflow tract or the central venous system. If a focal venous stenosis is identified, it is treated with angioplasty and/or stent placement; if endovascular treatment fails or a long-segment stenosis is identified, surgical revision is required.

8.3   Intervention

Thrombolysis

1. Cross catheters technique (Fig. 32.4)

   (a) Using a single wall puncture technique, a 6-Fr sheath is placed in arterial end directed towards venous end.
   (b) A venogram is performed to assure graft is salvageable.

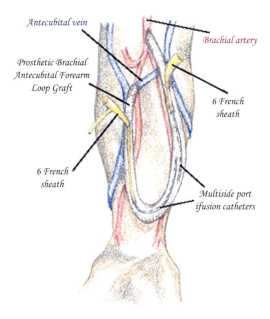

Fig. 32.4 Cross catheter thrombolysis technique

(c) Using a single wall puncture technique, a second 6-Fr sheath is placed in venous end directed toward arterial end.

(d) 0.035-inch hydrophilic wire is fed into the arterial sheath and guided into the venous outflow of the access.

(e) 0.035-inch hydrophilic wire is fed into the venous sheath and guided into the arterial inflow of the access.

(f) Multi-side port infusion catheters are fed over the hydrophilic wires and left in thrombosed portion of av access.

(g) 100,000 IU to 750,000 IU of urokinase mixed with 70 IU/kg of heparin is administered via infusion catheters using pulse-spray technique (12,500 IU urokinase/20 s).

(h) Balloon angioplasty (4–6 mm balloon) is performed to macerate any residual thrombi.

(i) A completion fistulogram/venogram is performed.

(j) Balloon angioplasty (6–10 mm balloon) is performed to treat any underlying stenosis.

(k) Recoil is treated with repeat angioplasty with prolonged balloon inflation (5–10 min) or use of a cutting balloon.

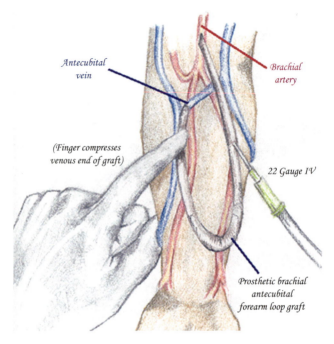

Fig. 32.5 Lyse-and-wait thrombolysis technique

    (l) Stents are reserved for residual stenosis >30% after all angio-
        plasty techniques have failed.

    (m) Sheaths are left in place and used for immediate postproce-
        dure dialysis.

2. Lyse-and-wait technique (Fig. 32.5)

    (a) In peri-operative holding, a 22-gauge IV catheter is placed in
        arterial end directed toward venous end.

    (b) 250,000 IU of urokinase mixed with 70 IU/kg of heparin is
        administered through the IV catheter over 2 min while arterial
        and venous ends of access are compressed.

    (c) Pt is taken to operating room after 30–90 min of waiting.

    (d) The 22-gauge IV is exchanged for a 6-Fr sheath which is
        directed toward the venous end.

    (e) Using a single-wall puncture technique, a second 6-Fr sheath
        is placed in venous end directed toward arterial end.

    (f) A completion fistulogram/venogram is performed.

    (g) Balloon angioplasty (6–10 mm balloon) is performed to treat any underlying stenosis.

    (h) Recoil is treated with repeat angioplasty with prolonged balloon inflation (5–10 min) or use of a cutting balloon.

    (i) Stents are reserved for residual stenosis >30% after all angioplasty techniques have failed.

    (j) Sheaths are left in place and used for immediate postprocedure dialysis.

Percutaneous Mechanical Thrombectomy (PMT)

1. Using a single-wall puncture technique, a 6-Fr sheath is placed in arterial end directed at venous end.
2. A venogram is performed to assure access is salvageable.
3. 70 IU/kg of heparin is administered through IV.
4. Venous end is treated with PMT; multiple devices are available.

    (a) AngioJet rheolytic catheter (Possis Medical, Inc.)

    (b) Arrow-Trerotola device (Arrow International)

    (c) Amplatz percutaneous rotational device (Microvena Corp.)

    (d) Trellis catheter (Bacchus Vascular Inc.)

5. Using a single wall puncture technique, a 6-Fr sheath is placed in venous end directed at arterial end.
6. Arterial end is treated with PMT.
7. A completion fistulogram/venogram is performed.
8. Balloon angioplasty (6–10 mm balloon) is performed to treat any underlying stenosis.
9. Recoil is treated with repeat angioplasty with prolonged balloon inflation (5–10 min) or use of a cutting balloon.
10. Stents are reserved for reserved for residual stenosis >30% after all angioplasty techniques have failed.
11. Sheaths are left in place and used for immediate postprocedure dialysis.

9 Postprocedure Management and Follow-up

After percutaneous intervention, the AV access is again monitored routinely while on dialysis, with physical examination and monthly determinations of access flow.

10 Complications and Management

10.1 Pulmonary Embolism

Symptomatic pulmonary embolism is seen rarely after endovascular thrombolysis/thrombectomy; however, asymptomatic pulmonary embolism, documented by nuclear medicine perfusion scans, is reported as high as in 70% of patients undergoing this procedure; patients likely remain asymptomatic due to the small size of the emboli; however, the ultimate fate of these pulmonary insults is largely unknown. Prevention and treatment are similar, infusion of IV or intragraft heparin.

10.2 Arterial Embolism

Arterial embolism may occur to the main arterial trunk, presenting as acute limb threatening ischemia, or distally, presenting as trashed or painful digits. Similar to pulmonary embolism, arterial embolism may be prevented with infusion of IV or intragraft heparin. Limb-threatening ischemia is treated immediately with endovascular techniques, such as thrombolysis or PMT; if endovascular intervention fails, open surgical repair is required. Trashed or painful digits are clinically monitored and usually resolve over several weeks time.

10.3 Vessel Rupture

Due to repeated high-pressure balloon angioplasties, the anastomoses or native vessels may rupture; this is treated with immediate covered stent placement, if endovascular intervention fails, open surgical repair is required.

11 Outcomes

Primary technical success rates have been reported as high as 96% for all methods of endovascular thrombolysis/thrombectomy; however, 6-month primary patency rates are 32%, 41%, and 31% after a 1st,

2nd, and 3rd procedure, respectively. Given these patency rates, in particular with forearm prosthetic AV access, placement of new autogenous AV access should be considered to avoid multiple repeat thrombolysis/thrombectomies procedures, which may lead to damage of the outflow vein and inability to place upper arm autogenous AV access.

References

1. http://www.kidney.org/professionals/KDOQI/guidelines.cfm
2. Sidawy AN, et al. Recommended standards for reports dealing with arteriovenous hemodialysis accesses. J Vasc Surg. 2002;35:603–10.
3. Sidawy AN, et al. The Society for Vascular Surgery: Clinical practice guidelines for the surgical placement and maintenance of arteriovenous hemodialysis access. J Vasc Surg. 2008;48(S):2–25.
4. Padberg FT, et al. Complications of arteriovenous hemodialysis access: recognition and management. J Vas Surg. 2008;48(S):55–80.
5. Mansilla AV, et al. Patency and life-spans of failing hemodialysis grafts in patients undergoing repeated percutaneous de-clotting. Tex Heart Inst J. 2001;28(4):249–53.
6. Kinney TB, et al. Pulmonary embolism from pulse-spray pharmacomechanical thrombolysis of clotted hemodialysis grafts: Urokinase versus Heparinized saline. JVIR. 2000;11(9):1143–52.

Chapter 33
Uterine Fibroid Embolization

Justin S. Lee and James B. Spies

1 Introduction

Uterine artery embolization has three major indications:

1. Management of uncontrolled postpartum hemorrhage
2. Prophylactic embolization of larger uterine tumors prior to surgical resection
3. Primary treatment of uterine leiomyomata.

The first description of UAE was in 1979 [1] for the management of uncontrollable postpartum hemorrhage. UAE as an alternative to hysterectomy is an efficacious and minimally invasive treatment of massive postpartum hemorrhage with few complications [2]. UAE offers an advantage over hysterectomy by preserving the uterus for future fertility.

UAE has been utilized in the preoperative setting to reduce arterial flow prior to hysterectomy for patients with large uterine or pelvic tumors in an effort to control operative blood loss.

The most common indication for UAE is the treatment of symptomatic uterine fibroids. The first report of uterine fibroid embolization (UFE) was in 1995 by Ravina et al. [3]. Several comparative

J.S. Lee, M.D. • J.B. Spies, M.D., M.P.H. (✉)
Department of Radiology, Georgetown University School of Medicine,
3800 Reservoir Rd. NW, CG 201, Washington, DC 20007-2113, USA
e-mail: jsl108@gunet.georgetown.edu; spiesj@gunet.georgetown.edu

A. Kumar and K. Ouriel (eds.), *Handbook of Endovascular Interventions*, 457
DOI 10.1007/978-1-4614-5013-9_33,
© Springer Science+Business Media New York 2013

randomized trials of UFE versus surgery and a large fibroid registry have solidified the procedure as a safe and effective intervention in the management of leiomyomata, which has been endorsed by the American College of Obstetricians and Gynecologists [4–7].

2 Anatomy

(a) *Arterial anatomy*

   1. Classically, the uterine artery is described as a medial branch of the anterior division of the internal iliac artery. The anterior division supplies the obturator, umbilical, vesicle, uterine, vaginal, middle rectal, and inferior gluteal arteries, and the posterior division gives rise to the iliolumbar, lateral sacral, and the superior gluteal arteries. The uterine artery is generally the first branch of the inferior gluteal artery. Commonly, the origin of the uterine artery can arise from a genitourinary trunk sharing an origin with the vaginal and middle rectal branches. The origin of a common trunk is generally just beyond the superior and inferior gluteal bifurcation. A significant degree of variation may exist.
   2. The uterine artery is described as having a "U-shaped" course that travels medially into the pelvis. In general, the artery is enlarged in patients with significant fibroids and large pelvic malignancies. In the case of hemorrhage, the vessel may be quite thin due to hypovolemia-related vasospasm. Occasionally, the vessel may be hypoplastic or absent on one side with an enlarged contralateral branch. If hypoplasia or absence is present on one or both sides, usually there is associated hypertrophy of other arteries supplying the pelvis and adnexa, primarily the ovarian arteries.

(b) *Uterine anatomy*

   1. Uterine leiomyomas are classified by their location within the myometrium as submucosal, intramural, and subserosal. Intramural and submucosal fibroids tend to be responsible for bleeding symptoms, while subserosal fibroids become symptomatic due to mass effect on adjacent pelvic organs. As the number and size of the fibroids increase, they cause uterine

enlargement, resulting in abdominal wall distortion, pelvic pressure, and discomfort as well as lower urinary tract symptoms.

2. A subtype of fibroid is the pedunculated fibroid, which can be submucosal, or subserosal. Pedunculated fibroids extend from the myometrium attached by a stalk that may be thick or narrow. Submucosal pedunculated fibroids protrude into the endometrial canal while subserosal fibroids may project into the abdomen or pelvis.

3   Disease Definition

(a) *Postpartum hemorrhage*:

1. Postpartum hemorrhage can be defined as primary or secondary. Primary postpartum hemorrhage occurs within the first 24 h following delivery and is usually a result of vaginal, cervical or uterine tears and/or uterine atony. Secondary postpartum hemorrhage occurs 24 h to 6 weeks after delivery and is usually due to retain placental fragments.

2. Embolization is considered when conservative measures including uterotonic agents such as oxytocin and uterine packing have failed.

(b) *Preoperative embolization*:

1. Preoperative embolization prior to hysterectomy or pelvic surgery is performed at the discretion of the gynecologist. Generally, it is considered in larger tumors when the potential for high-volume blood loss exists. Embolization alone is never a treatment for malignancy.

(c) *Uterine Fibroids*:
Uterine fibroids or more formally, leiomyomas are the most common benign neoplasm of women, affecting 30% of women in their premenopausal years. Fibroid growth is linked to estrogen, progesterone, and a number of growth factors. Fibroids will eventually regress in menopause, they commonly cause symptoms requiring intervention prior to menopause. Several hormonal medical therapies exist but are limited in widespread use due to

poor side-effect profiles. Typical indications for intervention are as follows:

1. *Heavy menstrual bleeding*: Heavy menstrual bleeding or menorrhagia is caused by intramural and submucosal fibroids tendency to distort the endometrial cavity. Submucosal fibroids grow into the endometrial cavity and also cause interperiod (metrorrhagia) bleeding. Serosal fibroids and smaller intramural fibroids rarely cause menorrhagia because they do not distort the endometrial cavity. Patients who present with complaints of heavy bleeding with serosal fibroids should be evaluated for other causes of bleeding such as adenomyosis, endometrial polyps, or bleeding diatheses.

2. *Pelvic Pressure*: Pelvic pressure is the most common bulk symptom. Patients may describe heaviness or bloating that is particularly worse around menstruation.

3. *Pelvic pain*: Pelvic pain is often cramping or low-grade pain. Occasionally shooting or severe pain may be described. If severe pain is the predominant symptom, other etiologies should be considered such as endometriosis. When evaluating pain symptoms, fibroid distribution should be considered. If a patient complains of pain in a particular spot, this should be correlated with the MRI or ultrasound. If fibroid distribution does not correspond to the pain location, other causes should be evaluated.

4. *Urinary symptoms*: Fibroids commonly compress the urinary bladder and contribute to many urinary problems. Urinary symptoms such as urgency, frequency, incontinence, retention, and hydronephrosis are related to the mass effect of large fibroids. Incontinence is a less frequent symptom and often multifactorial. Urinary retention is the least frequent presenting symptom. Embolization may exacerbate retention requiring urinary catheter placement. Hydronephrosis is caused by a significantly enlarged fibroid uterus and is often incidentally found during the work-up. Follow-up renal ultrasound 4–6 weeks following embolization should be performed to ensure resolution.

4 Diagnosis: Clinical and Laboratory

Success with uterine artery embolization depends on complete history, appropriate physical examination and relevant imaging. Failure to adequately evaluate a patient may lead to ineffective or inappropriate embolization delaying definitive treatment.

(a) *Clinical Evaluation*

1. *Postpartum hemorrhage*: Determine the cause of hemorrhage. Is it primary or secondary? Did the patient undergo vaginal delivery or c-section? Does the obstetrician suspect a site of bleeding? What measures have been performed to control bleeding? Hemodynamic stability, transfusion requirements, correction of coagulopathies, and patient counseling/consent are important components of the evaluation.

2. *Preoperative embolization*: Discussion with the surgeon is necessary to plan the timing of embolization and to gain an understanding regarding the planned surgery. A careful evaluation of the preoperative imaging is required to evaluate potential collateral blood flow that may need to be investigated and embolized.

3. *Uterine Fibroid Embolization*: A thorough gynecologic history should be obtained. The patient should have had a gynecologic examination by a gynecologist within 1 year of the consultation. Confirming that the primary symptom can be attributed to the patient's fibroids is essential. An assessment of uterine size in weeks is helpful in comparison to the imaging findings.

(b) *Laboratory evaluation*:

1. For fibroid patients, a current PAP smear should be normal. Endometrial biopsy should be considered with prolonged menstrual bleeding (menstrual periods greater than 10 days) or when menstrual cycles occur more frequently than every 21 days. In these circumstances, endometrial abnormalities increase in likelihood.

2. Complete blood count, serum electrolytes and a urine or serum pregnancy test should routinely be performed. In the case of postpartum hemorrhage, the pregnancy test will be positive.

3. A coagulation panel is not routinely performed except in patients with a history of coagulopathy or those on anticoagulation medication. Postpartum patients with large transfusion requirements should have coagulation parameters evaluated and corrected if possible.

(c) *Imaging Evaluation*

1. Postpartum hemorrhage patients do not require preprocedural imaging except in rare circumstances. Secondary or delayed postpartum hemorrhage patients may have imaging such as a CT or ultrasound, which may identify highly vascular residual placental tissue, but in general, obtaining imaging may delay definitive treatment.

2. Preoperative embolization of pelvic neoplasms should always have some form of imaging to evaluate the uterus and adnexa. Cross-sectional imaging such as MRI or contrast enhanced CT is helpful to evaluate for potential collateral vessels supplying the tumor. It is not rare for a pelvic tumor to recruit branches of the inferior mesenteric artery.

3. UFE patients must have preprocedural imaging. Contrast enhanced MRI is preferred to allow accurate assessment of fibroid burden, size, and location. Contrast enhancement is crucial to demonstrate viability of fibroids as unenhanced fibroids are already devascularized and will not respond to embolization. MRI is also useful to detect other abnormalities that may contribute to symptoms such as adenomyosis and endometriosis. Transabdominal and transvaginal ultrasound may be substituted for an MRI if one cannot be obtained, realizing that ultrasound lacks the same degree of accuracy in fibroid evaluation, particularly in assessing fibroid perfusion. Ultrasound is excellent to identify endometrial abnormalities particularly when performed as a sonohysterogram.

5 Management/Preprocedural Preparation

(a) *Postpartum hemorrhage*: Assessment of the appropriateness of embolization cannot be made without prompt patient evaluation. Evaluation of measures already performed should be completed prior to angiography to determine if steps such as uterine artery ligation were already attempted. The hemodynamic stability of the patient should be assessed as well as an evaluation of the coagulation status. Patients who have received multiple transfusions may need further correction of their coagulation factors. If the patient is hemodynamically compromised, adequate venous access should be obtained prior to arterial access, which can be performed in the angiography suite. Patients with hemodynamic compromise should be evaluated for renal insufficiency secondary to shock, which is also an indirect measure of the adequacy of resuscitation and will provide an understanding about contrast limitations.

(b) *Preoperative embolization*: A procedure performed on an elective basis prior to surgery has limited evaluation and management steps. Review of the relevant laboratory data and imaging is still critical.

(c) *Uterine fibroid embolization*: The success of the procedure is dependent on a thorough preprocedural consultation. Goals of the consultation are to ensure that the symptoms are adequately explained by fibroids, review the imaging findings, and discuss the expectations and available treatment options. Identifying patients who are the best candidates for embolization requires all of the above components. Patients with a single large dominant fibroid seeking to become pregnant may be a better candidate for myomectomy. Patients with significant adenomyosis and no future plans for fertility may have better symptom resolution with a hysterectomy. Although, UAE may be effective and durable in many patients. Patients wishing to become pregnant with significant distortion of the endometrial cavity may be better suited for myomectomy.

6 Contraindications

(a) *Absolute contraindications*:

1. Pregnancy: every patient should have a urine or serum pregnancy test on the day of the procedure or within a few days prior to the procedure.
2. Suspected Leiomyosarcoma, endometrial, cervical, or ovarian malignancy should be adequately excluded with imaging.

J.S. Lee and J.B. Spies

UFE should never be considered a definitive treatment for malignancy.

(b) *Relative contraindications*:

1. Desire for pregnancy within 2 years: Patients can become pregnant and have term pregnancies, although rates may be lower after UFE compared to myomectomy. Patient should be adequately counseled about the uncertainties regarding fertility rates after UFE [7].
2. Renal insufficiency: The use of iodinated contrast may exacerbate renal insufficiency. Preprocedural hydration, the use of n-acetyl cysteine, and limiting the volume of contrast used are all steps that may be taken to limit the impact on renal function.
3. Allergy to iodinated contrast: patients can be pretreated with corticosteroids to reduce severe allergic reactions.
4. Coagulopathy or anticoagulation use: Postprocedural bleeding risks are similar to surgery. The risks can be reduced with the use of a closure device and performing the procedure through a single arterial puncture.

(c) *Patient preparation*:

1. Patients should be NPO 6 h prior to the procedure.
2. A Foley catheter should be placed prior to the procedure to ensure that excreted contrast in the bladder does not obscure evaluation of the uterus.
3. UFE patients should be given instructions on the use of a patient controlled analgesia pump for postprocedure pain management, and pain management protocols should be clearly delineated to the nursing staff. Preoperative embolization patient should be given a PCA pump if the surgical procedure is not going to occur immediately after embolization.
4. A single dose of prophylactic antibiotics may be given, although no evidence exists that this has any impact on postprocedure infection rates.
5. Conscious sedation using a protocol of fentanyl and midazolam is routinely used during the procedure with a nurse continuously monitoring the patient. However, patients with sleep apnea or potential for airway compromise may need an anesthesia consult for airway management.

7   Operative Alternatives

(a) *Hysterectomy*

  1. UAE for postpartum hemorrhage patients is generally used if the desire for future fertility exists. Hysterectomy remains the gold standard in the treatment of postpartum hemorrhage, although increasingly UAE is becoming a viable first-line alternative.

(b) *Myomectomy*

  1. Myomectomy is a good alternative to hysterectomy for the treatment of uterine fibroids, particularly, when future fertility is the goal and if there are a small number of fibroids present. The procedure may be performed open or laparoscopically. Submucosal fibroids may be removed via a vaginal approach, hysteroscopically. While myomectomy is quite safe with a skilled surgeon, a potential complication is hysterectomy if bleeding cannot be controlled during the procedure. Rarely, embolization may be needed to control postoperative bleeding in a patient after myomectomy.

(c) *High-Frequency Ultrasound*

  1. High-frequency ultrasound (HIFU) is not a surgical option, but rather a completely noninvasive method of treating fibroids. Briefly, a focused ultrasound beam is directed at the fibroid with the guidance of MRI causing heat necrosis of the fibroids. At this time, HIFU is limited in application and can only be used to treat fibroid that is located anteriorly. Usually, HIFU only treats 1 or 2 fibroids and only half the volume of each treated fibroid is ablated. It is currently not covered by most insurance plans.

8   Intervention

(a) *Uterine artery catheterization*

  1. Unilateral or bilateral femoral artery puncture can be performed with placement of a five French sheath in each vessel.

Table 33.1 Imaging system position for optimal visualization

Vessels	View
Internal iliac	Opposite oblique
Uterine artery	Opposite oblique

2. Bilateral puncture allows for visualization of both uterine arteries during arteriography and embolization. The advantage of simultaneous embolization and angiography is a decrease in radiation dose. A less quantitative advantage is the ability to identify a dominant uterine artery allowing for embolization to be concentrated on the side supplying the most flow to fibroids.

3. A pelvic angiogram can be performed prior to selection of the internal iliac arteries (Table 33.1). This is not required and forgoing a pelvic angiogram can reduce radiation dose. However, in cases of pelvic hemorrhage, a routine pelvic or even abdominal aortogram may be warranted to evaluate for collateral vessels supply pelvic structures.

4. A cobra, Rim or a reverse curve catheter such as a Roberts catheter is advanced over the bifurcation and into the contralateral internal iliac artery.

5. From this position using the opposite oblique positioning, a digital roadmap should be performed to identify the uterine artery origin. If the origin is not well identified in the contralateral oblique position, it may be necessary to try a roadmap in the ipsilateral oblique position. Visualization of the uterine artery is critical for successful catheterization.

6. Using a 0.027 microcatheter and microwire, the uterine artery is selected and catheterized. The uterine artery is tortuous and passage of the catheter may take several attempts. Unfortunately, the artery is prone to spasm and care must be taken in its selection. The artery has a "U-shaped" as it turns medially along its course toward the uterus. The microcatheter should be advanced beyond the cervicovaginal branches when possible to reduce the risk of nontarget embolization.

7. Spasm of the vessel can be avoided with careful technique. Spasm may be flow limiting, which can lead to under embolization and a false endpoint. If spasm is encountered intra-arterial nitroglycerin or papavarine may be used. Often the only option is to retract the catheter and wait for the vessel spasm to resolve.

8. If simultaneous bilateral embolization is going to be performed, the above steps are repeated to catheterize the opposite uterine artery. When both vessels are properly selected, angiography of the uterine arteries should be performed simultaneously to assess flow and fibroid distribution. Careful evaluation of the angiogram will help guide the selection of embolic material.

9. If a unilateral approach is used, after successful catheterization of the uterine artery, followed by embolization, a Waltman loop is used to remove the 5 Fr catheter over the aortic bifurcation.

9 Embolic Choice and Technique

(a) The goal of embolization for postpartum hemorrhage is rapid occlusion of the feeding arteries. Most often this can be accomplished with a gelatin sponge slurry which has advantages in that it is quick and considered a temporary agent. Coil embolization is generally not performed because it only provides proximal vessel occlusion. The tendency for collateral vessels in a gravid uterus will make such proximal occlusion inadequate. Particulate embolic material and microspheres should be avoided as it may lead to myometrial injury.

(b) Embolic materials used for preoperative and fibroid embolization should be permanent and be small enough to be carried to the distal circulation. Two well-studied materials are particle PVA (Contour, Boston Scientific; Natick, MA; Ivalon, Cook Inc. Bloomington, IN; others) and Embosphere® Microspheres, Biosphere Medical, Rockland, MA). Spherical PVA (Contour SE, Boston Scientific; Natick, MA) has been shown to be inferior in fibroid infarction and should not be used for UFE. Two newer products, acrylamido PVA hydrogel spheres (Bead Block™, Terumo, Somerset, NJ) and Polyzene F®-coated hydrogel spheres (Embozene™ Microspheres, Celanova Biosciences Inc., Newnan, GA), have not been studied in comparative trials.

(c) In UFE, embolic material is administered in small aliquots using the flow in the uterine vessels to carry the embolic material distally. The goal is <u>not</u> to occlude the entire uterine artery, but to leave it with slow flow or near stasis. Supplemental embolization with coils should not be performed, as this will completely occlude the uterine arteries preventing future embolization if the patient develops new fibroids. Occlusion also causes unnecessary ischemia of the normal myometrium, causing unnecessary pain and increases the risk of tissue injury.

10 Ovarian and Collateral Supply

(a) There is occasionally additional supply to the uterus and fibroids from the ovarian arteries. Although only present in about 5% of patients, this supply can impact outcome. Routine aortography after embolization is low yield but may be performed when there is clearly nonperfused tissue seen on uterine arteriography. An aortogram should be done to determine collateral supply in cases of postpartum hemorrhage and preoperative embolization.

(b) Ovarian embolization in fibroid patients has limited data. Consulting the patient about possible ovarian injury is appropriate prior to proceeding.

(c) Selective catheterization of the ovarian artery is best accomplished with a Mikaelsson catheter (Angiodynamics, Queensbury, NY). A microcatheter should be used and advanced into the vessel about one-third the distance to the ovary to ensure no reflux occurs into the aorta.

(d) Ovarian embolization is performed with particulate or spherical embolic material until the fibroid branches are occluded. Flow is generally very sluggish because of severe spasm typically encountered with ovarian catheterization. Embolization must be done very carefully to avoid reflux into the aorta and distal embolization to the feet.

11 Complications and Management

(a) Fibroid passage is the most common serious complication and presents as severe menstrual cramping, with or without discharge, tissue passage, or heavy bleeding. It may also have a more chronic presentation, with persisting vaginal discharge, often described as watery or clear mucous, which may become superinfected. It occurs most commonly 3 weeks to 6 months after the procedure and most frequently with large intracavitary fibroids or those large fibroids with a large submucosal interface.

1. Diagnosis is made by vaginal exam with either tissue in vagina or a dilated cervical canal with visible prolapsing tissue. Pelvic MRI examination will show tissue descending in the endometrial cavity, pointing to the cervix with occasional dilation of the internal cervical os. Advanced passage presents with tissue extending from the endometrial cavity into the vagina.
2. Fibroid passage can be managed conservatively but is the most common complication that requires reintervention, usually a D&C/hysteroscopic resection or manual extraction of the fibroid. If the fibroid cannot be extracted, hysterectomy may be required.
3. Fibroid passage with an open cervical os may result in superinfection requiring antibiotics.

(b) Pulmonary embolus

1. Most common life-threatening complication, with an incidence of 1 in 400.
2. Transient hypercoagulability occurs after UFE.
3. Use of intermittent pneumatic compression devices may reduce the risk. For high-risk patients, low molecular weight heparin prophylaxis should be considered.

(c) Missembolization

1. Missembolization occurs when embolic material is inadvertently administered or refluxes down a nontarget artery. Injury to other organs (other than the ovaries) or the skin necrosis can occur very rarely, likely less than 1 in 1,000 for experienced interventionalists.
2. Management is usually conservative, with local care of skin injuries. Bladder injuries may require urologic evaluation and occasionally intervention.

(d) Myometrial injury

1. Myometrial injury is very rare, about 1 in 500. Diagnosis should be suspected when pain is persisting and not improving after 4–5 days postembolization or when pain is severe

      enough to require readmission. Contrast-enhanced MRI will show nonenhancing area of myometrium.

    2. Management of this type of injury is conservative, with pain management. Severe uterine injury may require hysterectomy.

(e) Ovarian failure

    1. Ovarian failure after uterine embolization and is age dependent. Approximately 5% of women over 45 may have temporary or permanent amenorrhea after UFE. At age 40, the likelihood is closer to 1%.

    2. Management is conservative. Some women that become amenorrheic after UFE regain their menstrual cycles several months after embolization.

12 Outcomes

(a) Short-term outcomes

    1. For both menorrhagia and bulk-related symptoms (pain, pressure, and urinary symptoms) are improved in between 80 and 95% of patients, depending on the study reviewed [4–8].

(b) Reintervention is needed in approximately 5–10% of patients the first year due to lack of symptom improvement.

(c) UFE has been demonstrated to be effective compared to surgery in randomized trials at 24 months after treatment (2–4).

(d) There are insufficient data to determine whether myomectomy or UFE is better for women seeking to become pregnant. Results from one comparative trial suggest that there are better outcomes with myomectomy for those seeking pregnancy within 2 years of the procedure [9].

References

1. Brown BJ, Heaston DK, Poulson AM et al. Uncontrollable postpartum bleeding: A new approach to hemostasis through angiographic arterial embolization Obstet Gynecol. 1979;54:361–65.
2. Salazar GM, Petrozza JC, Walker TG. Transcatheter endovascular techniques for management of obstetrical and gynecologic emergencies. Tech Vasc Interv Radiol. 2009 Jun;12(2):139–47.

3. Ravina J, Herbreteau D, Ciraru-Vigneron N, Bouret J, Houdart E, Aymard A, et al. Arterial embolisation to treat uterine myomata. Lancet. 1995; 346:671–2.
4. Edwards RD, Moss JG, Lumsden MA, Wu O, Murray LS, Twaddle S, et al. Uterine-artery embolization versus surgery for symptomatic uterine fibroids. N Engl J Med. 2007;356:360–70.
5. Hehenkamp WJ, Volkers NA, Birnie E, Reekers JA, Ankum WM. Symptomatic uterine fibroids: treatment with uterine artery embolization or hysterectomy– results from the randomized clinical Embolisation versus Hysterectomy (EMMY) Trial. Radiology. 2008;246:823–32.
6. Mara M, Maskova J, Fucikova Z, Kuzel D, Belsan T, Sosna O. Midterm clinical and first reproductive results of a randomized controlled trial comparing uterine fibroid embolization and myomectomy. Cardiovasc Intervent Radiol. 2008;31:73–85.
7. Committee on Gynecologic Practice, American College of Obstetricians and Gynecologists. ACOG Committee Opinion. Uterine artery embolization. Obstet Gynecol. 2004 Feb;103(2):403–4.
8. Goodwin SC, Spies JB, Worthington-Kirsch R, Peterson E, Pron G, Li S, et al. Uterine artery embolization for treatment of leiomyomata: long-term outcomes from the FIBROID Registry. Obstetrics Gynecol. 2008;111:22–33.
9. Pinto I, Chimeno P, Romo A, Paul L, Haya J, de la Cal M, et al. Uterine Fibroids: Uterine artery embolization versus abdominal hysterectomy for treatment of symptomatic uterine fibroids: a prospective randomized, and controlled clinical trial. Radiology. 2003;226:425–31.

Chapter 34
Intracranial Arteriovenous Malformations

David Fiorella and Wendy Gaza

1 Anatomy

Arteriovenous malformations (AVMs) are an abnormal conglomeration of arteries and veins, which share a direct communication through a "nidus" of small irregular and friable blood vessels without an intervening capillary bed. The nidus is the anatomical convergence point of the inflow of multiple feeding arteries and outflow into one or more dilated draining veins. Anatomic variations can range from a predominantly fistulous malformation (with few sources of inflow which directly transition to one or more venous recipients for outflow) to those with a large and complex nidus (with multiple arterial feeders transitioning through an anatomically extensive nidus that empties into multiple draining veins).

D. Fiorella, M.D., Ph.D. (✉)
Department of Neurological Surgery, Cerebrovascular Center, Stony Brook
University Hospital, HSC T-12, Room 080, Stony Brook, NY 11794, USA
e-mail: David.fiorella@stonybrook.edu; dfiorell@gmail.com

W. Gaza, M.D.
Stony Brook University Hospital, Stony Brook, NY, USA

A. Kumar and K. Ouriel (eds.), *Handbook of Endovascular Interventions*,   473
DOI 10.1007/978-1-4614-5013-9_34,
© Springer Science+Business Media New York 2013

2 Disease Definition

AVMs are believed to be congenital lesions that can be found throughout the circulatory system. As AVMs grow, the feeding arteries and draining veins become hypertrophied. The fragility of these vessels can predispose them to hemorrhage. Flow-related aneurysms can also develop and lead to an increased risk of hemorrhage. Approximately 4–17 of AVMs are associated with aneurysms either involving the feeding arteries proximal to the AVM nidus or within the nidus itself. In general, AVMs pose an estimated 2–4 risk of hemorrhage per year. In AVMs that have already caused symptomatic hemorrhage, the rehemorrhage risk is roughly 6–18 during the first year and returns back to the baseline risk in the following 1–2 years. Other manifestations of AVMs include seizures, focal neurologic deficit, and headaches.

3 Disease Distribution

AVMs are uncommon lesions with a prevalence of 1.4–3.4 . Most frequently, patients present between the ages of 20–40, and children are rarely symptomatic. A majority of intracranial AVMs are supratentorial involving the surface and deep structure but can also be found in the cerebellum and brainstem. AVMs located in vascular border zones may contain arterial supply from multiple cerebral arterial branches. Additionally, adjacent dural structures can provide collaterals.

4 Classification

The Spetzler-Martin Grading Scale (Table 34.1) is a system utilized to estimate the risk of surgical intervention. There is a low operative morbidity and mortality for Grade I and Grade II AVMs estimated at <1 . Grade III AVMs are associated with a <3 operative risk, and in Grade IV and Grade V AVMs, the surgical risk significantly rises to approximately 31 and 50 , respectively. It is important to note that the Spetzler-Martin Grading Scale is not used for determining the appropriate endovascular treatment or the risk of hemorrhage untreated.

Table 34.1 Spetzler-Martin grading system

Feature		Points
Size	Small (<3 cm)	1
	Medium (3-6 cm)	2
	Large (>6 cm)	3
Eloquence of adjacent brain	Noneloquent	0
	Eloquent	1
Pattern of venous drainage	Superficial	0
	Deep	1

5   Diagnosis

Many AVMs are diagnosed after they have become symptomatic by intracranial hemorrhage, new onset seizure, or headaches. A definitive diagnosis is made through radiographic imaging.

6   Diagnostic Imaging

Noncontrast head CTs are often utilized as a first line imaging modality, to evaluate for acute hemorrhage. MRIs provide more detailed information about previous hemorrhage and anatomy of the AVM with respect to the underlying brain parenchyma. Conventional angiography is the gold standard for the diagnosis and evaluation of brain AVMs. Conventional angiography is particularly essential for lesions which have hemorrhaged such that high-risk features (e.g., deep venous drainage, nidal aneurysms, limited venous outflow) can be defined.

7   Management

Small, surgically accessible AVMs may be resected without prior embolization. Some operators are now attempting endovascular treatment of these smaller lesions with the goal of achieving a complete obliteration of the nidus with embolic agents. Anatomically, larger lesions are usually treated with preoperative emboilzation followed by surgical resection. Lesions with a nidus measuring less than 3 cm may be amenable to treatment with radiosurgery. Conservative management (no treatment) also represents an important option, and in many cases (particularly with larger or eloquent AVMs), this represents the best option. In patients who present with an acute large hemorrhage, surgical evacuation of the hematoma may be the first step in management. When the patient becomes more stable, and the hematoma resolves, the decision to proceed with elective endovascular therapy can be made on an individual basis. In cases of smaller hemorrhages, patients should undergo noninvasive imaging with a contrast MRI and MRA as well as diagnostic angiography.

Following hemorrhage, patients should be kept under tight blood pressure control with systolic blood pressure not exceeding 120 mmHg. Antiepileptic prophylaxis is generally not recommended; however, in those patients who present with parenchymal hemorrhage, seizures, or later develop seizures, antiepileptics should be continued throughout the course of the therapy.

8   List of Open Operative Choices

Treatment options are largely dependent on the risk of hemorrhage or other focal neurologic deficit. They include the following:

1. Radiosurgery—Used for total obliteration of smaller AVMs
2. Total surgical resection

Once an AVM has been surgically cured, there is little to no chance of recurrence.

9   Intervention

9.1   Principles

The embolic agents used most frequently are n-butylcyanoacrylate (NBCA) (Trufill NBCA Liquid Embollic, Cordis Corp) and more recently ethylene-vinyl alcohol copolymer (Onyx) (ev3, Irvine, California). NBCA was introduced in the late 1980s as a fast-polymerizing liquid adhesive and polymerizes upon direct contact with blood. Because of its thrombogenic nature, exquisite skill is required to avoid injection into the vein that can lead to outflow occlusion and hemorrhage.

Onyx is a liquid embolic agent that is nonadhesive and polymerizes by precipitation instead of ionic contact, thereby reducing the risk of catheter adherence to the polymer. Onyx has become increasingly used due to its more straightforward handling characteristics, more controlled injections, and nidus penetration. Onyx is available in various viscosities with Onyx18 and Onyx 34 available for the preoperative embolization of brain AVMs. In most cases, Onyx 18 is used through injections of small arterial feeders in order to obtain nidus penetration. It may be preferable to use the more viscous Onyx 34 for cases with high-flow nidus shunting.

The decision to use either NBCA or Onyx is operator dependent, taking into account the AVM flow dynamics, anatomy, and ultimate goal in endovascular treatment. In general, there are six options for neuroendovascular therapy as follows:

(a) *Preoperative embolization:* This is performed in single or multiple procedures prior to complete surgical resection. This is the most common method utilized in moderate to large AVMs. The goal is to gradually decrease the size of the AVM by 80–90 by embolizing arterial pedicles, or selective embolizations targeted at locations with difficult surgical access. Generally, embolizations are performed in a stepwise fashion to minimize the risk of hemorrhage from dynamic flow-related changes. Interval timing between embolization procedures varies among institution ranging from a few days to a few months.

(b) *Targeted therapeutic embolization:* This treatment strategy is generally reserved for AVMs not amenable to surgical resection (Grades IV and V) and is aimed at treated the bleeding source. Intranidal pseudoaneurysms may form as a result of AVM hemorrhage. Flow-related aneurysms and intranidal aneurysms also pose a risk for hemorrhage. It is often difficult to identify the hemorrhagic source within a large AVM nidus; however, superselective angiography can be useful for anatomical exploration and selective endovascular treatment of the aneurysm/pseudoaneurysm can be performed.

(c) *Preradiosurgery embolization:* Gamma-knife radiosurgery is most effective on small, <3 cm AVM nidus size. In cases involving dominant holohemispheric AVMs, preradiosurgery embolization is aimed at significantly reducing the AVM size. Although this provides a relatively high cure rate, between 80% and 88%, a longer latency period of 2–3 years continues to put patients at symptomatic risk during this time. Due to this latency period, patients selected for this therapy are those with AVMs that are relatively stable and have not hemorrhaged in the recent past.

(d) *Curative embolization* is an option for small AVMs with few arterial pedicles. The difficulty in curing larger, complex AVMs is in visualizing the arterial supply within the previous embolic casts. Additionally, with successive embolizations and changes in flow dynamics within the nidus, it can be more challenging to gain distal access into the arterial pedicles (Fig 34.1).

(e) *Palliative embolization* is aimed at alleviating symptoms attributed to shunting. AVMs are also thought to cause symptoms from the high-flow shunting away from the normal brain parenchyma leading to a "steal" phenomenon along the perinidal region. In surgically unresectable AVMs, partial embolization targeted at the arterial pedicles responsible for the symptomatic shunting has been reported. However, controversy surrounds the issue of partial embolization since there is an increased risk of subsequent hemorrhage.

(f) *No embolization* is an option for asymptomatic, incidentally discovered AVMs. They may also be managed conservatively in many cases, without any treatment at all. Small AVMs can sometimes be treated with open surgical resection or radiosurgery without preoperative embolization.

9.2   Technique

Patients are placed under general endotrachial anesthesia. The femoral artery is accessed and a 6-French sheath is inserted. A 6-French Neuron or a 6-French Envoy guide catheter is utilized to gain distal access. When using NBCA, microcatherization can be performed with flow-directed microcatheters. Superselective angiography is necessary to determine the arterial pedicle to be embolized as well as identifying en passant vessels, draining veins, and areas for safe reflux. When using NBCA, preparation should be performed in an area free of ionic solutions such as blood, contrast, and saline. NBCA

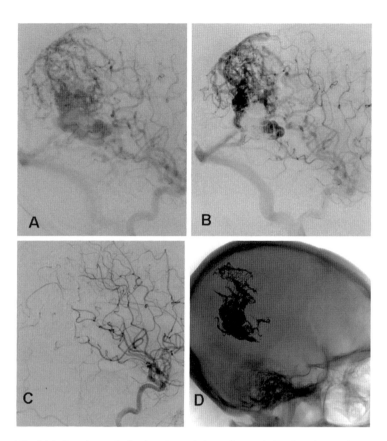

Fig. 34.1 Curative embolization. Lateral view of preembolization right parietal-occipital Grade IV AVM of a 46-year-old female who presented with a hemorrhage (**a**). Lateral view after one embolization procedure with Onyx (**b**), and after three embolization procedures with complete angiographic cure (**c**). Native unsubtracted view of Onyx cast after complete embolization (**d**)

is then diluted with ethiodol and sometimes is mixed with tantalum powder to increase the radiopacity of the mixture. The microcatheter is flushed with multiple syringes of 5 dextrose in water before injecting NBCA. Once the adhesive has been adequately delivered or there is radiographic evidence of reflux, the microcatheter should be rapidly removed and discarded. In AVMs with high-flow fistulas, it may be useful to first deploy coils within the arterial pedicle followed by NBCA injections.

When using Onyx, microcatherizations can be performed with DMSO-compatible microcatheters such as the Marathon, Echelon, UltraFlow, or Rebar (ev3, Peripheral Vascular, Plymouth, MI). The dead space of the microcatheter must first be flushed with dimethyl-sulfoxide (DMSO), the solvent for liquid delivery of Onyx. An air-tight interface between DMSO and Onyx should be obtained at the microcatheter hub. Biplane fluoroscopy with blank roadmapping is utilized to evaluate for reflux. Onyx is generally injected slowly first forming a plug at the catheter tip. This may take a few seconds to a few minutes. Slow, controlled injections can then be performed to fill the nidus without occluding the venous drainage. When removing the microcatheter, the Onyx syringe should be aspirated while slowly retracting the catheter from the Onyx cast. Rapid removal of the catheter can increase the risk of hemorrhage.

10   PostProcedure Management and Follow-up

After embolization procedures, patients are kept under strict blood pressure control (SBP usually maintained around 100 mmHg) and admitted to the ICU for close observation. Patients may undergo postembolization MRIs to evaluate for hemorrhage and peri-nidal edema as well as percentage of residual nidal filling. Patients are administered dexamethasone (4 mg every 6 hours) overnight and are discharged on a tapering dose [If there is evidence of postprocedure peri-nidal edema]. For patients who have undergone surgical resection of the AVM, an immediate post-op angiogram can be performed while under anesthesia in order to ensure complete resection of the AVM.

11   Complications and Management

Endovascular embolization procedures carry significant risk. Complications include hemorrhage, vessel dissection/perforation, thromboembolism and ischemia, vasospasm, and microcatheter entrapment.

(a) Intraprocedure intracranial hemorrhage can result from vessel perforation or tearing from the microcatheter or microwire or resulting from tension placed upon the microcatheter during removal after glue injections. Sometimes, the perforation is angiographically occult; however, in some cases, contrast extravasation can be seen angiographically. An acute elevation in systemic blood pressure and heart rate may also sentinel a perforation or hemorrhage. The perforated vessel can be tamponaded with a balloon, infused with NBCA or Onyx or occluded with detachable coils. Normal pressure perfusion breakthrough syndrome can occur after AVM embolization when the blood flow previously going to the AVM is then diverted to the normal brain parenchyma leading to hyperperfusion and hemorrhage. This can be limited by strictly controlling blood pressure during and immediately after the procedure. Inadvertent venous occlusion or venous stasis can also lead to intracerebral hemorrhage. Large hemorrhages require emergent surgical evacuation.

(b) Ischemic complications can result from thrombotic emboli from the microcatheter or from the embolic material itself.

(c) Microcatheter retention can occur especially with excessive reflux, particularly if there is proximal vessel tortuosity. When this occurs, it is usually safer to leave the catheter in place rather than make multiple attempts to retrieve it. The catheter can be cut by the operator at the groin sheath. Patients can be placed on antiplatelet medications usually without significant clinical sequelae.

12 Outcomes

Definitive treatment of an AVM is historically based on total surgical resection of the lesion. Recently, improved obliteration rates have been reported with the use of nBCA and Onyx (sometimes in concert with adjunctive radiosurgery). The overall morbidity and mortality rates with embolization range from 6 to 8 and 1 to 2 , respectively.

References

1. Ondra SL, Troupp H, George ED. The natural history of symptomatic arteriovenous malformations of the brain: A 24-year follow-up assessment. J Neurosurg. 1990;73:387–91.
2. Graf CJ, Perrett GE, Torner JC. Bleeding from cerebral arteriovenous malformations as part of their natural history. J Neurosurg. 1983;58:331–7.

3. Hamilton MB, Spetzler RF. The prospective application of a grading system for arteriovenous malformations. Neurosurgery. 1994;34:2–7.

4. Fiorella DJ, Albuquerque FC, Woo HH, McDougall CG, Rasmussen PA. The role of neuroendovascular therapy for the treatment of brain arteriovenous malformations. Neurosurgery. 2006;59(S3):163–77.

5. Hauck EF, Welch BG, White JA, Purdy PD, Pride LG, Samson D. Preoperative embolization of cerebral arteriovenous malformations with Onyx. AJNR Am J Neuroradiol. 2009;30:492–5.

6. Katsaridis V, Papagiannaki C, Almar E. Curative embolization of cerebral arteriovenous malformations (AVMs) with Onyx in 101 patients. Neuroradiol. 2008;50:589–97.

7. Wikholm G, Lundqvist C, Svendsen P. Embolization of cerebral arteriovenous malformations: Part I—Technique, morphology and complications. Neurosurgery. 1996;39:448–59.

8. Frizzel RT, Fisher 3rd WS. Cure, morbidity, and mortality associated with embolization of brain arteriovenous malformations: A review of 1246 patients in 32 series over a 35-year period. Neurosurgery. 1995;37:1031–40.

Chapter 35
Coronary Angiography

Samir Kapadia and Evan Lau

1 Anatomy

The left main coronary artery takes off from the posterior part of the left aortic sinus and bifurcates into the left anterior descending (LAD) and left circumflex (LCx) arteries. The LAD gives off septal branches, which penetrate into the interventricular septum, as well as diagonal branches, which come off laterally. The LCx gives rise to obtuse marginal branches. The RCA originates from the anterior portion of the right aortic sinus. It gives rise to RV marginal branches and usually sends branches to the posterior left ventricular wall. "Dominance" refers to the side from which the posterior descending artery (PDA) originates. Approximately 80% of the population is right dominant, with the PDA arising from the RCA. The following are some of the more common anomalies of the coronary arteries:

(a) Absence of left main, with separate origins of LAD and LCx from the aorta (incidence 0.41%).
(b) High takeoff of the RCA (incidence 0.15%)
(c) LCX arising from the right coronary sinus, coursing posterior to the aorta (incidence 0.37%)

S. Kapadia, M.D. (✉) • E. Lau, M.D.
Sones Cardiac Catheterization Laboratory, Cleveland Clinic,
9500 Euclid Ave, J2-3, Cleveland, OH 44195, USA
e-mail: kapadis@ccf.org

A. Kumar and K. Ouriel (eds.), *Handbook of Endovascular Interventions*,   483
DOI 10.1007/978-1-4614-5013-9_35,
© Springer Science+Business Media New York 2013

(d) RCA originating from the left aortic sinus, or the left coronary arteries originating from the right aortic sinus. This may have important clinical implications, particularly if the artery takes a course in between the aorta and pulmonary artery; such anomalies are associated with angina and sudden death and may require surgical correction.

2   Disease Definition

The vast majority of stenotic lesions are consequences of atherosclerosis. Distinct pathologic entities that may also cause stenotic disease include coronary vasospasm, in-stent restenosis, transplant vasculopathy, radiation vasculopathy, and vasculitis.

3   Disease Distribution

It is well known that coronary artery disease (CAD) is the leading cause of mortality worldwide. As life expectancy increases in developing countries, along with the greater adoption of the Westernized diet, the burden of coronary artery disease also rises. In the USA, CAD risk factors continue to be prevalent and under treated in many segments of the population. Although mortality associated with CAD is decreasing in the USA, it continues to be the leading cause of death.

4   Diagnosis: Clinical and Laboratory

As in atherosclerotic disease of other arterial beds, the earliest stages of coronary artery disease are asymptomatic. It is clear that early atherosclerotic lesions grow in the vessel wall without impinging on the lumen, classically described as the Galgov Phenomenon. Stenotic disease does not usually become apparent until there is significant flow limitation of blood supply to myocardium distal to a lesion, which happens at 50–70% diameter stenosis in the coronary circulation. The hallmark manifestation is angina or chest discomfort, which typically has the following characteristics: poorly localizable, pressure or burning sensation, radiating to the jaw/throat/arms, provoked by exertion, and palliated by sublingual nitroglycerin. However, many patients do not present with typical symptoms. Other common manifestations include dyspnea, atypical chest pain, or no pain (silent ischemia).

Patients with coronary artery disease largely present in one of three clinical circumstances: acute coronary syndrome, chronic stable angina, and silent ischemia.

Acute coronary syndromes manifest as new onset angina, anginal pain at rest, and/or increase in the severity of preexisting angina. The pathophysiology of these clinical entities involves atherosclerotic plaque rupture or plaque erosion with intraluminal thrombosis. There are three clinical syndromes that fall under the rubric acute coronary syndrome.

(a) Unstable angina—The clinical syndrome mentioned above, with or without ECG changes, and without the presence of cardiac markers.
(b) Non-ST elevation myocardial infarction (NSTEMI)—the clinical syndrome, with or without ECG changes, and with the presence of cardiac biomarkers.
(c) ST elevation myocardial infarction (STEMI)—the clinical syndrome with the presence of new ST elevation on the ECG. This presentation implies the presence of an acute occlusion of a coronary artery.

The ECG and cardiac biomarkers are important tools in the diagnosis and management of acute coronary syndromes. ECG changes supportive of an acute coronary syndrome include ST elevation, Q wave formation, ST depression, and T wave inversions. Several biomarkers are elevated in the context of myocardial infarction. The most commonly used biomarkers include creatine kinase (CK), the isoenzyme creatine kinase-MB (CK-MB), and troponin. Measurement of serum troponin represents the most sensitive assay for myonecrosis.

Patients with chronic stable angina, the second predominant presentation of coronary artery disease, demonstrate a stable pattern of provocable angina, usually with a stereotypic level of exertion or emotional stress. As opposed to acute coronary syndrome, the pathophysiology of chronic stable angina entails supply/demand mismatch of oxygen delivery to myocardium distal to a fixed coronary stenosis.

Although the fixed stenosis may have been created by the process of plaque rupture, thrombosis, and healing, the presentation of chronic stable angina implies a stable process at the level of the atherosclerotic plaque.

In chronic stable angina, the ECG may show transient ST depression or even ST elevation at times of stress. Cardiac biomarkers are not elevated.

Silent ischemia patients have positive stress tests with no clear anginal symptoms. They may have stable or unstable plaques, and their outcome is typically worse than stable angina patients but better than patients with unstable angina/non-ST elevation myocardial infarction patients. Diagnosis can also be made by ST segment analysis of Holter monitoring.

5 Diagnostic Imaging

Diagnostic imaging of coronary artery disease falls into two major paradigms: noninvasive imaging and invasive imaging. Examples of noninvasive imaging modalities include:

(a) Radionuclide/Nuclear Imaging—assessment of blood flow as measured by myocardial uptake of radionuclide tracers during rest and stress.

(b) Echocardiography—assessment of blood flow as measured by myocardial functioning (wall motion) at times of rest and stress.

(c) MRI—assessment of blood flow as measured by both wall motion abnormalities as well as myocardial perfusion of gadolinium. Magnetic resonance coronary angiography may also be performed; however, it does not have the spatial resolution to accurately detect and quantitate luminal narrowing of coronary arteries. It is useful in identifying anomalous coronary arteries.

(d) Coronary CT Angiography—Although it does not yet meet the spatial resolution of fluoroscopic angiography to define the severity of coronary lesions, it has excellent negative predictive value. Image quality can be impeded by coronary calcification as well as metallic objects such as stents. Although decreasing with "step-and-shoot" techniques, radiation exposure still remains a concern.

Table 35.1 Diagnostic catheter selection

Artery	Catheter	Comments
Left main	JL4	Most often used
	JL3.5	Small aortic root
	JL5, JL6	Enlarged aortic root
	AL-1,2	Posterior takeoff, separate ostia
RCA	JR 4 or modified JR-4	Most often used
	3D RCA	Anterior takeoff
	AR-1,2	Distorted aortic root
	AL-1,2	Anterior takeoff
Aorto-coronary bypass	JR4	Convenient, left- and right-sided grafts
	LCB	Left-sided grafts, upward takeoff
	MP, AL-1	Dilated aorta, longer reach
	RCB	Right-sided grafts
	MP, AR-1	Right-sided grafts, downward takeoff
LIMA	IMA	Acute caudal takeoff
	IMA—special	Curved subclavian
RIMA	IMA	

JL Judkin's Left, *AL* Amplatz Left, *JR* Judkin's Right, *3D RCA* 3 dimensional Right coronary Artery, *AR* Amplatz Right, *LCB* Left Coronary Bypass, *MPB* Multipurpose, *RCB* Right Coronary Bypass, *IMA* Internal Mammary Artery

The other major paradigm of coronary artery assessment involves invasive imaging. Invasive modalities include coronary angiography (using traditional fluoroscopy), fractional flow reserve (FFR), and intravascular ultrasound (IVUS). Diagnostic Angiography is the gold standard in luminal assessment and the diagnosis of coronary artery disease. A schematic of the technique is as follows:

(a) Obtain femoral, radial, or brachial arterial access. Sheath sizes for diagnostic angiography usually range from 4 F to 6 F.
(b) Advance coronary catheters (most commonly JL4 or JR4 via femoral approach) into the aortic root, using a J-tipped guide wire. Table 35.1.
(c) Engage coronary ostia.
(d) Inject contrast (iso or low osmolar contrast) via hand injection or assist device.
(e) Cine images are commonly recorded on 16 cm and 22 cm magnification. Ideally, images from multiple angulations are taken of each artery in order to visualize important segments in at least two, perpendicular planes (Table 35.2, Fig. 35.1)
(f) Repeat steps (a)–(e) for both right and left coronary arteries, aortocoronary grafts, and mammary grafts (when applicable).

Table 35.2 Angiographic views for specific coronary segments

Vessel	Angulation	Segments
LM	LAO 50^0/CAU 30^0	Bifurcation of the LAD/LCx
	RAO 20^0/CAU 20^0	Proximal and mid LM
LAD	LAO 50^0/CAU 30^0	Proximal LAD
	PA/CRA 45^0	Mid and distal LAD
	RAO 30^0/CRA 30^0	Diagonals
	LAO 50^0/CRA 40^0	Mid and distal LAD
LCx	LAO 50^0/CAU 30^0	Proximal, mid, distal LCx, proximal OM
	RAO 20^0/CAU 20^0	Mid and distal LCx, Mid/distal OM
	PA/CAU 35^0	Proximal, mid, and distal LCx, Proximal OM
RCA	LAO 30^0 CRA 20^0	Proximal, mid, distal RCA
	RAO 30^0	Mid, distal RCA, PDA
	PA/CRA 30^0	Bifurcation of PDA/PLV

LAO left anterior oblique, *RAO* right anterior oblique, *CRA* cranial, *CAU* caudal, *LM* left main, *LAD* left anterior descending, *LCx* left circumflex, *RCA* right coronary artery, *OM* obtuse marginal, *PDA* posterior descending artery, *PLV* posterior left ventricular branch

The techniques of fractional flow reserve and intravascular ultrasound provide adjunctive information to diagnostic angiography:

(a) Fractional Flow Reserve (FFR)—involves the use of a wire with a mounted pressure transducer. Measurements are taken proximal (within the guide catheter placed in the aorta) and distal to a coronary lesion. The fractional flow reserve is the ratio of the mean distal over the mean proximal pressure, taken during times of maximal hyperemia (i.e., adenosine administration). Flow-limiting stenoses have an FFR of ≤0.75–0.80.

(b) Intravascular Imaging Modalities—involves the use of a catheter mounted with various imaging elements, which allow for interrogation of the vessel and its wall from within the lumen. These technologies include the following:

   1. Intravascular ultrasound (Gray scale IVUS)—uses a catheter mounted with an ultrasound transducer. The tissue resolution is able to differentiate the three layers of a normal artery as well as detect changes related to atherosclerotic plaque. Its use includes determination of reference vessel diameter, cross-sectional area of a stenosis, plaque morphology, adequacy of stent deployment, presence of dissection, etc.

Left Ventriculogram with Right and Left Coronary Arteries

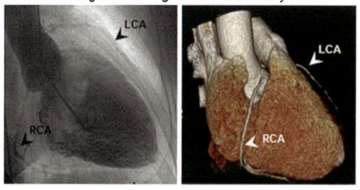

RAO CAUDAL (Left Coronary Artery)

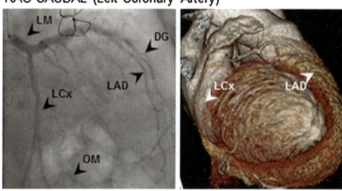

CTA image flipped horizontally

LAO CAUDAL (Left Coronary Artery)

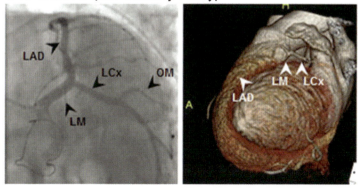

Fig. 35.1 Selected angiographic view with corresponding 3D CTA reconstructions

PA CRANIAL (Left Coronary Artery)

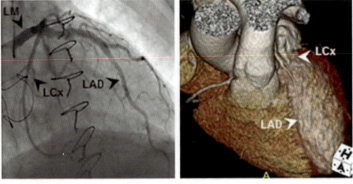

LAO CRANIAL (Left Coronary Artery)

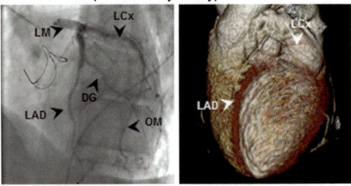

RAO – right anterior oblique; LAO – left anterior oblique; LCA – left coronary artery; RCA – right coronary artery; LM – left main; LAD – left anterior descending; LCx – left circumflex; OM – obtuse marginal; DG – diagonal

Fig. 35.1 (continued)

2. Virtual Histology—adjunct to IVUS, which uses analysis of radiofrequency scatter to determine plaque composition. The various components are given a color coding: fibrous tissue (green), fibro-fatty tissue (light green), necrotic core (red), dense calcium (white).

3. Optical Coherence Tomography—creates tomographic images using fiberoptics and reflection of infrared light.

Produces pictures with better spatial resolution than IVUS, although the depth of penetration is limited. Requires continuous displacement of blood in order to produce images.

4. Spectroscopy—analyzes plaque composition by using differential tissue absorption of wavelengths of light.

5. Thermography—detection of "vulnerable" plaque by the increase in temperature associated with macrophage-rich plaque. May be detected by direct measurement of temperature or by infrared imaging.

6 Management Paradigm and Indications as Well as Timing of Treatment

(a) Acute Coronary Syndrome

1. ST elevation MI—immediate revascularization, either by the administration of systemic thrombolytics or percutaneous coronary intervention, when available.

2. Unstable angina/NSTEMI

- High risk—early invasive management with diagnostic angiography ± revascularization
- Low risk—conservative management, with diagnostic angiography ± revascularization only if recurrent ischemic symptoms or positive stress testing.

(b) Chronic Stable Angina

1. Revascularization after failure of optimal medical therapy.

7 Open Operative Choices

Coronary artery bypass and percutaneous coronary intervention are the two major modalities of revascularization. Coronary artery bypass has the advantage of durability, while PCI represents a less invasive modality. In general, CABG is preferred for:

(a) Left main or ostial LAD disease
(b) Multivessel disease (usually involving LAD)
(c) Multivessel disease with depressed EF

(d) Diabetics with 2-vessel disease.
(e) Contraindication to dual antiplatelet therapy.

8 Intervention: Technique and Pitfalls

(a) Pretreatment—Patients scheduled to undergo percutaneous coronary intervention should receive antiplatelet therapy pretreatment as early as possible. This would include aspirin 325 mg and plavix 600 mg (at least 2 h before procedure). For emergent procedures, oral antiplatelet therapy should be given as soon as possible.

(b) Periprocedural antithrombotic therapy—There are several possible regimens depending on the scenario. This should be initiated at the start of the procedure (often given before or immediately after arterial access is obtained).

   1. Heparin (60–100 units/kg bolus)—to goal ACT 250–350 for the duration of the procedure only. This may be used for low-risk patients, typically receiving PCI for chronic stable angina.
   2. Heparin (50–70 units/kg bolus)+glycoprotein IIB/IIIA inhibitor—goal ACT 200–250 for the duration of the procedure only. To be used for high-risk patients, including STEMI, unstable angina/NSTEMI, inadequate technical result, inadequate antiplatelet pretreatment. Several GP IIB/IIIA inhibitors are available

      • Abciximab (0.25 mg/kg bolus; 0.125 mcg/kg/min infusion×12 h). Used particularly in STEMI.
      • Eptifibatide (180 mcg/kg bolus, maximum 22.6 mg, followed by repeat 180 mcg/kg bolus 10 min later; 2 mcg/kg/min, maximum 15 mg/h×18 h). If creatinine clearance <50 mL/min, dose adjustment should be made (bolus unchanged, 1 mcg/kg/min×18 h).
      • Tirofiban (0.4 mcg/kg/min×30 min, followed by 0.1 mcg/kg/min×12–24 h post PCI). If creatinine clearance <30 mL/min, reduce dose by 50%.

   3. Bivalirudin (0.75 mg/kg bolus, 1.75 mg/kg/h infusion)—goal ACT 250–350. Equivalent efficacy to heparin+GP IIB/IIIA inhibitor, in some studies. Less bleeding risk but potentially higher postprocedural MI risk.

(c) Femoral access. Intervention may be performed via brachial and radial access. Minimum 5 F catheter is required. Radial access is better for bleeding complications although size-related issues may be important for bifurcation lesions.

(d) A guiding catheter is directed to the aortic root over a 0.035 in J-tipped guidewire (Fig. 35.2).

1. Left coronary guide catheters

   - XB 3.5—commonly used, "hugs" the lesser curvature of the aorta, helpful for LAD interventions
   - XB 4 or XB 5—when lesser curvature is elongated
   - JL4—less support for coronary intervention
   - AL 1, AL 2—Excellent for support, useful for LCx interventions

2. Right coronary guide catheters

   - JR 4—Less support
   - AR 1, AR 2, AL 1, AL 2—better support, sometimes difficult to prevent deep engagement
   - Hockeystick—Upward takeoff of RCA

3. Aortocoronary bypass guide catheters

   - JR—For left-sided bypasses
   - LCB—For more upward takeoff of left bypasses
   - MPB, AR 1—for right coronary bypass grafts with downward angulation
   - MPB and AL 1—Also useful for left bypasses with dilated aorta

4. Left internal mammary artery guide catheter

   - IMA or JR4
   - The guide catheter's distal end is connected to a Y adaptor, allowing for simultaneous connection to a manifold for contrast injection, as well as access to the central lumen for insertion of interventional equipment.

(e) Coronary wire—once the ostium of the intended vessel is engaged with the guide catheter, a coronary interventional wire

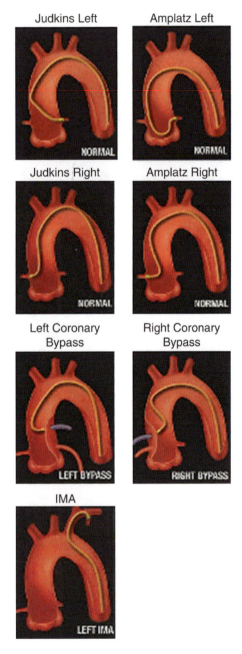

Fig. 35.2 Selected coronary catheters

is passed through the guide catheter, into the target vessel, and across the lesion. The following are commonly used wires:

1. Work horse wires for most lesions - Prowater®, Asahi soft®, BMW®, Runthrough®
2. Tortuous arteries—Runthrough®, Reflex®
3. Extra support—BHW®, Platinum plus®, GrandSlam®
4. Severe lesions (hydrophilic wires)—Whisper®, PT2®, Choice PT®, Schoenobi®
5. Total occlusion—Miracle Bro 3, 4.5, 6, 12®; Confianza® and Confianza pro®
6. Specific applications—Filters for SVG interventions, Roto-floppy®, and Roto Extra-Support® for rotational atherectomy
   The wire will serve as a platform for the delivery of balloons, stents, and other interventional equipment.

(f) Predilation—Predilation is performed to facilitate delivery of a stent, and/or to make sure that a severely calcified lesion will allow proper stent expansion. The predilation balloon diameter is typically undersized by a millimeter compared to vessel size, and attention is paid not to predilate segments that are not ultimately covered by a stent. Compliant balloons are used for predilation.

(g) Stent deployment—bare metal stent (BMS) vs drug-eluting stent (DES) is chosen based on patient and lesion characteristics. For small arteries (<3.0 mm), long lesions (>15 mm), chronic occlusions, restenotic lesions, unstable lesions, bifurcation, or ostial lesions, DES is better than BMS. For diabetic patients, DES is preferred in patients that can tolerate long-term dual antiplatelet therapy. The size of the stent should be matched or slightly oversized to the expected width of the native vessel (measured by width of undiseased vessel). The length of the stent should be minimized, but long enough to bridge undiseased vessel segments proximal and distal to the lesion. The location of the stent should be confirmed via cine imaging, just prior to stent inflation. Stent is typically deployed at high pressures of at least 12–14 atm.

(h) Postdilation—subsequent balloon inflations, with noncompliant balloons at high pressure, are typically performed. This is done to ensure full expansion of the stent to the desired width of the native vessel.

(i) Postsurveillance—cine images are generally taken after intervention, to ensure that the vessel has not been injured (dissection or perforation). Usually, this includes a cine image with the coronary wire in place (in case an intervention is required) and a second with the wire removed. IVUS is frequently used to ensure adequate stent expansion or to assess angiographic "haziness."

8.1 Special Circumstances

(a) Difficult to cross lesions—On occasion, lesions may be difficult to cross, with a wire or with a balloon. There may be difficulty in delivering the stent to the intended segment, related to tortuosity of the vessel/lesion, calcification of the lesion, and/or severity of the luminal narrowing. There are several methods to employ in these circumstances:

1. Hydrophilic wires or wires without transition may help
2. Over the wire balloon to support wire in the proximal artery may allow better torque transmission.
3. Increase wire tip stiffness—if a lesion cannot be crossed with one wire, stiffer-tipped wires may be successful, especially in totally occluded arteries. There is a greater risk of perforation with a stiffer-tipped wire. If a lesion has already been crossed by a wire and there is difficulty in delivering devices, exchange to a stiffer bodied wire may provide a sturdier platform for equipment delivery.
4. Better guide catheter support—the angulation of guide catheter engagement may need adjustment for better support. Alternatively, a different or larger caliber guide catheter (i.e., 7 or 8 F) may be required for appropriate support.
5. Predilation with larger balloons may change the luminal morphology enough to allow for stent delivery
6. Stent choice—a stent with lower profile struts, or with a more flexible morphology, may be required to cross a tortuous, narrow lesion.
7. Buddy wire technique—a second interventional wire may be passed across the lesion. The stent may be delivered over one of the wires, with the second wire creating a barrier between one side of the stent and the vessel wall. This may change the coefficient of friction enough to allow for stent delivery.

8. Rotational atherectomy—In severely calcified lesions rotational atherectomy helps to prepare the lesion for stent delivery and expansion.

(b) Saphenous Vein Graft Intervention

Lesions located in saphenous vein grafts are associated with greater risk of periprocedural complications and restenosis when compared to native coronary vessels. The use of embolic protection devices has been shown to decrease periprocedural myocardial infarction and distal embolization resulting in no-reflow phenomenon. Filters and distal or proximal occlusion devices are used for this purpose. Longer stents are preferred in SVG, and postdilation is typically not performed, so as to prevent distal embolization.

(c) In-stent restenosis

In-stent restenosis (ISR) lesions can be treated with balloon angioplasty using a noncompliant balloon or a cutting balloon. Mechanism of ISR should be investigated with IVUS to make sure that stent expansion is adequate. In some circumstances, a second stent will be placed within the first stent, particularly if the lesion involves ISR of a bare metal stent or the stenosis involves the edges of the primary stent. If the initial stent is a drug-eluting stent, the second stent used may be of a platform with a different anti-roliferative agent. In-stent restenosis lesions which already have two layers of stenting are not amenable to a third layer.

9 Postprocedure Management and Follow-up Protocol

Following percutaneous coronary intervention, patients are typically observed as inpatients at least overnight. If radial artery access is used, the sheath is pulled immediately after the procedure and hemostasis is achieved with an external compression device. Femoral artery access can be managed with immediate sheath removal with the use of a closure device. If a femoral sheath is to be managed with manual compression, a PTT <50 is usually required prior to sheath removal.

Patients are required to take lifelong aspirin therapy with 81 mg daily. The duration for dual antiplatelet therapy with clopidogrel (75 mg daily) depends on the type of stent used. Prasugrel is a new thienopyridine agent that may replace clopidgrel in specific situations. For bare metal stents, the minimum requirement for dual antiplatelet therapy is 1 month when the intervention is for stable angina and 12 months after stent placement for an acute coronary syndrome. For the first-generation drug-eluting stents, the minimum requirement is 12–24 months, with a recommendation for longer use if tolerated. Some second-generation drug-eluting stents may require a shorter duration of clopidogrel administration; however, this is extremely controversial and under active investigation.

Patients should have clinical follow-up for recurrence of symptoms, which may herald progression of native artery disease or in-stent restenosis. The average asymptomatic patient does not require routine diagnostic imaging follow-up to assess stent patency.

10 Complications and Management

(a) Access site complications

1. Bleeding—occurs within the first 24 h. This may be a result of arterial or venous bleeding and may lead to significant anemia and hemodynamic instability. Large femoral hematomas can lead to femoral nerve compression and damage. Rapid hematoma expansion can often be controlled with manual compression. Pseudoaneurysms may be managed with manual compression or more commonly ultrasound-guided thrombin injection. Surgical consultation should be considered for large pseudoaneurysms and hematomas.

2. Retroperitoneal (RP) Hemorrhage—May be the result of arterial or venous bleeding. High index of suspicion should be maintained in the postprocedural setting, particularly for patients with unexplained hypotension or anemia. If hemodynamically stable, diagnosis may be most easily confirmed with a noncontrast CT scan. Often times, RP bleeds resolve with conservative management, but severe hemorrhage, particularly from an arterial source, may sometimes require surgical correction.

3. Arterial-venous fistula—consider surgical consultation, though small ones are largely managed conservatively.

(b) Renal Failure—In the first 2–3 days following a catheterization procedure, renal failure is usually related to contrast nephropathy. In appropriately selected patients, the risk of renal failure may be attenuated by n-acetylcysteine administration and hydration prior to contrast administration.

(c) Stroke—the risk of stroke in diagnostic procedures is 0.03–0.3%. The risk is slightly higher in interventional procedures (0.3–0.4%).

(d) Coronary Complications

   1. Distal embolization—occasionally, angioplasty and stenting of a coronary lesion may lead to distal embolization. This most commonly occurs with saphenous vein graft interventions. Distal embolization is manifested as "no-reflow" phenomenon, which is demonstrated by slow or inadequate contrast passage in a patent epicardial vessel. The underlying mechanism may be related to small vessel obstruction and/or spasm as a result of embolized plaque material. The efficacy of intra-arterial vasodilators in treating this phenomenon is unknown.

   2. Dissection—Intimal tearing may be the result of catheter or wire manipulation, or balloon/stent expansion. This usually necessitates further stenting to cover the segment of dissected vessel.

   3. Perforation—Can be treated with reversal of anticoagulation and prolonged balloon inflation. However, can occasionally cause life-threatening tamponade especially with periprocedural IIbIIIa inhibitor use. Coiling, covered stents or surgery may be required

(e) Thrombocytopenia

   1. Platelet counts should be monitored early after a procedure in which GP IIB/IIIA inhibitors are used (particularly abciximab), as these may cause severe, idiosyncratic thrombocytopenia.

11 Outcomes

The use of percutaneous coronary intervention has improved on the outcomes of death and reinfarction in patients with myocardial infarction. The advent in the use of stents, and subsequently the introduction of drug-eluting stenting, has improved upon the need for target lesion revascularization. In the most recent meta-analysis, bare-metal stenting results in ~20% need for target lesion revascularization at 4 years. This number has been reduced to 6–8% for the first-generation drug-eluting stents.

References

1. Boden WE, O'Rourke RA, Teo KK, et al. Optimal medical therapy with or without PCI for stable coronary disease. N Engl J Med. 2007;356(15):1503–16.
2. Grines CL, Browne KF, Marco J, et al. A comparison of immediate angioplasty with thrombolytic therapy for acute myocardial infarction. The Primary Angioplasty in Myocardial Infarction Study Group. N Engl J Med. 1993;328(10):673–9.
3. Grines CL, Cox DA, Stone GW, et al. Coronary angioplasty with or without stent implantation for acute myocardial infarction. Stent Primary Angioplasty in Myocardial Infarction Study Group. N Engl J Med. 1999;341(26):1949–56.
4. Mehta SR, Cannon CP, Fox KA, et al. Routine vs selective invasive strategies in patients with acute coronary syndromes: a collaborative meta-analysis of randomized trials. JAMA. 2005;293(23):2908–17.
5. Stettler C, Wandel S, Allemann S, et al. Outcomes associated with drug-eluting and bare-metal stents: a collaborative network meta-analysis. Lancet. 2007;370(9591):937–48.

Chapter 36
Vascular Access Closure Devices

Lina Vargas and Vikram S. Kashyap

In 2002, an estimated six million interventional cardiology and endovascular procedures were performed in the USA, and that number exceeded 10.5 million in 2009. In most of these procedures, the common femoral artery is used as the cardiac access site. For each of these cases, vascular access management is a critical aspect to determining a successful outcome without complications. For many decades, manual compression has been the "gold standard" for postprocedure vascular access management. With the development of endovascular procedures, larger sheaths and more intense anticoagulation measures are now routinely employed. These factors place greater demands on the safe performance of vascular access. In addition, many patients are likely to undergo repeated angiographic procedures over time, most frequently using the femoral artery as the vascular entry point. Site selection, puncture and closure must be optimized to avoid access site complications, primarily related to bleeding. Vascular Closure Devices (VCDs) were designed to decrease time to achieve hemostasis, as well as access site bleeding, thus permitting shorter time to patient ambulation, and increased patient comfort compared with manual compression.

L. Vargas, M.D.
Department of Vascular Surgery, Cleveland Clinic, Cleveland, OH, USA

V.S. Kashyap, M.D. (✉)
Division of Vascular Surgery, University Hospitals Case Medical Center,
11100 Euclid Ave, LKS 7060, Cleveland, OH 44106, USA
e-mail: Vikram.kashyap@uhhospitals.org

A. Kumar and K. Ouriel (eds.), *Handbook of Endovascular Interventions*,   501
DOI 10.1007/978-1-4614-5013-9_36,
© Springer Science+Business Media New York 2013

1 Anatomy

When available, previous catheterization procedures including femoral angiography can be useful to review the anatomy and location of the common femoral artery and its bifurcation, the inferior epigastric artery, and the femoral head. In the majority, the femoral bifurcation will be at or below the femoral head. The target area for arterial puncture is from the center to the bottom of the femoral head. If the bifurcation is located more cephalad, the safest area for skin puncture will be slightly higher to allow common femoral artery access.

Localization of the ideal arteriotomy site in every patient is facilitated by routine use of fluoroscopy to identify the bony landmarks. Puncture over the lower half of the femoral head is essential to have a "fixed" structure against which to compress the arteriotomy site, as well as to avoid the femoral artery bifurcation. The use of ultrasound guidance has gained popularity and is critical in situations where the femoral artery pulse is absent or the vessel is diseased. In addition, utilization of a micropuncture kit allows safe access without the risk of creating a large arterial puncture that cannot be cannulated. These kits are especially important in patients with difficult anatomy in whom multiple sticks are anticipated.

Immediately after sheath placement, a femoral artery angiogram should be done to confirm puncture site location, and to assess femoral artery anatomy and presence of atherosclerotic disease that would contraindicate use of a VCD due to increased risk of complications. Furthermore, VCDs are usually contraindicated in patients with significant atherosclerotic femoral arterial disease and high sheath insertions (above the inferior epigastric artery). Given the increased risk of retroperitoneal hematoma in patients with high sticks, urgent surgical consultation should be obtained for possible open closure of the external iliac artery.

2 Device Listing

A. Angio-Seal (St Jude Medical, Inc., St. Paul, MN) (Table 36.1)

Invasive, active approximation, intraluminal, thrombosing, temporary/resorbable.

Table 36.1 Vascular closure device characteristics

Closure device	Sheath sizes	Time till hemostasis	Permanent implant	Immediate repuncture
Angio-Seal	6,8	Short	No	No
Perclose	Perclose 5–8 Prostar XL 8–10	Short	Yes	Yes[a]
Starclose	5,6	Short	Yes	Yes[a]
Catalyst	5,6,7	Intermediate	No	Yes
Mynx	5,6,7	Intermediate	No	No
Exoseal	5,6,7	Short	No	No

[a]Not approved by FDA

Angio-Seal comprises two hemostatic mechanisms: active approximation and thrombosis. Initially, the arteriotomy site is approximated between an intra-arterial T-shaped resorbable anchor and an extravascular **collagen** plug, held together by a suture. The second hemostatic mechanism is the thrombosing effect of collagen. This device is considered highly effective, with one of the highest primary success rates among VCDs. All three components are absorbed within 90 days.

The Instructions for use (IFU), states that it can be immediately repunctured. In addition, for diagnostic cases it is labeled for 20-min ambuation and 60-min discharge for diagnostic cases

B. Perclose (Abbott Vascular, Santa Clara, CA) (Table 36.1)

Invasive, active approximation, intraluminal, nonthrombosing, permanent/nonresorbable.

The first suture-mediated VCD to be approved by the FDA was the Perclose device, which allows the insertion of a nonresorbable suture (**monofilament polypropylene**) directly into the arterial wall adjacent to the arteriotomy, which straddles the surrounding intima. Although not approved by the FDA, for this specific indication, this device is amenable to immediate repuncture.

C. Starclose (Abbott Vascular, Santa Clara, CA) (Table 36.1)

Invasive, active approximation, extraluminal, nonthrombosing, permanent/nonresorbable.

This device consists of a nitinol clip designed to be deployed outside the arterial lumen, in the media. The Starclose nitinol clip is nonresorbable, has no thrombosing effect, and has a theoretical decreased risk of infection attributed to the absence of a thrombosing plug. This device is also amenable to immediate repuncture, although the FDA has not yet approved this indication.

D. Catalyst (Cardiva Medical, Mountain View, CA) (Table 36.1)

Invasive, passive approximation, nonthrombosing/sealing, no foreign body.

The Catalyst closure device has the advantage of being delivered **through the procedural sheath**. Compression of the arteriotomy site occurs from inside the artery with a nitinol disk that is removed afterward through the fresh clot, leaving no "footprint" inside the artery. This temporary hemostasis allows the arteriortomy site to recoil to the size of an 18-gauge needle. The spring mechanism of the nitinol disk maintains traction at the puncture site from inside the vessel, but after removal, compression is required to achieve complete hemostasis, but for a shorter period of time than would be required for the original arteriotomy. In addition, the Catalyst has topical agents that help promote hemostasis when exposed to the tissue track during removal.

Catalyst III is indicated for use in patients receiving heparin as it is coated with protamine sulfate.

This VCD is amenable to repuncture.

E. Mynx (Access Closure, Mountain View, CA) (Table 36.1)

Invasive, passive approximation, sealing, temporary/resorbable.

Passive approximation of the arteriotomy site is achieved with a sealing (nonthrombosing) agent outside the artery, **polyethylene glycol**, that is delivered through the **procedural sheath** used; this last characteristic makes this VCD one of the best tolerated by patients. This is also beneficial when considering a decreased infection risk and avoidance of upsizing the track by using the existing sheath. The sealant dissolves within 30 days.

F. Exoseal (Cordis Corporation, Miami Lakes, FL) (Table 36.1)

Invasive, active approximation, intramural, thrombosing, temporary/resorbable.

The arteriotomy site is sealed by the deposition of an absorbable plug (**polyglycolic acid**) on the extravascular surface. The device is deployed through the **procedural sheath**. The plug is completely absorbed in 60–90 days.

3   Technique for Deployment: Use of Common Closure Devices

The commonly used VCDs are fairly straightforward to use and are packaged with a complete IFU (Instructions for Use). However, each device requires a learning curve of at least 5–10 cases to obtain optimal results. Each device has approximately 3–5 steps for safe deployment. Listed below is a summary of the steps. The IFU of each device should be reviewed for the full-procedural method as well as for specific troubleshooting.

3.1   *Perclose*

A guide is inserted and advanced through the sheath. This guide contains needles, suture, and a footplate that helps the precise placement of needles around the arteriotomy site. The sutures are captured after the needles are deployed, the plunger is retracted and a knot is advanced with the help of the knot pusher. The knot is tightened after the device is completely removed, and finally, the suture tails are cut below the skin surface.

3.2   *Starclose*

After a 5-mm skin incision is made; the subcutaneous tunnel is dilated with a blunt dissector. Exchange the intervention sheath with the sheath provided with the closure device. Subsequent steps are based upon a CLICK system, as follows:

1. Click 1: Occurs after the device is passed through the sheath and the Sheath Hub and the Clip Applier connect. While introducing the Clip Applier through the sheath, ensure that the angle of introduction is the same as that of the tissue tract.
2. Click 2: After ensuring that the front of the device is facing upward, retract the device back 3–4 cm. Then push the Plunger with your thumb holding the device steady. A second click will then be heard at the end of the plunger introduction. This allows the Locator Wings to open and lock. Current devices have a

numbering system (number 2 for this step), which identifies each step's completion.

3. Click 3: Assume a syringe grip on the device and advance the Thumb Advancer. This will deliver the clip to the arteriotomy site while splitting the sheath. Once again the newer devices have a numbering system (number 3 for this step), which will be visible once the step is completed.

4. Click 4: Raise the body of the device to a 60–75° angle and while maintaining downward pressure, depress the Deployment Button. This allows the release of the arteriotomy closure clip while simultaneously collapsing the Locator Wings.

At the completion hold pressure for a few seconds and withdraw the entire system.

3.3 Mynx

The catheter with a nonthrombogenic sealant, polyethylene glycol, is delivered through the same procedural sheath. A balloon is inflated and placed against the anterior wall of the femoral artery to achieve temporary hemostasis while the sealant is deployed. This avoids intra-arterial placement. The plug seals both the arterial puncture and the tissue tract.

3.4 Exoseal

This device is deployed through the existing sheath used for the intervention. The steps are as follows:

1. Introduce the device through the sheath. Continue insertion till such time you see blood coming from the drip hole translucent tubing. Stop any further insertion at this point and start pulling the device back till such time the blood stops coming from the drip hole.

2. Next pull the sheath back till you hear the click of the sheath hub and the device locking.

3. Pull the entire system (sheath locked with device) back slowly till you see the indicator bars turning black. If they turn red then you have retracted too much.

4. At this point (black indicator), press the deployment green button and slowly retract the entire device. Hold gentle pressure till hemostasis is achieved.

4   Postprocedure Management and Follow-up Protocol

Patients at risk for complications include those who are obese, with known atherosclerotic disease, or on anticoagulation; other risk factors can be related to the procedure and include use of large catheters or sheaths. In addition to the local site, careful attention should be paid to ensure that the distal pulse exam is at baseline preprocedure status.

Regardless of individual patient risk factors and procedure-related factors, all patients are required to complete an established period of bed rest before attempting ambulation. The duration varies with the device used. All should be closely monitored for significant changes in vital signs, pulse examination, and access site bleeding or significant hematoma formation—external or internal (retroperitoneal or preperitoneal)

All patients need to receive printed information about the type of closure device used to achieve hemostasis. In addition, patients need to be instructed on postprocedure care, restrictions, and signs and symptoms that might indicate possible complications.

5   Complications and Management

5.1   Hemorrhage

Most common complication after arterial access. Pressure over the puncture site might be enough to obtain control, but surgical exploration might be required in cases of uncontrolled hemorrhage or expanding hematoma. Location of bleeding and hematoma formation depends on the location of the arterial puncture. If above the inguinal ligament, retroperitoneal bleeding and hematoma can occur and should be suspected in patients with hypotension and back pain after diagnostic or interventional percutaneous procedures. An outline of the management plan for cases of hemorrhage is given in Fig. 36.1.

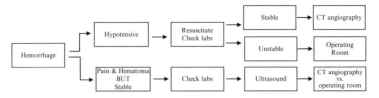

Fig. 36.1 Management of Hemorrhage

5.2 Pseudoaneurysm

The hematomas that may occur after diagnostic or interventional procedures usually resolve spontaneously and, therefore, may only require observation and follow-up. If a partially thrombosed hematoma (i.e., pseudoaneurysm) persists or enlarges, further management may be required, especially if there is evidence of skin compromise, pressure necrosis, compression of neighboring structures (femoral vein or nerve with secondary DVT or neuropathy), distal hypoperfusion, or infection. Pseudoaneurysms less than 1.5–2 cm can be observed, while those between 2 and 3 cm will likely need thrombin injection, while those larger than 3 cm are best treated with surgical repair. Concomitant factors such as use of anti-coagulants as well as antiplatelets also have an impact in this management algorithm. Proximal arterial control is indicated before attempting surgical repair usually as primary repair.

5.3 Arteriovenous Fistulas

Postprocedural Arteriovenous Fistulas (AVFs) may be observed, especially if small. In general, AVFs should be addressed by open repair, especially when large, or when the common femoral artery is involved.

5.4 Arterial Obstruction

This may occur secondary to embolization, vessel spasm, or most commonly disruption of atherosclerotic plaque. Femoral exploration is warranted in cases of occlusion or stenosis evidenced by duplex ultrasound or angiography, and embolectomy may be required in cases of symptomatic embolization. All foreign bodies must be removed, and if open, the wound should be irrigated with antibiotic solution.

5.5   Device Specific Complications

5.5.1   Angio-Seal

Infrequent, but possible complications with use of Angio-Seal include arterial obstruction secondary to, or embolization of, the intra-arterial anchor, causing lower extremity ischemia. Another rare complication of this VCD is infection initiated in the resorbable collagen plug that extends from the arteriotomy site to the skin. If anchor embolization leads to ischemia, it has to be treated appropriately by open means.

5.5.2   Perclose

Infection risk is decreased with monofilament polypropylene suture instead of braided sutures. Femoral artery laceration or posterior wall dissection caused by the footplate are other complications.

5.5.3   Starclose

Mal-deployment of clip. Increased risk of oozing, especially in fully anticoagulated patients.

5.5.4   Catalyst

Inadvertent dislodging of the device with bleeding. Does not obviate manual compression and discomfort from this.

5.5.5   Mynx

Polyethylene glycol may not seal. It is also important to mention that sealing agents are considered to be potentially less effective at preventing bleeding from arteriotomy site, especially in anticoagulated patients, but this has never been formally studied.

6 Outcomes

Many factors relating to the patient, physician, staff, and hospital impact access management for patients. Problems with the arterial puncture site remain the single-most important impediment to early ambulation, early hospital discharge, and risk of postprocedure complications like bleeding, arterial injury, infection, hematoma, pseudoaneurysm, and arteriovenous fistula. Complication rates range from 0.1 to 12 % depending on the study cited and some of these complications even lead to death. Moreover, certain complications such as bleeding can be predictors of early mortality, which increases the importance of managing vascular access sites to avoid certain complications. In addition, more complicated postintervention antiplatelet regimes heighten the need for optimal vascular site management. To improve the outcomes in patients undergoing endovascular procedures, preventing access site complications is critical. The careful use of vascular closure devices can help in this aim.

References

1. Schnyder G, Sawhney N, Whisenant B, et al. Common femoral artery anatomy is influenced by demographics and comorbidity: implications for cardiac and peripheral invasive studies. Cathet Cardiovasc Interv. 2001;53:289–95.
2. Dauerman H, Applegate R, Cohen D. Vascular closure devices – The second decade. J Am Coll Cardiol 2207;50:1617-1626
3. Tiroch KA, Arora N, Matheny ME, et al. Risk predictors of retroperitoneal hemorrhage following percutaneous coronary intervention. Am J Cardiol. 2008;102:1473–6.
4. Fitts J, Ver LP, Hofmaster P, et al. Fluoroscopy-guided femoral artery puncture reduces the risk of PCI-related vascular complications. J Interv Cardiol. 2208;21:273-278
5. Koreny M, Riedmuller E, et al. Arterial puncture closing devices compared with standard manual compression after cardiac catheterization. JAMA. 2004;291(3):350–7.

Chapter 37
Endovascular Treatments in the Field

Neil G. Kumar and David L. Gillespie

1 Role of Endovascular Treatments in the Field

The use of endovascular techniques to treat traumatic vascular injuries was first reported by Marin et al in 1993. In this report, seven vascular injuries to the superficial femoral artery or subclavian arteries were treated using transluminally placed covered stents. These grafts were successfully inserted percutaneously or through open arteriotomies that were remote from the site of vascular trauma. Endovascular treatment of these traumatic injuries resulted in decreased blood loss, reduced requirements for anesthesia, and limited need for extensive dissection in the traumatized field.

2 Endovascular Suite: Field Requirements

The minimum requirements to successfully perform endovascular therapies in an austere environment are a form of imaging (usually a c-arm), an imaging table, and an adequate supply of disposable

N.G. Kumar, M.D. • D.L. Gillespie, M.D. (✉)
Division of Vascular Surgery, University of Rochester,
School of Medicine and Dentistry, Rochester, NY 14642, USA
e-mail: David_gillespie@urmc.rochester.edu

A. Kumar and K. Ouriel (eds.), *Handbook of Endovascular Interventions*,   511
DOI 10.1007/978-1-4614-5013-9_37,
© Springer Science+Business Media New York 2013

products such as sheaths, wires, catheters, stents, etc. In most civilian hospitals, this issue is managed effectively through hospital logistics and resupply by the individual product vendors. In the field environment however, resupply of materials is more challenging. In the US Military, resupply would be managed through the military's logistics system. This system however requires preidentification of the products needed and incorporation of them into a delivery platform.

To perform endovascular procedures successfully in any location, you must have excellent imaging. In the field environment, this is usually accomplished using a portable C-arm It must have digital subtraction angiography capabilities to facilitate imaging of the vascular structures without interference from bony structures. Imaging vascular software should also be included to allow performing accurate length, diameter, and angulation measurements intraoperatively to help the surgeon during endovascular therapies. You must have an operating table that is fluoroscopy compatible. In the field environment, considerations of space should be made in order to have enough clearance from the floor and ceiling to accommodate the image intensifier and X-ray source of the C-arm. The table should have controls for height and tilt. The table should meet all space and mobility constraints dictated by the field environment and delivery platform. A power injector is required for improved image quality.

The endovascular suite must be large enough to accommodate the endovascular team c-arm, power injector, and fluoro table. The storage of endovascular supplies requires a separate location and a method of accessing the inventory such as hanging hooks so that supplies can be accessed quickly and efficiently. In the US Military platforms, the OR iso-shelter can be configured to house either two standard OR tables or a single fluoro table with a c-arm (Figs. 37.1, 37.2 and 37.3).

Space considerations also relate to radiation safety in that the level of radiation is reduced by the square of the distance to the source (inverse square law). As such, as the endovascular suite becomes larger, they become safer and more comfortable, but at the expense of mobility and maximizing the resource of space. The repeated use of fluoroscopy requires the endovascular team to monitor potentially unsafe levels of radiation. This risk is reduced by monitoring radiation levels, wearing protective shielding, and minimizing fluoroscopy time. In the civilian hospital, great care is also taken to verify that radiation levels outside the suite are negligible. Patient safety should not be overlooked in the development of the endovascular suite.

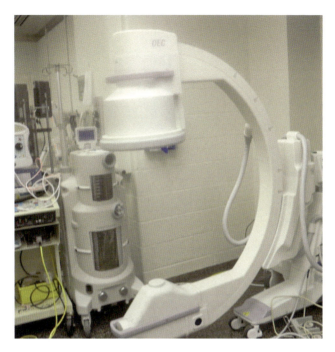

Fig. 37.1 Portable C-arm. Note the ability to move the C-arm away from the operating table for non-endovascular operations. PICTURE COURTESY OF: Colleen F. DeCarlis, RN, BS

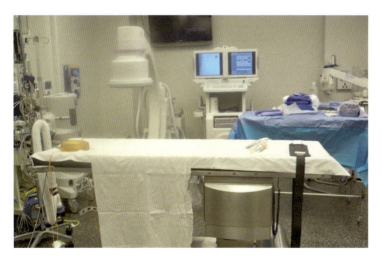

Fig. 37.2 Fluroscopy table. The fluoroscopy table can be imaged through and also has sufficient clearance to allow the C-arm to move freely. PICTURE COURTESY OF: Colleen F. DeCarlis, RN, BS

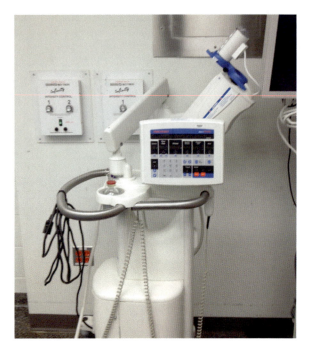

Fig. 37.3 Power injector. The power injector allows for improved image quality. PICTURE COURTESY OF: Colleen F. DeCarlis, RN, BS

Anesthesia is usually intravenous sedation with local supplementation. Cardiopulmonary monitoring is performed by an anesthesiologist, CRNA, or nurse using continuous electrocardiogram and intermittent blood pressure measurements.

3   Disease Distribution

In 2005, Fox et al published the first report of the distribution of vascular injuries seen in the current conflicts in Iraq and Afghanistan. From December 2001 through March 2004, all wartime evacuees evaluated at a single institution were prospectively entered into a database and retrospectively reviewed. Of 3,057 soldiers evacuated for medical evaluation, 1,524 (50%) sustained battle injuries. Known or suspected vascular injuries occurred in 107 (7%) patients, and these patients comprised the study group. Sixty-eight (64%) patients were wounded by explosive devices, 27 (25%) were wounded by gunshots, and 12 (11%) experienced blunt traumatic injury. The majority of injuries (59/66 [88%]) occurred in the extremities. Nearly half (48/107) of the patients underwent vascular repair in a forward hospital in Iraq or Afghanistan. Twenty-eight (26%) required additional operative intervention on arrival in the USA. Vascular injuries were associated with bony fracture in 37% of soldiers. Twenty-one of the 107 had a primary amputation performed before evacuation. Amputation after vascular repair occurred in eight patients. Of those, five had mangled extremities associated with contaminated wounds and infected grafts. Sixty-seven (63%) patients underwent diagnostic angiography. The most common indication was mechanism of injury (42%), followed by abnormal examination (33%), operative planning (18%), or evaluation of a repair (7%). The conclusions of this study were that wounding patterns reflected past experience with a high percentage of extremity injuries. Management of arterial repair with autologous vein graft remains the treatment of choice. Repairs in contaminated wound beds should be avoided. An increase in injuries from improvised explosive devices in modern conflict warrants the more liberal application of contrast arteriography. Endovascular techniques have advanced the contemporary management and proved valuable in the treatment of select wartime vascular injuries. This was confirmed in a later report by Clouse et al when they reported on their series of 408 arterial injuries managed in theater.

In 2006, Weber et al published a larger series on the modern military trauma experience with upper extremity trauma. In this report of 58 patients with upper extremity arterial wounds there were a total of 63 distinct arterial injuries. The axillary artery was injured in eight patients (13%). The brachial artery was injured in 33 patients (52%). The radial artery was injured in 16 patients (25%), and the ulnar artery was injured in six patients (10%).

The modern management of venous injuries suffered during military trauma was reported by Quan et al in 2006. In this report or 81 venous injuries in 65 patients, 43 (66%) patients suffered concomitant arterial injuries and 11 (17%) multiple venous injuries. Venous injury from improvised explosive devices was seen in 44 (67.7%) patients, gunshot wounds in 18 (27.7%), and motor vehicle accidents in 3 (4.6%). Extremity injuries accounted for a large number of wounds, comprising 64.2% of the cases, with 19.7% torso and 16.1% neck wounds. Ligation was the most common modality of treatment in combat zones. In a later report on venous injuries, Quan reported to find no difference in the incidence of venous thromboembolic complications between venous injuries managed by open repair versus ligation. Venous injuries were treated by ligation in 65 patients (63.1%) and by open surgical repair in 38 (36.9%). Postoperative extremity edema occurred in all patients irrespective of method of management. Thrombosis after venous repair occurred in 6 of the 38 cases (15.8%). Pulmonary emboli developed in three patients, one after open repair and two after ligation ($P > 0.99$).

4 Diagnosis

The diagnosis of vascular injuries still depends greatly on physical exam findings. Previous studies have shown little value in performing arteriography for proximity as a sole indication in civilian trauma. In general, performing ankle brachial indices can select out those patients at high risk for vascular injury that need arteriography. Patients with an ABI <0.9 has been shown to correlate with a higher incidence of vascular injury in civilian trauma patients. In contrast, occult vascular injuries requiring further intervention occur at a much higher frequency in combat. As such, liberal imaging is advocated, even in patients with a diffuse injury pattern and a normal physical exam. Recent combat casualties have stimulated a reassessment of the principles of management of high-risk extremity injuries with a normal vascular examination. Rapid evacuations have presented numerous US soldiers to the USA for evaluation in the early postinjury period. The liberal application of arteriography is a low-risk method to provide high-yield data in the delayed vascular evaluation of extremities injured from modern military munitions. Physical examination findings remain the most useful indicator, but a normal examination can be misleading and should not guide the decision for invasive imaging. Lesions are found and require further intervention at a higher rate than expected from the typical civilian trauma experience.

5   Diagnostic Imaging: Ultrasound/CT/MRI/ Diagnostic Angiography

The use of handheld Doppler during Vietnam as reported by Lavenson et al sets the standard for the field assessment of vascular trauma patients. Today duplex ultrasonography has extended the noninvasive diagnostic capabilities of trauma surgeons. The focused abdominal scan (FAS) has become the standard of care in both civilian and military trauma to date. Over time duplex ultrasonography has become easily portable and can be applied rapidly in most field hospital situations. For these reasons, ultrasound is well suited as an adjunct to physical exam in diagnosing vascular injury. However, its usefulness in the assessment of extremity vascular injuries can be limited. As in any situation, the accuracy of ultrasound is user dependent in diagnosing vascular injury.

Multislice (2–16) computed tomography (CT) (Fig. 37.4) is a technique that is now applied to many military combat support hospitals. It is currently designed to be deployed in its own iso-shelter as an adjunctive component. The usefulness of these low slice CT scans

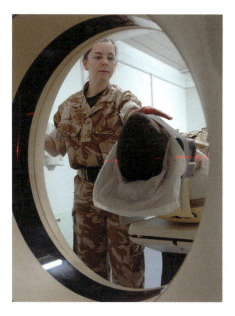

Fig. 37.4 Field Deployable Military CT Scanner. Image of a soldier undergoing CT imaging in a field hospitable. Image taken from http://www.armedforces-int. com/article/military-hospital-built-by-g3-systems.html

is, however, limited by their slow speed and the fact that metal artifact is created by bullet fragments and shrapnel commonly found in war military trauma. Newer generation 64 slice CT angiography, however, has been shown to be reliable in the diagnosis of occult vascular injury, even in the presence of bullet fragments, shrapnel and orthopedic hardware. CT also has the advantage that the entire arterial system can be imaged with a single, well-timed contrast bolus. This modality is quickly becoming the imaging method of choice in military evacuation and rear echelon hospitals.

Magnetic resonance imaging is not an option for use in the field at the current time. Bullet and metallic missile fragments preclude the use of this imaging modality in the majority of cases.

Due to its accuracy, and low comparative cost, digital subtraction angiography has become the method of choice for diagnosis of vascular injuries in the field. There are still, however, challenges regarding its portability. To date, this technology is only available in evacuation hospitals in the field. As detailed above, it requires a full OR iso-shelter for space and support considerations. The major advantage of DSA is the ability to not only diagnose vascular injuries but also potentially treat them using endovascular techniques (Figs. 37.5, 37.6 and 37.7).

The last diagnostic modality that is available in the field environment is digital fluoroscopy. This is simply a portable flat plate X-ray that uses digital technology for development. These machines are available for use in the far forward support hospitals. They are useful for any plain X-ray imaging such as chest X-rays or orthopedic imaging. They require little maintenance and can be used for vascular injury diagnosis with some effort.

6 Management

Vascular trauma in military injuries is treated (Fig. 37.9) differently than civilian vascular trauma due to the nature of the wartime injuries. Blast injuries sustained in military conflicts not only result in combined, nerve, artery, and bony injury but also destroy the majority of available autologous conduit for vascular reconstruction. As such, the emergent use of prosthetic grafts as a temporizing measure has been shown to be an effective limb salvage strategy. It allows time for patient resuscitation and transfer to the USA where elective revascularization can be undertaken with any remaining autologous vein conduits at a later date.

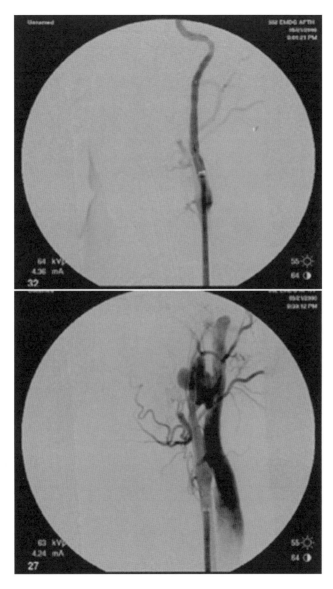

Fig. 37.5 Use of covered stents in the deployed environment for treatment of carotid jugular arteriovenous fistula

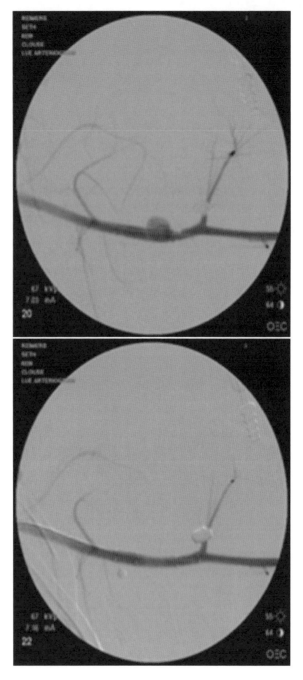

Fig. 37.6 Use of covered stents in the deployed environment for treatment of axillary artery pseudoaneurysm

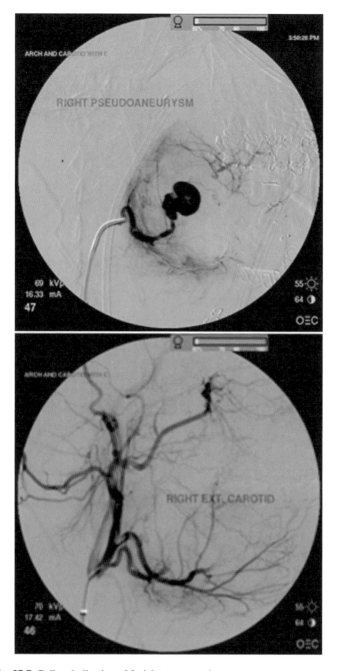

Fig. 37.7 Coil embolization of facial artery pseudoaneurysm

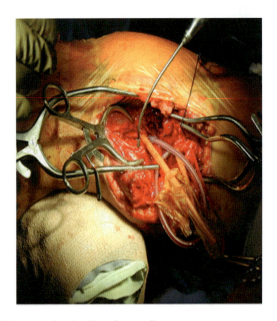

Fig. 37.8 Intravascular shunting of extremity trauma

The use of vascular shunts (Fig. 37.8) as a damage control adjunct has been described in several series from civilian institutions. In 2006, Rasmussen et al reported their experience using temporary shunting of military vascular injuries. There were 126 extremity vascular injuries treated. Fifty-three (42%) had been operated on at forward locations and 30 of 53 (57%) had temporary shunts in place upon arrival to our facility. The patency for shunts in proximal vascular injuries was 86% ($n=22$) compared with 12% ($n=8$) for distal shunts ($p<0.05$). All shunts placed in proximal venous injuries were patent ($n=4$). Systemic heparin was not used, and there were no shunt complications. All shunted injuries were reconstructed with vein in theater and early viability for extremities in which shunts were used was 92%. They concluded that temporary vascular shunts in proximal injuries have high patency rates compared with those placed in distal injuries. This vascular adjunct represents a safe and effective damage control technique and is preferable to attempted reconstruction in austere conditions.

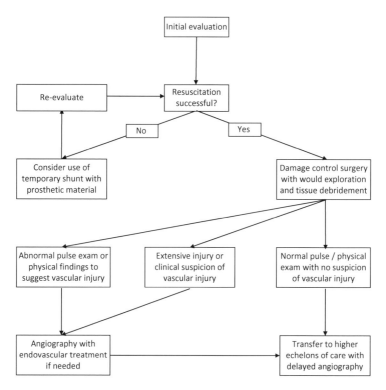

Fig. 37.9 Summary of the role of endovascular treatments in the field

7   List of the Open Operative Choices

The main indication for open surgery is in the acute setting where damage control is needed. Injuries involving difficult to access locations such as subclavian and high cervical vascular injuries have high morbidity associated with open repair. Endovascular repair has supplanted open treatment in such locations.

Removal of foreign bodies remains an area where open repair is used. However, even in the field environment, endovascular treatment including snare removal of the missile emboli has proven useful. Aidinian et al reported on the diagnosis and successful management of four arterial or venous injuries caused by missile emboli. In this report, all patients with venous emboli were treated with anticoagulation and those with arterial emboli were treated with standard embolectomy techniques with good result.

8 Complications and Management

Early experiences with endovascular treatments in the field are very promising. Procedure-related complications were low (3%) and mortality was low (1%) as well. The single death in their review was due to the lack of long-term dialysis capabilities for a soldier suffering from contrast-induced acute renal failure. Management of complications was most often corrected with open repair. However, as shown by the single death, management of expected complications is difficult in the field. Of the 150 catheter-based interventions in this report, 94 were diagnostic and 56 were therapeutic. Of the 56 therapeutic interventions, 39 were filter placements. Of the remaining therapeutic interventions, ten were embolization using coils or thrombotic material, five were covered stent placements, one was a bare metal stent placement, and one was a missile embolectomy. All ten of the embolization cases were effective in the short term, and none required open surgery to control hemorrhage. One patient undergoing embolization for hepatic injury and associated hemorrhage underwent open laparotomy 1 month after the initial injury and endovascular treatment to evacuate an infected perihepatic hematoma. All five covered stents were effective in controlling hemorrhage in the targeted vessel and were patient at the time of discharge from the combat hospital. The one patient who underwent balloon angioplasty and placement of a bare metal stent in an iliac artery to treat an anastomotic stenosis after open repair was discharged after 5 days. Finally, the one patient who underwent endovascular snare to retrieve a bullet lodged in a renal vein was discharged after 5 days as well. Importantly, this procedure saved the need for open repair. However, while these results are promising, long-term follow-up is lacking.

References

1. Marin ML, Veith FJ, Panetta TF, Cynamon J, Sanchez LA, Schwartz ML, Lyon RT, Bakal CW, Suggs WD. Transluminally placed endovascular stented graft repair for arterial trauma. J Vasc Surg. 1994;20:466–72. discussion 472–463.
2. Rasmussen TE, Clouse WD, Peck MA, Bowser AN, Eliason JL, Cox MW, Woodward EB, Jones WT, Jenkins DH. Development and implementation of endovascular capabilities in wartime. J Trauma. 2008;64:1169–76. discussion 1176.

3. Fox CJ, Gillespie DL, O'Donnell SD, Rasmussen TE, Goff JM, Johnson CA, Galgon RE, Sarac TP, Rich NM. Contemporary management of wartime vascular trauma. J Vasc Surg. 2005;41:638–44.
4. Clouse WD, Rasmussen TE, Peck MA, Eliason JL, Cox MW, Bowser AN, Jenkins DH, Smith DL, Rich NM. In-theater management of vascular injury: 2 years of the balad vascular registry. J Am Coll Surg. 2007;204:625–32.
5. Weber MA, Fox CJ, Adams E, Rice RD, Quan R, Cox MW, Gillespie DL. Upper extremity arterial combat injury management. Perspect Vasc Surg Endovasc Ther. 2006;18:141–5.
6. Quan RW, Adams ED, Cox MW, Eagleton MJ, Weber MA, Fox CJ, Gillespie DL. The management of trauma venous injury: Civilian and wartime experiences. Perspect Vasc Surg Endovasc Ther. 2006;18:149–56.
7. Quan RW, Gillespie DL, Stuart RP, Chang AS, Whittaker DR, Fox CJ. The effect of vein repair on the risk of venous thromboembolic events: a review of more than 100 traumatic military venous injuries. J Vasc Surg. 2008;47:571–7.
8. Gillespie DL, Woodson J, Kaufman J, Parker J, Greenfield A, Menzoian JO. The role of arteriography for blunt or penetrating trauma in proximity to major vascular structures. Ann Vasc Surg. 1993;7:145–9.
9. Johansen K, Lynch K, Paun M, Copass M. Non-invasive vascular tests reliably exclude occult arterial trauma in injured extremities. J Trauma. 1991;31:515–9. discussion 519–22.
10. Johnson ON, Fox CJ, O'Donnell S, Weber M, Adams E, Cox M, Quan R, Rich N, Gillespie DL. Arteriography in the delayed evaluation of wartime extremity injuries. Vasc Endovascular Surg. 2007;41:217–24.
11. Lavenson G RN: The use of doppler for vascular trauma assessment. Am J Surg 1977
12. White PW, Gillespie DL, Feurstein I, Aidinian G, Phinney S, Cox MW, Adams E, Fox CJ. Sixty-four slice multidetector computed tomographic angiography in the evaluation of vascular trauma. J Trauma. 2009;68:96–102.
13. Vertrees A, Fox CJ, Quan RW, Cox MW, Adams ED, Gillespie DL. The use of prosthetic grafts in complex military vascular trauma: a limb salvage strategy for patients with severely limited autologous conduit. J Trauma. 2009;66:980–3.
14. Eger M, Golcman L, Goldstein A, Hirsch M. The use of a temporary shunt in the management of arterial vascular injuries. Surg Gynecol Obstet. 1971;132:67–70.
15. Howe Jr HR, Pennell TC. A superior temporary shunt for management of vascular trauma of extremity. Arch Surg. 1986;121:1212.
16. Andreev A, Kavrakov T, Karakolev J, Penkov P. Management of acute arterial trauma of the upper extremity. Eur J Vasc Surg. 1992;6:593–8.
17. Reilly PM, Rotondo MF, Carpenter JP, Sherr SA, Schwab CW. Temporary vascular continuity during damage control: intraluminal shunting for proximal superior mesenteric artery injury. J Trauma. 1995;39:757–60.
18. Cox MW, Whittaker DR, Martinez C, Fox CJ, Feuerstein IM, Gillespie DL. Traumatic pseudoaneurysms of the head and neck: early endovascular intervention. J Vasc Surg. 2007;46:1227–33.
19. Aidinian G, Fox CJ, Rasmussen TE, Gillespie DL: Varied presentations of missile emboli in military combat. J Vasc Surg 2009

Chapter 38
Hypercoagulable States

**Guillermo A. Escobar, Peter K. Henke,
and Thomas W. Wakefield**

1 Thrombophilia

Defined by the WHO as "a tendency toward thrombosis." Inherited
thrombophilia is "the presence of an inherited factor that by itself
predisposes towards thrombosis but… requires interaction with other
components … before onset of the clinical disorder."

1.1 Coagulation Pathway

1. *The extrinsic pathway*
   Extravasated factor VII (FVII) is activated by perivascular tissue
   factor (from vascular smooth muscle cells, pericytes, and adventitial fibroblasts). FVIIa then activates factors FX and FIX. The
   latter ignites the intrinsic pathway, while FXa converts prothrombin (FII) to thrombin (FIIa), which then polymerizes fibrin (FI)

G.A. Escobar, M.D. • P.K. Henke, M.D.
Section of Vascular Surgery, University of Michigan Health System,
Ann Arbor, MI, USA

T.W. Wakefield, M.D. (✉)
Section of Vascular Surgery, 5463 Cardiovascular Center,
University of Michigan Health System, 1500 E. Medical Ctr Dr., THCC 2210,
Ann Arbor, MI 48109 SPC 5867, USA
e-mail: thomasww@umich.edu

A. Kumar and K. Ouriel (eds.), *Handbook of Endovascular Interventions*,   527
DOI 10.1007/978-1-4614-5013-9_38,
© Springer Science+Business Media New York 2013

and activates platelets. Activated platelets expose surface GPIIb–IIIa receptors which bind inactive FII while clots are formed. This helps concentrate FII within the thrombus to help form a stable clot scaffold interlaced with activated platelets. The phospholipid surfaces on platelets also accumulate coagulation factors FXa and FVa, which can each activate the intrinsic pathway. Once the extrinsic cascade is started, several activated factors (FVIIa, FIXa, and FXa) can subsequently activate FVII and thus amplify itself as a positive-feedback loop and also activates the intrinsic pathway.[1]

2. *The intrinsic pathway*
   Activated platelets, prekallikrein, high molecular weight kininogen, or negative charges activate FXIIa (Hageman's factor). FXI can be activated by several activated factors (FXIIa, FVIIa, FXa, and FIIa), including itself (FXIa), which then can activate circulating FVIII (which is usually bound to VonWillebrand's factor). FVIIIa then serves as the cofactor for FIX that is membrane bound. Together, with calcium, they form the *intrinsic Xase complex* (calcium, FVIIIa, and FIXa). This activates FX and allows FXa to activate, and form a complex with membrane-bound FV to form the *prothrombinase complex* (FXa-FVa) which can robustly activate FII. Fibrin is subsequently polymerized by FIIa and cross-linked by FXIII (fibrin-stabilizing factor).

1.2 Coagulopathic Conditions (Including Platelet Disorders)

A. *List*
   Von Willebrand's disease—Deficient Von Willebrand's factor (vWF)
   Bernard-Soulier syndrome—Abnormal/deficient glycoprotein Ib-IX-V complex
   Thrombocytopenia
   Hemophilia A, B, and C (deficiency of factors VIII, IX and XI respectively)
   Acquired antibodies to coagulation factors (factor VII and VIII are the most common)
   Disseminated intravascular coagulation (DIC)

B. *Tests and interpretation*

Von Willebrand's disease—vWF antigen assay to measure levels of vWF and glycoprotein Ib binding assay measures the functionality. Ristocetin test reveals platelet activation at lower than normal amounts of ristocetin.

Bernard-Soulier syndrome—Measure platelet function. Genetic testing confirmatory—autosomal recessive disorder.

Thrombocytopenia—Measure platelet count. Spontaneous bleeding usually occurs in counts <20,000/cc

Hemophilia A, B, and C—Measure levels of coagulation factors VIII, IX, and XI, respectively. If low, then genetic investigation for mutation: X chromosome for hemophilia A and B and hemophilia C is autosomal recessive.

Acquired antibodies to coagulation factors: Patients have prolonged PTT and/or INR. Detection of low levels of the involved coagulation factors. Serial dilutions of the plasma with serial clotting times will reveal normalization of clotting times and rapid reversal of the prolonged clotting times when mixing with coagulation factor-rich plasma. Usually in patients with a history of repeated transfusions of plasma and/or concentrated coagulation factors (e.g., leukemia, massive blood resuscitations, or hemophilias).

DIC—Low platelets, prolonged coagulation times, elevated fibrin split products, elevated D-dimers, and low fibrinogen. Clinically, the patient is bleeding excessively from multiple sites.

1.3 Systemic Conditions Predisposing to Hypercoagulable States (Table 38.1)

A. <u>Cancer:</u> Mucin-producing adenocarcinoma (lung cancer, colorectal cancer, and ovarian cancer especially) is a higher risk for venous thromboembolic events (VTE).

B. <u>Age:</u> Statistically alone, age confers a thrombophilic state because most risk factors for thrombophilia (atherosclerosis, surgery, paralysis, cancer etc.) are commonly associated with older populations. Patients >50 years also has high antiphospholipid antibody counts of unknown significance. Animal models have also demonstrated age that may lead to higher concentrations of

Table 38.1 Conditions associated with spontaneous thrombosis

Arterial

Intravascular foreign bodies

Unstable atherosclerotic plaques

Malignancies, especially mucin-producing adenocarcinomas

Antibody-mediated hypercoagulable states (Lupus, antiphospholipid syndrome)

Myeloproliferative syndromes (Polycythemia Vera and Essential
    Thrombocytosis)

Berger's syndrome

Kawasaki's syndrome

Aneurysms

Venous

Intravascular foreign bodies

Compression syndromes (May-Thurner, Paget-Schroetter, etc.)

Oral contraceptives

Malignancies, especially mucin producing adenocarcinomas

Genetic disorders (Factor V Leiden mutation, antithrombin III mutation, protein
    C deficiency, protein S deficiency, etc)

Antibody-mediated hypercoagulable states (Lupus, antiphospholipid syndrome)

Myeloproliferative syndromes (Polycythemia Vera and Essential
    Thrombocytosis)

Trauma and surgery

Prolonged immobility

Advanced age

Varicose veins

Arterial and venous

Intravascular foreign bodies

Malignancies, especially mucin producing adenocarcinomas

Antibody-mediated hypercoagulable states (Lupus, antiphospholipid syndrome)

Myeloproliferative syndromes (Polycythemia Vera and Essential
    Thrombocytosis)

Advanced age

P-selectin and less inflammatory cells involved in fibrinolysis which may also contribute to age-related thrombophilia[2].

C. Heparin induced thrombocytopenia (HIT): HIT usually occurs 5–14 days after being exposed to heparin and is defined as a 50% drop in platelets associated with a recent exposure to any heparin. Typically it presents as a thrombotic, rather than a hemorrhagic, syndrome due to either a platelet-heparin complex which is benign and short lived (HIT Type I) or an antibody-mediated thrombocytopenia due to IgG versus heparin-platelet factor IV complex (HIT

Type II). Antibody formation in patients undergoing cardiac surgery may occur in 25–50% of patients, but only 1–5% may develop HIT. This syndrome is estimated to occur in 50,000–250,000 cases a year in the United States. Depending on its manifestations, as many as 30% may die, 20% may require amputation and up to 50% may present with vascular occlusion[4, 5].

Both hemorrhagic and thrombotic manifestations occur when platelets are <20,000/cc. Antibody complexes and platelet activation may result in DVT, renal failure, peripheral embolization, and even stroke. Empiric treatment and heparin avoidance must immediately follow any suspected case. Antigenic and functional confirmatory tests (HIT antibody ELISA and serotonin release assay respectively) should be done upon suspicion. The HIT ELISA detects antibodies in the patient's blood, and the serotonin release assay detects abnormal activation of the patient's platelets upon exposure to heparin. The syndrome is initially treated with nonheparin anticoagulants to limit hypercoagulable complications. According to the eighth ACCP guidelines, the following should be used as a continuous infusion with their associated grades of recommendations: Danaparoid [Grade 1B], lepirudin [Grade 1C], argatroban [Grade 1C], fondaparinux [Grade 2C], or bivalirudin [Grade 2C].[6] The authors use Argatroban (if liver function is normal) or a hirudin inhibitor such as Lepirudin or Bivalirudin (if renal function is normal). They are titrated to a PTT 1.5–2 times normal. When platelet counts are >150,000/cc then oral vitamin K antagonists (VKAs) may be commenced for 6–8 weeks without stopping the intravenous anticoagulation until the goal INR is reached and then continued for five days after this (ACCP Guidelines Grade 1B). Because of several case reports of fondaparinux having cross-reactivity in cases of HIT, the authors do not use it for treatment of HIT.

Argatroban will falsely elevate the INR, and in order to determine if patients are therapeutic, if the INR is reported to be greater than 4, it may be necessary to stop the infusion for 4 h to determine the true INR while on VKA. Patients with type II HIT should avoid heparin thereafter and only be anticoagulated with thrombin inhibitors in the future.

D. Essential Thrombocytosis (ET) and polycythemia vera (PV):
Essential thrombocytosis and polycythemia vera are chronic Philadelphia-negative myeloproliferative disorders that are associated with a high risk of arterial and venous thrombosis of

both the small and the large vessels. The incidence of thrombotic events is unknown but may be as high as 50% upon diagnosis of either disease, but likely closer to 15–20%. Arterial thrombosis is more common in older patients with PV, and venous clots are more prevalent in those with ET and high hemoglobin concentrations, particularly if either have a history of a previous thrombotic event. The presence of leukocytosis at diagnosis has been suggested to play a role or predict the risk of clot formation, but its association has been questioned by recent studies[7]. There is also a higher risk of arterial thrombosis in patients with ET that have a JAK2V617F mutation. Cytoreduction is the key to lowering thrombotic risk in these patients, and low-dose aspirin may also be useful, but the Cochrane group's meta-analysis of aspirin use shows no statistically significant benefit in patients with PV and there are no randomized trials available in ET.

E. Pregnancy: Pregnancy and oral contraceptives are known risk factors for developing thromboembolic events. The overall incidence of venous thromboembolic event (VTE) during pregnancy is about 1/1,000 deliveries. It may be due to an increase in the amount of heparin-binding proteins, factor VIII, and fibrinogen in the setting of acquired activated protein C resistance.

Pregnancy may also unmask other inherited or antibody-mediated procoagulant disorders such as factor V Leiden, Protein C deficiency or antiphospholipid syndrome.

F. HIV—AIDS: HIV has an increased risk of spontaneous thrombosis. It affects about 0.26–7% of HIV + patients and has become an emerging issue not previously noted. It may manifest as venous thromboembolic complications (>60%) or even acute myocardial infarction. There have been reports of increased anticardiolipin (antiphospholipid) antibodies as well as decreased protein S (anticoagulant) which may account for this. Epidemiological studies have implicated protease inhibitor antiretrovirals. Patients with AIDS are also prone to develop malignancies which may also contribute to the increased risk of thrombosis.

G. Sepsis: Infectious systemic inflammatory response syndrome is nearly always associated with some sort of hypercoagulable state. Clinically significant abnormalities occur in half to three quarters of patients with severe infections, and up to 35% will have DIC criteria. The etiology seems to be associated with an elevation of acute-phase reactants such as fibrinogen, C5a, and other compliment levels. Additionally, it is suspected that sepsis may uncover otherwise clinically dormant, inherited hypercoagulable conditions such as factor V Leiden as well as Protein C and S deficiencies with a decreased survival. This has led to a large amount of research and even consensus statements that advocate modulating the anticoagulant pathway using infusions of activated protein C as a way to improve survival in septic shock[8].

H. Noninherited thrombosis:

May-Thurner Syndrome

Iliac vein compression syndrome (May-Thurner syndrome) is venous outflow obstruction or thrombosis of the lower extremities due to venous compression by the overlying right iliac artery. It is more common in females and on their left iliac vein. Rarely it affects the right iliac vein and vena cava in patients with a high iliac artery bifurcation or left-sided IVC.

Ilio-femoral thrombosis per-se was traditionally treated with anticoagulation alone. However, it may be better treated with catheter-directed lysis/thrombectomy, and in May-Thurner syndrome, a closed-cell stent is placed in the compressed vein to diminish postthrombotic syndrome and maintain patency[3].

The randomized, multicenter Acute Venous Thrombosis: Thrombus Removal With Adjunctive Catheter-Directed Thrombolysis (ATTRACT) trial (ClinicalTrials.gov identifier: NCT00790335) is planned to evaluate the outcomes of anticoagulation alone versus the use of pharmacomechanical thrombus removal in iliofemoral DVT.

If the thrombus extends below the inguinal ligament, then open thrombectomy and an arteriovenous fistula may be required. All cases of thrombosis are followed by anticoagulation with VKA and a follow-up venogram if stenting was performed.

Paget-Schrotter Syndrome (Stress Thrombosis)

Thrombosis of the axillary-subclavian veins, commonly associated with repetitive motion of the affected arm in young athletes (baseball, volleyball, swimming, etc.). This is due to hypertrophy and lateral insertion of the subclavius muscle which compresses the subclavian vein. Treatment includes anticoagulation and removal of the first rib and anterior scalene muscle. Endovascular thrombolysis and recanalization of the subclavian vein in Paget-Schroetter syndrome precedes surgical decompression, which is done either during the same hospitalization or after a few days to weeks. Angioplasty or stenting alone (without decompression) fails as neither can overcome the musculoskeletal compression of the subclavian vein.

Vascular Trauma and Intravascular Foreign Bodies

Damage to the endothelium leads to activation of platelets and coagulation factors. Any patient with vessel wall irritation from intraluminal foreign bodies such as stents or in-dwelling catheters is thrombophilic. Two thirds to three quarters of upper extremity deep venous thrombosis (DVT) are associated with central venous catheters.

Vena Cava Filters: Permanent and Temporary Filters

Inferior vena cava (IVC) filters lower the risk of pulmonary embolism (PE) in patients that have a DVT unable to be anticoagulated or who recur during anticoagulation. The 2008 ACCP conference guidelines state that IVC filters do not replace anticoagulation and should only be used in patients with contraindications or failures to anticoagulant therapy, not as prophylactic in those without a recent DVT or PE.[9] Filters do not increase overall survival (just the rate of PE). Complications include vena cava thrombosis (2–14% depending on the filter used), renal vein thrombosis, erosion into bowel, and/or aorta.

Retrievable filters are for patients with temporary contraindications to anticoagulation. Poor long-term follow-up leads to poor removal rates of temporary filters, and because they have a much higher rate of strut fracture compared to Greenfield filters, they should only be used only when planning to remove them. Permanent filters endothelialize after 2–3 weeks, and thus attempts to remove them should be carefully considered.

There is no randomized trial assessing the utility of superior vena cava (SVC) filters for upper extremity DVT. Well over half of patients with SVC filters will die of their underlying diseases within 2 months of SVC filter placement, [10] and the rare SVC filter perforation or migration result in a high mortality secondary to tamponade. Once an SVC filter is in place any blind attempt to insert a central catheter may dislodge the filter or entangle the guidewire. Therefore, the benefit of SVC filters is still unclear.

Surgery

May be associated with a VTE rate of 15–40%. It is thought to be
due to an increase of procoagulant and inflammatory cytokines
associated with surgical trauma; in addition to postoperative
inactivity. Procedures that require immobility during and after
the procedure (such as hip replacements) have the highest risk
of deep venous thrombosis (40–60). Sequential compression
devices (SCDs) and low molecular weight anticoagulation
each decrease the risk of VTE by half when each was compared to no therapy. For this reason, all patients undergoing
surgery should have pharmacologic prophylaxis and/or perioperative SCD prophylaxis according to their risk.[9]

2   Endovascular Procedures: Stents, Balloons, Duration of Procedure, etc.

2.1   *Endogenous Inhibitors of Coagulation*

Antithrombin III (AT III) binds to factor Xase complex and FIIa
Activated proteins C inactivates FVa and FVIIIa
Protein S is a cofactor for protein C and increases its affinity to FVa
and VIIIa
Endogenous heparin binds to AT III and increases its affinity to FVa
and VIIIa

2.2   *Non-Antiplatelet Antithrombotic Agents*

A. *Agents and administration route*
   Heparin/LMWH—Intravenous or subcutaneous
   Warfarin—Oral
   Fondaparinux and biotinylated idraparinux—Subcutaneous
   Hirudin derivatives (lepirudin, bivalirudin)—Intravenous
   Argatroban—Intravenous
   Rivaroxaban and Apixaban—Oral
   Dabigatran etexilate—Oral

B. *Mechanism of action*

Heparin (all forms): Potentiate antithrombin III (AT III) inhibition of factor Xa.

Warfarin: Inhibits production of vitamin K-dependent coagulation factors (II, VII, IX, and X) by interfering with vitamin K epoxide reductase which stops gamma carboxylation of the coagulation factors. It also inhibits the formation of anticoagulant proteins C and S (also vitamin K dependent).

Fondaparinux and biotinylated idraparinux: Pentasaccharide inhibits FXa

Hirudin derivatives: Inhibit thrombin (FIIa)

Argatroban: Inhibits thrombin (FIIa)

Rivaroxaban and Apixaban—Inhibits FXa

Dabigatran etexilate—Inhibits thrombin (FIIa)

C. *Indications for use*

Heparin: Any thrombotic syndrome. Intraoperative anticoagulation and DVT prophylaxis. Unfractionated heparin requires a continuous intravenous infusion and routine aPTTs every 6 h. Low molecular weight heparin (LMWH) may be used as an outpatient subcutaneously and is ideal for prophylaxis or treatment of DVT in pregnancy.

Warfarin: Long-term maintenance of anticoagulation. Used mainly in an ambulatory patient. Requires close monitoring of INR and stable diets. Its effective use is modified and made difficult by many drug and food interactions.

Fondaparinux and biotinylated idraparinux: Generally used as a heparin alternative for DVT prophylaxis and treatment via subcutaneous administration.

Hirudin derivatives: Treatment for HIT or used in patients requiring anticoagulation who have a history of HIT.

Argatroban: Treatment for HIT or used in patients requiring anticoagulation who have a history of HIT.

Rivaroxaban and Apixaban: Oral drugs that are actively being studied as substitutes for warfarin that do not require frequent lab monitoring.

Dabigatran etexilate: Oral drug that is actively being studied as a substitute for warfarin that does not require frequent lab monitoring

D. *Contraindications*

Heparin: History of HIT. LMWH is contraindicated in renal failure

Warfarin: Pregnancy. Severe liver failure

Fondaparinux and biotinylated idraparinux: Liver failure. Fondaparinux has reported cross reactivity in patients with HIT. Biotinylated idraparinux is currently in clinical trials.

Hirudin derivatives: Liver failure

Argatroban: Renal failure

Rivaroxaban and Apixaban: (still in clinical trials)

Dabigatran etexilate: (still in clinical trials)

E. *Method of reversal*

Heparin: Protamine (even low molecular weight heparin may be reversed)

Warfarin: Rapid reversal- Plasma transfusion. Slow reversal: Administration of vitamin K

Fondaparinux: None known.

Biotinylated Idraparinux: May be reversed with avidin.

Hirudin Derivatives: None known

Argatroban: None known

Rivaroxaban and Apixaban: None known

Dabigatran etexilate: None known

2.3 Thrombolytic Agents

A. *Plasmin activators*

1. *Streptokinase*

Purified from Streptococcus in 1933. Inexpensive but leads to antigenicity which may be mild or severe (anaphylactic). Rarely used in developed countries.

2. *Urokinase*

Purified in 1947 from the urine and produced by renal tubular cells. The FDA stalled production years ago, so it fell out of favor in the USA. However, is still the primary thrombolytic agent in Europe.

3. *Tissue Plasminogen Activator (tPA)*

Naturally found in the body. Extracted from 5 kg of uterine tissue in 1979 to get 1 mg of TPA. Since then, is purified from a melanoma cell line or from recombinant technology and is the primary thrombolytic in the USA. Is the most expensive of the three previous lytics.

4. *Reteplase*

Is a TPA that is modified to have less affinity to endothelium and monocytes, thus prolonging its half-life and faster lysis.

Mechanism of Action

Streptokinase: Forms an active complex with plasminogen known as "plasminogen activator" which can then activate plasminogen to form plasmin (plasminogen is the rate-limiting cofactor and substrate). The half-lives of the complex per-se and the lytic activity are 16 and 83 min.

Urokinase: Is a serine protease which cleaves two amino acids off plasminogen (Arg560-Val561) and activates it. The half-life is 14 min.

tPA and Reteplase: Are also serine protease activators of clot-bound plasminogen. The half-life of rTPA is 4–7 min. Reteplase has a half-life to 14–18 min

Indications for Use (Including FDA Approval for/Not): FDA indications for the use of thrombolytics include acute myocardial infarction, massive pulmonary embolus, acute thrombotic stroke, and unclotting central catheters. Common off-label uses include treatment of peripheral vessel/graft thrombosis and extremity DVT.

Contraindications: Surgery less than 6 weeks, high risk of bleeding, allergy to the lytic, thrombocytopenia. Should not be used on patients with acute limb ischemia with motor weakness. (Rutherford Class IIIb or IV ischemia should receive immediate revascularization and not wait for lytics to work.)

B. *Thrombolytic Devices*

Most have incorporated simultaneous thrombolytic infusions, which minimize the time to lysis and the total amount of lytic required to achieve lysis. No large head-to-head trial has been attempted between the devices, only versus catheter-directed thrombolysis alone.

1. AngioJet (Medrad, Inc): Multiple high-pressure jets come out of side holes at 10,000 psi to fracture clots up to 12 mm in diameter. The jets produce a low-pressure zone that removes the fractured thrombus. It is often used with a dilute lytic solution and uses a 0.035-inch guidewire over a 6-F sheath.
2. Trellis (Bacchus Vascular, Inc): Balloon containment of thrombus with chemical and mechanical thrombolysis. Mechanical thrombolysis is done with a battery-powered motor which moves a wire at 3,000 rpm. Requires an 8F sheath and uses a 0.035-in. guidewire. Lengths include 80 and 120 cm with treatment areas between 10, 15, and 30 cm.
3. Ekos (Ekos Corporation): Originally designed to improve the response to thrombolytics in strokes. It requires a lytic infusion and uses 2 MHz ultrasonic waves to destabilize clots and fibrin cross-linking to expose plasmin active sites for the lytic to work better. It is mounted on a 5.2-F catheter and is available in 106 cm and 135 cm catheter lengths and 6–50 cm treatment zones. The central lumen allows passage of a 0.035-in. wire and saline coolant while the side ports dispense the lytic. The disposable control unit can adjust the speed of the oscillating catheter and the position of the Sin wave to maximize the response.
4. Arrow-Trerotola (Arrow international Inc.): This is a purely mechanical, motor-driven nitinol cage mounted on a wire that spins to break up clots. Due to the risk of winding itself up in the struts of stents, it should not be used near them, or around other, loose guidewires. There are 5 F and 7 F cages with lengths of 65 and 120 mm, respectively.

3 Conclusion

With all the above factors to consider in a patient presenting with thrombosis, presented below is an adapted version of an international consensus guideline formed to standardize who need testing.

1. Any first, spontaneous thromoboembolic event (TE) without risk factors
2. TE in patients under the age of 50, even with a transient predisposing factor

3. Patients whose only risk factor is estrogen therapy or pregnancy
4. Recurrent TE regardless of risk factors (even superficial phlebitis if not associated with cancer or varicosities)
5. TE in patients <50 years, in uncommon sites (intra-abdominal, retinal etc.)
6. Warfarin-induced skin necrosis and purpura fulminans (when not associated with sepsis)
7. Two consecutive abortions, three nonconsecutive, or one fetal death after 20 weeks
8. Asymptomatic first-degree relatives of others with proven thrombophilia
9. Sever pre-eclampsia
10. Children with TE

These should be screened as a starting point with the following tests:

Collect <u>before</u> initiating anticoagulation: PTT, INR, antithrombin (AT), protein C and S levels.

Anticoagulation does <u>not affect</u>: Complete blood count (CBC), Factor V Leiden, Factor II G20210A mutation, anticardiolipin, anti-beta 2gp I, and fasting homocysteine levels.

References

1. Mackman N, Tilley RE, Key NS. Role of the extrinsic pathway of blood coagulation in hemostasis and thrombosis. Arterioscler Thromb Vasc Biol. 2007;27:1687–93.
2. McDonald AP, Meier TR, Hawley AE, et al. Aging is associated with impaired thrombus resolution in a mouse model of stasis induced thrombosis. Thromb Res. 2010;125:72–8.
3. Knipp BS, Ferguson E, Williams DM, et al. Factors associated with outcome after interventional treatment of symptomatic iliac vein compression syndrome. J Vasc Surg. 2007;46:743–9.
4. Rice L. Centers for Disease Control and Prevention ICD-9-CM Coordination and Maintenance Committee Meeting- Diagnosis Agenda. In: Prevention CfDCa, ed.; 2007.
5. Prechel M, Walenga JM. The laboratory diagnosis and clinical management of patients with heparin-induced thrombocytopenia: an update. Semin Thromb Hemost. 2008;34:86–96.
6. Warkentin TE, Greinacher A, Koster A, Lincoff AM. Treatment and prevention of heparin-induced thrombocytopenia: American College of Chest Physicians Evidence-Based Clinical Practice Guidelines (8th Edition). Chest. 2008;133:340S–80S.

7. Gangat N, Wolanskyj AP, Schwager SM, Hanson CA, Tefferi A. Leukocytosis at diagnosis and the risk of subsequent thrombosis in patients with low-risk essential thrombocythemia and polycythemia vera. Cancer. 2009;115:5740–5.
8. Dellinger RP, Levy MM, Carlet JM, et al. Surviving sepsis campaign: international guidelines for management of severe sepsis and septic shock: 2008. Crit Care Med. 2008;36:296–327.
9. Kearon C, Kahn SR, Agnelli G, Goldhaber S, Raskob GE, Comerota AJ. Antithrombotic therapy for venous thromboembolic disease: American College of Chest Physicians Evidence-Based Clinical Practice Guidelines (8th Edition). Chest. 2008;133:454S–545S.
10. Usoh F, Hingorani A, Ascher E, et al. Long-term follow-up for superior vena cava filter placement. Ann Vasc Surg. 2009;23:350–4.

Chapter 39
Simulators in Endovascular Treatment

Javier E. Anaya-Ayala, Jean Bismuth, Mark G. Davies, and Alan B. Lumsden

1 Introduction

Training in Vascular and Endovascular Surgery faces enormous challenges as a consequence of rapidly evolving technology and changes in postgraduate medical education (e.g., restriction of working hours thereby effectively reducing operative time). Traditionally, Vascular Surgery training has distinguished itself by being a low-volume/high-complexity specialty, systematically focused on case load to determine its adequacy. As new training paradigms are being developed and assessed for vascular residents, simulator-based training will become crucial to the trainee's proficiency.

The authors have no competing interests to declare and received no financial contributions.

J.E. Anaya-Ayala, M.D.
The Methodist Hospital Research Institute, The Methodist Hospital,
Houston, TX, USA

J. Bismuth, M.D. • M.G. Davies, M.D., Ph.D., M.B.A. (✉) • A.B. Lumsden, M.D.
Division of Vascular Surgery, Department of Cardiovascular Surgery,
The Methodist DeBakey Heart & Vascular Center, The Methodist Hospital,
6550 Fannin Street, Suite 1401, Houston, TX 77030, USA
e-mail: mdavies@tmhs.org

A. Kumar and K. Ouriel (eds.), *Handbook of Endovascular Interventions*,   543
DOI 10.1007/978-1-4614-5013-9_39,

2 What Is a Simulator?

Simulation is used in many contexts, including the modeling of natural systems or human systems in order to gain insight into their functioning. Virtual reality (VR) simulations have long been used as training and evaluation tools in aviation and other professions. Medical simulation is defined as a "person, device or set of conditions which attempts to present education and evaluation of problems authentically." Simulation-based training in medicine and surgery has only recently become generally accessible. The broad consensus is that the new technologies will become an integral part of how vascular surgeons acquire new procedural skills and are assessed for proficiency and maintenance of competency.

Endovascular therapy is increasingly being applied to all territories of the vascular system, and a different set of skills is required when compared with open surgery. Simulations represent an excellent opportunity for training in procedures and management of potential complications; although it does not replace clinical training, it completely avoids the risks of patient injury and medicolegal liability associated with hands-on training in patient care settings. Rather, it offers a means for mentored instruction in a more realistic way than can be provided with demonstration, and it is more efficient (more cases can be practiced), more realistic (human anatomy and physiology are modeled), and less expensive than training in large-animal models.

3 Types of Simulators

Simulations are categorized into two broad groups:

1. Low fidelity (LF)
2. High fidelity (HF)

LF simulations use materials and equipment that are different from those used for the task being considered. HF simulations use realistic materials and equipment to reproduce or represent the setting task. HF endovascular procedure simulators provide real-time interactive simulation, two-dimensional graphic displays of angiographic anatomy and mechanical interfaces with guide wires, sheaths, and catheters, which provide some degree of haptic feedback.

3.1   The Available Simulation Models for Endovascular Skills Are as Follows

A. Synthetic: These models range from low fidelity solid plastic models to high fidelity systems with fluoroscopy and pulsatile flow. This is relatively inexpensive and benefits from being portable, simple to set up, and radiologic screening is not often required; among its disadvantages is the fact that they cannot fully replicate the dynamic behavior of the human arterial circulation in terms of the elasticity of arterial walls or blood flow.

B. Large animal models offer highly realistic training options for advanced interventions with the possibility of artificially inducing blood vessel lesions by endothelial injury and sutured patches. On the other hand, some of the disadvantages are the fact that the use of animal models is limited by expense, legal and ethical issues and the requirement for specialist facilities as well as the knowledge of the anatomical and size differences compared to human bodies.

C. Human Cadaveric models have also been described to offer highly realistic conditions for testing endovascular devices and training. These allow full procedures to be performed including arterial puncture and closure though preserved cadaveric tissue differs in feel and deformation from living tissue. Garrett described the process of establishing pulsatile flow in the arterial tree of a human cadaver following a thrombolytic process using fresh frozen human cadavers. The antegrade arterial flow was established by pumping fluid into an inflow cannula placed in the descending aorta via the axillary artery and an outflow cannula in the superficial femoral artery. Limitations are availability and high cost as well as the fact that preserved cadaveric tissue differs in feel and deformation from living tissue.

Early experience has shown that simulation is well accepted by trainees, performance on simulators improves with training and practice and simulation prior to the first endovascular procedures can improve clinical performance. Endovascular procedure simulators that offer hands-on procedural training with visual, haptic (relating to or based on the sense of touch), and aural feedback are now more widely available. Although they have notable differences in design and features, all of the commercially available VR endovascular procedure simulators are categorized as high-fidelity simulators because they include haptic, aural, and visual interfaces and provide a pseudorealistic representation of the clinical situation. Dawson et al. subjectively evaluated how vascular surgery residents and program directors perceived simulation in the acquisition of endovascular procedural skills, with the conclusion being that simulation training was judged to be most beneficial for vascular residents early in their endovascular experience, to facilitate the transition to complex procedures.

D. Virtual Reality Simulation

VR simulation uses a computer-generated three-dimensional model of the vascular tree allowing the user to interact with simulation through an interface device. Recent developments in computer power and volume rendering techniques enable a high degree of realism in simulated fluoroscopic images. Patient specific simulation is also possible which may allow rehearsal of a procedure prior to performing the real case. HF VR simulation is available.

The devices are still prone to technical failure and require regular calibration and maintenance. Despite the cost, computer-based simulation may be an attractive option for endovascular training. Trainees can repeatedly perform a procedure or indeed a maneuver until proficiency has been demonstrated. The use of standardized task may allow the development of a proficiency-based curriculum with subjects demonstrating a predetermined benchmark level of expertise prior to interventions on patients.

3.2 Commercially Available VR Endovascular Simulators

Currently available endovascular simulators include Procedicus VIST™ (Mentice, Gothenburg, Sweden), Animator (Simbionix Corporation, Denver, CO), and Endovascular Accutouch (Immersion Medical, Gaithersburg, MD). The **Procedicus VIST simulator** comprises a mechanical unit housed within a plastic mannequin cover, a high-performance desktop computer, and two display screens. The term haptic relates to tactile feedback which is created by a series of motorized carts which lock onto the inserted instrument allowing the subject to manipulate the simulated instrument, in real-time with force-feedback. Commercially available simulation modules include occlusive arterial disease in the coronary arteries, intracranial vessels, carotid, renal and ileo-femoral regions, as well as aortic aneurysm and some management of venous disease. The subject is able to select appropriate instruments and perform interventional procedures using the simulated fluoroscopic screen. Performance is measured using metric parameters such as volume of contrast fluid used, fluoroscopy time, and markers of stent placement accuracy. The **Angiomentor Ultimate endovascular trainer** has a similar range of arterial procedures to the VIST and also boasts advanced haptic technology. It differs from the VIST in that there is greater emphasis on patient monitoring, drug administration, and response to physiological disturbance, for example, administration of atropine to correct bradycardia induced by carotid sinus stimulation and appropriate therapeutic responses to chest pain or breathlessness. Two cheaper and more portable editions have become available, the Angiomentor Express and the Angiomentor Mini with similar simulation packages but less peripheral attachments such that the Mini can fit into a handheld case. The **SimSuite** is a larger simulator system with up to six interactive screens to facilitate multidisciplinary training. Similar to the Angiomentor system, response to patient physiology features substantially in the simulation. Additionally though, appropriate case selection and management are also taught. The **Endovascular Accutouch simulator** also boasts peripheral arterial, carotid, and coronary simulation modules with metric based-assessment. The reliability of simulator devices remains problematic, and there is a significant requirement for regular maintenance and calibration. One of the main problems with the use of computer-based simulation is keeping the simulators up and running. Regular calibration is required to ensure optimum levels of force-feedback. This needs to be checked daily and is dependent on environmental temperature which needs to be stable. Inserted tools are detected by the haptic interface using an optic mechanism which distinguishes both the presence and the diameter of the instrument allowing the selected tool to be simulated. This part of the unit requires calibration less frequently but is subject to interference from dust particles and debris. Calibration and maintenance tasks require skilled technical support for heavy usage periods especially involving more challenging cases such as carotid artery stent procedures. Simsuite (MSC), on the other hand, retains responsibility for servicing their machines as part of their lease agreement. With regard to endovascular tools, real-life tools can be used but the floppy tips of guide wires, stents, or embolic protection device need to be removed.

4 Outcomes with Simulators

The learning curve used in the context of skills training refers to the time taken and/or the number of procedures an average practitioner needs to be able to perform a procedure independently with an acceptable outcome. Two types of variables are generally used: measures of **patient outcome** such as complications and survival or measures of **surgical process** such as blood loss and operative time. Endovascular practitioners have a procedure-related learning curve. The outcomes of sequential groups of patients undergoing carotid artery stenting have been analyzed in several studies and have demonstrated decreased procedure-related complications, fluoroscopic time, and contrast volume used with increased physician experience. Studies tend to suggest that inexperienced subjects in particular derive significant benefit in terms of improved performance on the simulator with repetitive practice compared with expert subjects, who also have a short learning curve as they become familiar with the simulator. The suggested benefit of simulation-based practice is that subjects gain basic psychomotor skills that become automated by the time they perform procedures in real patients. Before widespread adoption of simulators into the endovascular curriculum, it is necessary to demonstrate transfer of endovascular skill to real procedures. Recent evidence of skills transfer using VR simulation for endovascular skills training is encouraging, with improved performance in the catheterization lab demonstrated in vivo. Berry et al. performed a randomized trial comparing a live porcine model with VR simulation training to perform an iliac artery angioplasty task. Total score (combined global rating scale and task-specific checklist) improved significantly with repetitive practice in both the porcine and VR groups. Notably, this improvement was shown to transfer from the VR simulator to the porcine model.

5 Accreditation

The trend in medical skills training is a move toward using objective assessment tools to demonstrate technical competence. However, objective measures of skills performance are not well reported in endovascular interventions yet. A number of assessment tools are available including time-action analysis, error analysis, global rating scales and procedure-specific checklists, motion analysis, and, perhaps most promising, VR simulators. Time-action analysis has been used as a method of objective assessment of performance in open and minimally invasive surgery. This method can be reapplied to real life or simulator performance and involves breaking down the procedure into a series of steps with performance analyzed by how long an individual takes to complete each step. This procedure is, however, manpower intensive in terms of setup and video analysis time. In addition, the amount of time taken to complete an individual procedural step does not offer any measure of quality of performance. Therefore, time-action analysis may be more useful as a research tool, offering an insight into instrument design and procedural efficiency.

6 Conclusion

Simulator training offers significant benefits in the context of a competence or proficiency-based training program because these can be used early on in the learning experience to acquire and reinforce basic wire and catheter handling skills prior to learning on patients. The available evidence tends to suggest that inexperienced subjects are able to improve their endovascular skills performance with repetitive practice using VR simulation. However, further work to validate VR simulators as assessment tools is required especially to examine the question of skills transfer from simulation to real life if they are to fulfill their potential to provide a HF training experience and objective assessment of endovascular skill. In particular, the transfer effectiveness of VR endovascular training is not established.

There is need for continuous update of education content, which can expensive and time consuming. The cost of the simulators, particularly VR, ranges from $100,000 to 250,000 with additional maintenance costs and usually from a limited education budget. In addition, the proprietary components for training on new devices may be present on a simulator but access prohibited from general use and controlled by the device company which paid for the development of the module.

Although simulation-based training is unlikely to replace real-life experience, it is an adjunct for training to allow novices to learn basic skills away from the patient leading to a shorter and flatter learning curve. Despite rapid progress in the development of simulator technology, in particular, computer-based simulation, there is still a considerable gap in knowledge about how best to make use of this technology. What device is required at various stages of training is yet to be established. Task analysis is required to determine what core skills are required as well as how they are best delivered by the available modalities of training. Advanced simulation may not be necessary early in the learning curve. Basic skills tasks such as wire and catheter manipulation may be effectively taught by relatively cheap synthetic models prior to performing complete procedures using VR simulators or anesthetized animals. Preprocedure review of an angiogram usually allows identification of difficult anatomy; however, using VR simulation for rehearsal affords the opportunity to experiment with different catheter shapes to selectively cannulate the target artery and size the stent and embolic protection device. This may improve procedure efficiency and also reduce risk to the patient from catheter manipulation. Especially in the aortic arch or supraaortic trunks.

Nowadays, simulation-based training offers the opportunity to shorten the trainee's learning curve, improve patient safety, and reduce expense in terms of operating room time, but this does not remove the requirement for specialist supervision. In order to benefit fully from this new technology, training structures need to evolve to make use of the available technology.

References

1. Cronenwett JL. Vascular surgery training; is there enough case material? Semin Vasc Surg. 2006;19(4):187–90.
2. Kwolek CJ, Crawford RS. Training the next generation of vascular specialists: current status and future perspectives. J Endovasc Ther. 2009;16 Suppl 1:I42–52.
3. Lermausiaux P, Leroux C, Tasse JC, Castellani L, Martinez R. Aortic aneurysm: construction of a life-sized model by rapid prototyping. Ann Vasc Surg. 2001;15:131–5.
4. Dawson DL, Meyer J, Lee ES, Pevec WC. Training with simulation improves residents' endovascular procedure skills. J Vasc Surg. 2007;45(1):149–54.
5. Neequaye SK, Aggarwal R, Van Herzeele I, Darzi A, Cheshire NJ. Endovascular skills training and assessment. J Vasc Surg. 2007;46(5): 1055–64.

6. Lin PH, Bush RL, Peden EK, Zhou W, Guerrero M, Henao EA, Kougias P, Mohiuddin I, Lumsden AB. Carotid artery stenting with neuroprotection; assessing the learning curve and treatment outcome. Am J Surg. 2005;190: 850–7.
7. Van Herzeele I, Aggarwal R, Choong A, Brightwell R, Vermassen FE, Cheshire NJ. Virtual reality simulation objectively differentiates level of carotid stent experience in experienced interventionalists. J Vasc Surg. 2007; 46(5):855–63.

Chapter 40
Training Paradigms in Endovascular Surgery: Australasia, South America, South Africa, Europe

W. Richard Wilson, Robert Fitridge, Ricardo C. Rocha Moreira, Christian B. Liu, Barbara D. Moreira, Martin Veller, Konstantinos G. Moulakakis, Efthimios D. Avgerinos, and Christos D. Liapis

1 Australasia

1.1 History of Evolution of Training Paradigm to Its Present Status

During the last 15 years, there has been a dramatic change in the management of vascular disease with a marked increase in the utilisation of endovascular techniques for occlusive and aneurysmal disease. This exponential rise in the number and complexity of minimally invasive radiological procedures has resulted in the formal separation of vascular surgical training from general surgery.

W.R. Wilson, M.D., F.R.C.S.
Department of Surgery, The Queen Elizabeth Hospital, University of Adelaide, Woodville, South Australia, Australia

R. Fitridge, M.S., F.R.A.C.S. (✉) • B.D. Moreira, M.D.
University of Adelaide, Department of Vascular Surgery, The Queen Elizabeth Hospital Adelaide, Woodville Road, Woodville, South Australia, 5011, Australia
e-mail: Robert.fitridge@adelaide.edu.au

R.C.R. Moreira, M.D., Ph.D. (✉)
Department of Vascular Surgery Service, Hospital Universitario Cajuru da PUCPR, Rua Bruno Filgueira 369 conj 201, Curitiba, PR 80240, Brazil
e-mail: ina@onda.com.br

A. Kumar and K. Ouriel (eds.), *Handbook of Endovascular Interventions*,   553
DOI 10.1007/978-1-4614-5013-9_40,
© Springer Science+Business Media New York 2013

In Australasia, vascular surgery is one of the nine independent specialties of the Royal Australasian College of Surgeons. Peripheral vascular diseases are overwhelmingly managed by vascular surgeons. Most vascular surgeons perform the majority of the endovascular procedures on their patients. More complex interventions are often performed in conjunction with interventional radiologists.

Selection into vascular, radiology or cardiology training programs is by competitive interview. Programs are open to registered medical graduates with 2 years' postgraduate experience in an approved hospital as an intern/resident. The vascular surgery, radiology and cardiology programs for Australia and New Zealand are managed by single Boards in each specialty and trainees are rotated to different units throughout the 5-year program.

1.2 Current Certification Requirements for Endovascular Therapy in Australia

The requirement for a consistent approach to certification/credentialing in endovascular therapy led to a collaborative approach between the Royal Australasian College of Surgeons, Royal Australasian College of Radiologists and the Cardiac Society of Australia and New Zealand. The Conjoint Committee for the Recognition of Training in Peripheral Endovascular Therapy developed guidelines covering both technical and cognitive aspects of endovascular therapy. Details

C.B. Liu, M.D.
Hospital Nossa Senhora das Graças, Curitiba, Brazil

M. Veller, M.D. (✉)
Department of Vascular Surgery, University of Witwatersrand, 27 Eton Road
Parktown, PO Box 3100, Saxonwold 2132 Johannesburg, South Africa
e-mail: acv@icon.co.za

K.G. Moulakakis, M.D.
Department of Vascular Surgery, Attikon University Hospital,
1 Rimini Street, 124-62 Chaidari, Athens, Greece
e-mail: konmoulakakis@yahoo.gr

E.D. Avgerinos, M.D. • C.D. Liapis, M.D. (✉)
Department of Vascular Surgery, Attikon University Hospital, 1 Rimini
Street,124-62 Chaidari, Athens, Greece
e-mail: efavgerinos@gmail.com; liapis@med.uoa.gr

of the guidelines may be found at http://www.surgeons.org. The key elements include performance of 100 angiograms and 50 interventions (at least 50% performed as principal operator), undertaking an approved radiation safety/fluoroscopy course, maintaining and submitting a logbook of procedures performed (1).

1.3   Training Paradigms to Fulfill the Above

The current minimum period of specialist training in vascular surgery, radiology and cardiology is 5 years. Trainees must rotate between several certified hospital departments, providing a variety of experience and exposure. A logbook of procedures must include clinical indications, assessment of procedural risk, outcomes, and complications, and indicate for which procedure the trainee was the primary operator. Participation in research, audit and attendance at national and international courses and meetings is a prerequisite.

(a) *Vascular and Endovascular Surgery*
All trainees in the Vascular Surgical training program will complete endovascular training as a core component of their program. Each trainee must complete an on-line curriculum module in vascular imaging during the first 2 years of the program. This module covers the principles of vascular ultrasound, CT and angiography (including the biological effects of radiation and radiation safety). Subsequent modules are focussed on regions of the body and include relevant endovascular management, e.g., the module "Thoracic and Abdominal Disorders" will include EVAR, TEVAR and renovascular interventions as core elements of this module.

Completion of the on-line curriculum modules, submission of adequate open and endovascular logbook numbers, completion of ultrasound requirements and satisfactory mentor assessments are required prior to trainees being "signed-off" by the Board to sit the exit examination in vascular surgery. This examination must be passed prior to undertaking independent vascular practice (2).

1. *Certification requirements in open surgery*
The minimum requirements for open surgery are 50 abdominal aortic aneurysms with (20 as primary operator), 40 carotid endarterectomies (20 as primary operator); 60 renal access

procedures (30 as primary operator), and lower limb bypass (20 top/20 bottom ends as primary operator).

2. *Certification requirements in endovascular surgery*
The minimum requirements for endovascular procedures are: 100 percutaneous arterial cases and 50 peripheral interventions. They must also undertake 50 endoluminal grafts (20 as primary operator).

3. *Certification requirements in ultrasound imaging*
Vascular trainees spend 100 h in ultrasound training both scanning and scan reporting. The trainee must complete ten ultrasound-based clinical case reports.

(b) *Interventional Radiology*
The Royal Australian and New Zealand College of Radiologists specifies all trainees in general radiology must receive training in all aspects of imaging including computed tomography, ultrasound, nuclear medicine, MRI, angiography and basic interventional techniques. Certification as an Interventional Specialist requires a dedicated fellowship in the final year of training (3).

1. *Certification requirements in basic interventional techniques*
Performance of 100 angiographic and interventional radiological procedures including fine needle and core biopsies; abscess drainage and biliary procedures, renal procedures, central venous catheter placement and angiographic studies.

2. *Certification requirements as an interventional radiologist*
Performance of 300 peripheral angiograms under accredited supervision including 50 peripheral/renal angioplasties (25 as primary operator and at least ten using an antegrade femoral approach), 30 vascular stents (15 as primary operator), 20 cases of peripheral vascular thrombolysis (10 as primary operator), 10 cases of peripheral catheter guided thrombus aspiration (5 as primary operator), and ultrasound-guided vessel puncture (20 cases as primary operator).

(c) *Cardiology*
Cardiac Society divides coronary catheterisation training into two component parts: Diagnostic Coronary Angiography (DCA) and Percutaneous Coronary Intervention (PCI). A significant portion of training should be spent at a unit with on-site surgery. DCA training is undertaken during or after core training in Cardiology.

PCI training follows completion of core FRCAP training in Cardiology and after completion of DCA training (4,5).

1. *Certification requirements in Diagnostic Coronary Angiography*
   Participation in 400 DCAs under accredited supervision with 150 as primary operator.

2. *Certification requirements in Percutaneous Coronary Intervention*
   Participation in 400 PCIs under accredited supervision including 100 complex cases (such as chronic occlusions, bifurcation lesions, multilesion/multivessel intervention, acute intervention) and 200 cases as primary operator.

(d) *Interventional Neuroradiology*
Training in interventional neuroradiology requires a 1-year interventional neuroradiology fellowship after general radiology training or following neurosurgery training. This is predominantly undertaken by radiologists in Australia and New Zealand (6).

1. *Certification requirements for interventional neuroradiology*
   Performance of 150 supra-aortic selective cerebral angiograms under direct supervision and training in adjunctive neurointerventional rescue techniques including intracranial thrombolysis and neuroimaging.

2. *Certification requirements for carotid and subclavian angioplasty and stenting*
   Completion of a 1-year interventional neuroradiology fellowship or supervised performance of 150 supra-aortic selective angiograms including, 50 selective carotid angiograms, 30 carotid stents (15 as primary operator), and 50 peripheral interventions as primary operator. If a carotid practitioner is not trained in neurointerventional rescue techniques, then a certified interventional neuroradiologist must be available on site.

1.4   Demographics of Trainees in Australasia

(a) *Vascular Surgery*
   Number of trainees in Australasia—53
   Number of trainees finishing per year—9–11

(b) *Cardiology*
Number of trainees—151
Number of trainees finishing per year—30

(c) *Radiology*
Number of trainees—314
Number of General Interventional Fellowships—7
Number of Vascular Radiology Fellowships—1
Number of Interventional Neuroradiology Fellowships—3
Number of trainees finishing per year—60

1.5 Funding of Training Programs

Training is publicly funded by the various Australian state Health Departments and the New Zealand Health Authority. Trainees are responsible for an annual college registration fee to support each training program.

1.6 International Opportunities for Graduates

Training in an overseas department is granted to registrars who have successfully completed their exit examination. Requests for approval should be submitted not less than 2 months prior to proposed departure.

1.7 List of Societies in the Region Which Are a Forum for Endovascular Interventional Discussion/Presentations

(a) Australia, New Zealand Society of Vascular Surgery (http://www.anzsvs.org.au)
(b) International Endovascular Society (http://www.ies2009.com.au)
(c) The Cardiac Society of Australia and New Zealand (http://www.csanz.edu.au)
(d) Royal Australian and New Zealand College of Radiologists (http://www.ranzcr.edu.au)

(e) Australian New Zealand Society of NeuroRadiology (http://www.ranzcr.edu.au/affiliatedgroups/anzsnr)
(f) Interventional Radiology Society of Australasia (http://www.irsa.au)

1.8   Future Developments in Training Underway

The recently developed curriculum for Vascular Surgical training in Australasia may be used as a template for training in Vascular and Endovascular surgery internationally (1).

1.9   Landmark Papers on the Topic

1. Conjoint Committee for the Recognition of Training in Peripheral Endovascular Therapy
    http://www.surgeons.org/Content/NavigationMenu/Education Training
2. Fitridge RA, Quigley F, Vicaretti M. Should we develop a core international curriculum for Vascular and Endovascular Surgery? European Journal of Vascular and Endovascular Surgery 2010; in press.
3. Guidelines for Credentialling for Interventional Radiology
    http://www.ranzcr.edu.au/educationandtraining
4. Guidelines for Competency in adult diagnostic cardiac catheterisation and coronary angiography
    http://www.csanz.edu.au/Education/Guidelines/Trainingand CompetenceFiles
5. Guidelines for competency in percutaneous coronary intervention (PCI)
    http://www.csanz.edu.au/Education/Guidelines/Trainingand CompetenceFiles
6. Guidelines for Accreditation and Credentialling in Interventional Neuroradiology
    http://www.ranzcr.edu.au/documents/download.cfm/ RANZCR_ANZSNR_IRSA

2   South America

2.1   Background

A technical revolution has swept the worldwide vascular community over the past 15 years. In Brazil and other South American countries, the so-called "endovascular revolution" has transformed both vascular practice and education. In the pre-history of endovascular surgery in Brazil, the vast majority of vascular surgeons had no experience with catheter-based diagnostic or therapeutic procedures. Only a few radiologists and vascular surgeons were then performing diagnostic angiograms and simple interventions, such as balloon angioplasty. The single most important innovation that has spurred the development of endovascular surgery in Brazil was the invention of the endograft for aortic aneurysms by Parodi in the early 1990s. All of a sudden, most vascular surgeons were interested in acquiring skills to perform endovascular grafting. The demand for acquiring such skills led to changes in training content at the residency level and the creation of part time endovascular training for those surgeons already in practice.

The "endovascular revolution" has coincided with a dramatic change in vascular diagnosis: the introduction of new imaging modalities, such as CT angiography, Doppler ultrasonography and, more recently, MR angiography. This coincidence has brought remarkable changes as to who practices vascular radiology and endovascular surgery in Brazil. Radiology residents have been attracted to these fascinating new diagnostic tools and have lost interest in therapeutic intervention. While the number of radiology residents seeking training in interventional radiology has dwindled over the years, hundreds of vascular surgeons have gone after opportunities for endovascular training. Currently, for each radiologist entering the subspecialty of interventional radiology in Brazil, there are more than ten vascular surgeons being certified in vascular radiology and endovascular surgery. As a logical consequence, the large number of vascular surgeons trained on endovascular techniques have taken over most of the facilities dedicated to vascular intervention.

This chapter describes the peculiar shifts the "endovascular revolution" has brought upon vascular practice and education in Brazil and other countries of South America. It also covers the new training paradigms as well as certification requirements that are evolving as endovascular surgery becomes a routine activity for vascular surgeons.

2.2   Endovascular Training in Brazil

Endovascular training is the last step of a long and arduous road that leads from secondary education to medical practice. This form of advanced training is preceded by at least 10 years of university-level study. In Brazil and other South American countries that adopt the European continental system of higher education, there is no college. A high school graduate can go directly into medical school at the university, after passing a very competitive examination. The medical school course has a duration of six years, leading to a medical degree (equivalent to a M.D. degree in English-speaking countries). The new medical graduate must then take one of two pathways to endovascular training: either a vascular surgery or a radiology residency. A cardiology residency is not an option, for cardiology is not a parent specialty of the endovascular surgery certifying board.

2.2.1   The Making of a Vascular Surgeon in Brazil

The aspiring vascular surgeon must complete a 2-year general surgery residency, followed by 2 years of an accredited vascular surgery residency. After completing four years of postgraduate training, the newly trained vascular surgeon can sit for a certifying examination offered by SBACV—the Brazilian Society of Angiology and Vascular Surgery. About 140 surgeons come out of residency training in vascular surgery every year in Brazil. The certifying examination passing rate has been about 60%; hence, about 85 vascular surgeons receive the vascular surgery specialty certificate every year.

2.2.2   The Making of an Interventional Radiologist in Brazil

After graduation in medical school, the aspiring interventional radiologist must complete a 3-year residency in general radiology. It is also necessary to complete a two-year full time training program in interventional radiology, under the supervision of a member of the SOBRICE. As mentioned above, the number of radiology residents completing full training in interventional radiology has dropped significantly over the years. In 2008, only eight residents received interventional radiology certification in Brazil.

2.2.3   Other Specialties Involved in Vascular Interventions

Recently, a few residency programs of neurology/neurosurgery and neuroradiology have offered opportunities for endovascular learning to their trainees. The content of this training varies widely, depending on the characteristics of each program. Graduates from those specialties may apply to vascular radiology and endovascular surgery certification, on a case by case basis.

2.3   Development of Vascular Surgery in Brazil

Vascular surgery has developed over several decades as a branch of surgery. In Brazil, that branching occurred early on: in the 1950s, vascular surgery and angiology, its sister medical specialty, were already well-defined, independent medical fields, with full-time practitioners and a professional society, the Brazilian Society of Angiology [*Sociedade Brasileira de Angiologia*]. In 1958, the federal agency that regulates medical practice in Brazil officially recognised both Angiology and Vascular Surgery as distinct specialties. Over the following decades, as vascular surgical techniques evolved, a large number of young general surgeons were attracted to and trained in the field of vascular surgery, while the number of medical angiologists dwindled. By the 1980s, vascular surgeons vastly outnumbered medical angiologists and the Brazilian Society of Angiology was compelled to change its name to Brazilian Society of Angiology and Vascular Surgery [*SBACV—Sociedade Brasileira de Angiologia e Cirurgia Vascular*].

The number of physicians dedicated to vascular care has increased rapidly over the past 3 decades, thanks to the large number of trained vascular surgeons coming out of the residency programs. Data from the Brazilian Federal Council of Medicine show that 3,288 physicians were listed as vascular surgeons and medical angiologists in 2007. More than half of all vascular surgeons are also certified in angiology and indeed practice both vascular medicine and surgery.

One peculiar aspect of vascular practice in Brazil is the existence of a large number of vascular surgeons who dedicate themselves to the care of venous problems. Those so-called phlebologists—about 40% of all vascular specialists—do not perform any arterial operations, limiting their practice to the care of varicose veins and telangiectasias. Except for a few, phlebologists are neither trained nor perform endovascular procedures.

2.4   Certification in Vascular Radiology and Endovascular Surgery

In 2002, the Federal Medical Council/Brazilian Medical Association Joint Commission of Medical Specialties established a new sub-specialty: vascular radiology and endovascular surgery. A joint certifying board was formed by the Brazilian Society of Angiology and Vascular Surgery and by the Brazilian College of Radiology. The first certifying examination was held in 2003, with applicants coming from the two parent specialties: vascular surgery and radiology. Currently, the requirements for certification in vascular radiology and endovascular surgery are as follows:

1. Board certification in vascular surgery or general radiology.
2. For vascular surgeons: letter of reference signed by a full member of the SBACV, stating the applicant has performed a specified number of endovascular procedures under supervision and has access (professional privileges) to an endovascular facility in a hospital or clinic.

   For radiologists: completion of a fellowship-level training program in interventional radiology, under the supervision of a member of the Brazilian Society of Interventional Radiology and Endovascular Surgery (SOBRICE), a sub-specialty branch of the Brazilian College of Radiology.

   For applicants from other areas: board-certified specialists from neurology, neurosurgery and neuroradiology are also eligible, provided they fulfill the requirement of endovascular experience during their training, as required of vascular surgeons and radiologists.
3. Passing a two-part (written and oral) examination offered once a year by the joint board of examiners of vascular radiology and endovascular surgery.

As of December 2009, out of the 2,055 board-certified vascular surgeons practicing in Brazil, only 368 have been certified in vascular radiology and endovascular surgery. Some 75 radiologists, neurosurgeons and neuroradiologists have also been certified. The number of interventional cardiologists performing "extra-cardiac" vascular interventions is unknown, but estimated to be only a few.

2.5   Demographics of Applicants to Endovascular Surgery Training

Vascular surgery residents and, to a much lesser extent, radiology residents have formed the pool of applicants who undergo training in endovascular techniques. As mentioned before, there is no structured pathway for a resident in cardiology to obtain endovascular training in Brazil. Nevertheless, a few residents in interventional cardiology learn to perform what they call "extra-cardiac" procedures, especially carotid angioplasty, during their training in cardiac catheterisation labs.

2.5.1   Endovascular Training at the Residency Level

Currently, there are 75 accredited vascular surgery residency programs in Brazil, which offer 145 first-year positions. The total number of residents in training was 291 at the end of 2008. Almost all residency programs in Brazil now offer training in endovascular techniques as part of regular learning experience. Only in a few busy programs, however, the vascular surgical resident has the opportunity to participate in enough number of procedures to be properly trained. The solution found by some 15 programs has been to add a third year of residency training, with emphasis on endovascular procedures. The results of this approach are yet unknown.

In 2007, the Brazilian Society of Angiology and Vascular Surgery filed an application in the Federal Medical Council/Brazilian Medical Association Joint Commission of Medical Specialties to make a third year of residency training mandatory in all accredited vascular surgery residency programs. The objective was to provide the residents with more opportunities to develop endovascular skills. The application was provisionally rejected, but an appeal is now under consideration by the Joint Commission.

2.5.2 Endovascular Training of Practicing Vascular Surgeons

The endovascular revolution has created the need of additional training for vascular surgeons, both for recently board-certified and for those with many years of practice. This demand has been partially met by part-time mini-fellowships of 6–12-month duration, which have been created in hospitals with large volumes of arterial cases. All such programs, called "specialisation courses", are scheduled in 15–20 three-day modules, carried over weekends, where the trainee attends lectures, followed by hands-on experience of participating in interventions, under the supervision of the program endovascular staff. Currently, there are six such "specialisation courses" in Brazil, with about 150 trainees enrolling on those programs each year. The main criticism of this model is the fact that the content and quality of those programs are not uniform. The vascular and radiology societies do not formally recognise those mini-fellowships, even though cases performed by trainees are accepted as part of the endovascular board requirements.

2.6 Funding of Endovascular Training Programs

Funding has been a critical issue faced by vascular surgery educators in Brazil. Vascular surgery residency programs have been chronically underfunded: the residents receive a meagre stipend, barely enough to live modestly in a large city where most residency programs are located. Residency program staff (program directors and instructors) are not paid at all. All residency-level teaching in Brazil is voluntary and depends on the instructors´ enthusiasm and dedication.

The funding situation is even worse at the endovascular mini-fellowship programs: the endovascular trainees have to pay for their training. The average cost of an endovascular program of a few month's duration is U$ 20,000.00, a sizable amount for a young surgeon-in-training. The industry of endovascular materials has stepped in, offering endovascular "grants" to vascular residents who have recently completed a surgical residency and to practicing vascular surgeons in need of endovascular training. As a matter of fact, endovascular training in Brazil is wholly dependent upon industry support, despite the potential conflicts of interest created by this situation.

The problem of funding training in endovascular surgery remains unsolved. An indeterminate number of Brazilian certified vascular surgeons who are not yet performing endovascular operations will certainly need additional training over the next few years, in order to apply for certification. The vascular surgical community in Brazil is left with a twofold task: how to offer adequate endovascular surgery training to the 140 or so young vascular surgeons starting residency training every year, and how to teach endovascular techniques to over 2,000 vascular surgeons already in practice.

The solution to this huge problem will need the conjoined efforts of SBACV, the universities and teaching hospitals, as well as financial support from government agencies and the industry.

2.7 International Opportunities for Graduates

Meetings, congresses and symposia have provided the venues where vascular specialists exchange information and experiences from all over the world. The resulting international web of relationships has created opportunities for Brazilian vascular surgeons to obtain advanced training in endovascular surgery abroad. Virtually, all leading endovascular surgeons and interventional radiologist working in Brazil have spent time as vascular fellows abroad. Curiously, most vascular surgeons have trained in the USA, while interventional radiologists have preferred countries of Western Europe, especially France and Spain. The knowledge and experience brought back home by those specialists have been invaluable to the development of endovascular surgery in Brazil.

2.8 Training Paradigms in Other Countries of South America

Argentina is the only other South American country, besides Brazil, that has a sizable vascular community. It also has an honorable history of teaching, research and practice of vascular medicine. Indeed, Argentine vascular surgeons and radiologists have been responsible for some of the greatest innovations in endovascular surgery. Both Julio Palmaz, inventor of the Palmaz stent, and Juan Carlos Parodi, aortic endograft designer, hail from Argentina. A peculiar fact about vascular practice in Argentina is the close association between vascular and cardiac surgery. Indeed, most endovascular specialists in Argentina have been trained in cardiovascular surgery and practice their trade in cardiovascular institutions. Other than that, endovascular training and practice in Argentina are similar to those in Brazil. Medical schools and residency programs are similar, as are the training and certification requirements for endovascular surgery.

Scant information on endovascular training is available from other South American countries. Colombia and Chile have relatively small vascular communities, where endovascular training programs are just starting. No information is available from the other countries of the region (Bolivia, Ecuador, French Guyana, Guyana, Paraguay, Peru, Suriname, Trinidad and Tobago, Uruguay and Venezuela).

Reference

Moreira RCM. Critical issues in vascular surgery: Education in Brazil. J Vasc Surg 2008; 48:87S–89S.

3 South Africa

3.1 Current Certification Requirements for Endovascular therapy in South Africa

Other than being a registered medical practitioner with the Health Professions Council of South Africa (HPCSA), no specific additional certification is required to perform endovascular therapies in South Africa. Despite this, nearly all endovascular procedures are performed by individuals who have sub-specialist registration with the HPCSA in vascular surgery (as a sub-specialty of general surgery), cardiology (as a sub-specialty of internal medicine) or those that have an interest in interventional radiology because:

– The HPCSA stipulates that patient care should be performed by clinicians who are appropriately trained for the circumstances under which care is being delivered. For example, the performance of an emergency operation by a general practitioner with minimal surgical training will be considered to be appropriate if this is done in a remote rural setting where no more qualified clinician can be accessed within a reasonable time even if severe complications develop as a consequence of how the operation was performed. On the other hand, a minor procedure performed by the same individual in an elective setting within easy access of a specialist surgeon would be considered malpractice if only minor adverse consequences arise. In the latter example, the HPCSA has the ability to impose heavy fines and to erase a medical practitioner from the professional register.

– The majority of endovascular procedures are performed in tertiary hospitals. In the public health-care sector, these hospitals usually are large university hospitals while in the private sector patients demand a high quality of care and hospitals, in which such care is delivered usually have doctor bodies that have developed peer review mechanisms.

3.2   Training Paradigms

(a) *Vascular surgery*

As vascular surgery is a sub-specialty of general surgery, training can only be embarked on after completion of training in general surgery. This currently requires a minimum 4 years (and usually 5 years) full-time study and recognition of this training by the HPCSA. In addition, successful completion of three sets of examinations set by the College of Surgeons of South Africa is required.

Once this has been completed, training in vascular surgery can be embarked on and this consists of two years of full-time study in a recognised university vascular surgical unit. A further examination is required (set by the College of Surgeons under the auspices of the Vascular Society of Southern Africa). Part of this examination includes an evaluation of the candidate's experience in the form of a logbook, which includes an evaluation of the endovascular procedures performed or observed during the training period. As the training units are in public sector hospitals, funding restrictions result in modest numbers of endovascular procedures being performed in comparison to open vascular operations. This is particularly true for the more expensive procedures, while endovascular interventions for vascular trauma and occlusive disease are being performed in greater numbers. Despite these limitations, all recently qualified vascular surgeons will perform peripheral endovascular interventions after completion of their training.

(b) *Cardiology*

Training in cardiology is similar to that in vascular surgery but requires three years to complete (after a 4-year training in internal medicine). During this time, most training units are able to expose their trainees to a some diagnostic and basic cardiac endovascular interventional procedures. Few peripheral interventions are, however, performed in these units. The examination and other requirements are similar to those listed above for vascular surgery. Further sub-specialist registration in interventional cardiology is not recognised, in South Africa, and as a consequence, while the majority of cardiologists will perform cardiac interventional procedures, it is estimated that fewer than 1 in 5 perform peripheral endovascular interventions.

(c) *Interventional radiology*

Registration as a sub-specialist in interventional radiology is not possible in South Africa. As a consequence, a small number of endovascular procedures are performed by interventional radiologists other than in the teaching hospitals where frequent access to interventional radiology suites is controlled by the radiologists.

3.3 Demographics of Applicants

(a) Total number of programs:

Six of the 8 South African universities, which have faculties of health sciences, train vascular surgeons and cardiologists. These universities also include some interventional radiology in the training of radiologists.

(b) Average number of annual graduates:
     In recent years, three vascular surgeons have graduated annually,
     while in cardiology, there have been 6–8 per year.

(c) *Population requirements*
     Accurate estimates are difficult to come by as a result of modest
     data on vascular disease prevalence and difficulty in determining
     what is needed for a developing country such as South Africa.
     Added to this are the uncertainties caused by the quadruple bur-
     den of disease currently affecting South Africans (HIV/AIDS,
     tuberculosis, trauma and diseases associated with poverty).

     Recent work done to estimate the numbers of general sur-
     geons needed in South Africa suggests that this number should
     be in the region of 1,000 for the current population of 48 million
     (this would require more than a doubling of current numbers).[1,2]
     Assuming that 10—20% of these should be vascular surgeons
     we would require at least 100 compared to the current number of
     less than 40 practicing vascular surgeons. In order to achieve this
     in the foreseeable future, at least 12 vascular surgeons should be
     graduating annually.[3]

     Similar data have not been developed for cardiology. Currently
     approximately 160 cardiologists are registered in South Africa,
     and the consensus is that this is not enough to meet the demand for
     their services. The current number of trainees is also not enough
     to maintain the current number available. The estimate is that the
     current number of training posts should also at least be doubled.

3.4   Funding of Training Programs

All clinical training in South Africa is government funded. Modest
additional money is available through donations for specific projects.

3.5   International Opportunities for Graduates

Limited fellowships are available for additional training in specialist
units in other countries. No formal exchanges are currently in place.

3.6 List of Societies Which Are a Forum for Endovascular Interventional Discussions and Presentations

– Vascular Society of Southern Africa (VASSA)
– Interventional Radiological Society of South Africa (IRSSA)
– South African Society of Cardiovascular Intervention (SASCI)

A cooperative venture between the above societies, the South African Endovascular Working Group (SAEWG), has been formed to facilitate communication and to help guide the above professions.

3.7 Regional Paradigms for Endovascular Training vis-á-vis Africa

Limited interaction currently exists with other African countries. This is due to the perception that peripheral vascular pathologies are rare in Africa and because of the vast basic health care needs of the substantially underserved populations in most of the regions north of South Africa.

Other than in some countries bordering the Mediterranean, no other regional or country based vascular surgical society exists in Africa.

The Pan African Society of Cardiology unites a number of African cardiac societies. During their previous meeting, little emphasis was placed on endovascular therapies.

3.8 History of Paradigm to Its Present Status

From a peripheral endovascular perspective, endovascular treatment has usually been considered to be part of vascular surgery. As a consequence when vascular surgery became a recognised sub-specialty in 1994, it was considered that training in vascular surgery should always include endovascular training. Cardiology, which has been a recognised sub-specialty for much longer, started introducing cardiac endovascular training into formal training in the 1980s, but as stated above a few of the training units train cardiologists to perform peripheral interventions.

The current structure of the training units in South Africa and the lack of competition in these units for patients result in very little cross-disciplinary training occurring. This has resulted in few cardiologists performing peripheral vascular interventions. In addition, the formation of the SAEWG has ensured that if this does occur that these are usually performed by appropriately trained interventionists for appropriate reasons.

3.9   Future Developments in Training Underway

The national curricula in both cardiology and vascular surgery are being modified to more accurately define the endovascular therapy skill levels required by trainees. This is evoking much debate regarding the minimum skill levels required and how these will be assessed by the examining bodies. In addition, more formal accreditation of training units and credentialing of endovascular interventionists is being considered.

At a national level, there is a concern that there are too many interventional suites in the private sector. This has initiated a debate which is considering limiting the number of endovascular units with the view that this will improve on the efficiency and quality of care delivered. In the public sector, there is no doubt that the number of units should be dramatically increased.

References

1. Khan D, Pillay S, Veller M, Panieri E, Westcott MJR. General surgery in crisis—the critical shortage. South Afr J Surg. 2006;44:88–95.
2. Khan D, Pillay S, Veller M, Panieri E, Westcott MJR. General surgery in crisis—factors that impact on a career in general surgery. South Afr J Surg. 2006;44:108–13.
3. Veller M. Education in vascular surgery—critical issues: a Southern African perspective. J Vasc Surg. 2008;48:84S–6S.
4. Degiannis E, Oettle GJ, Smith MD, Veller MG. Surgical education in South Africa. World J Surg. 2009;33:170–3.

4   Europe

4.1   Introduction

Vascular surgery has changed rapidly during the last 2 decades with an enormous evolution and an obvious diversion in endovascular techniques. As a consequence, modern vascular training becomes demanding and challenging. Modern educational residency programs are being re-established towards traditional open vascular surgery and cutting-edge endovascular—interventional surgery. In addition, the possibility of free movement of citizens and specialist doctors within the European Union (EU) has raised the necessity to harmonise rules and revise specialist training programs between the different European countries. The changing face of vascular surgery demands a proportional modification of vascular training, and this becomes particularly important and potentially complicated considering the two European directives that inevitably have altered the current status of vascular practice [1,2]. The European working time directive 93 104 EC (48-h week) has raised questions on the efficacy of training, while the "Recognition of Professional Qualifications" directive has raised questions on the actual ability of vascular professionals to practise in countries other than their own with diplomas and qualifications issued in their home country [1,2].

4.2   Current Certification Requirements for Vascular and Endovascular Surgery in Europe

Throughout Europe, the history of vascular surgery as a speciality is relatively short. Vascular surgery is a recognised sub-specialty in Europe since the foundation of the Division of Vascular Surgery (initially incorporated in the European Board of Surgery) in 1993 and a recognised full specialty since its recognition by UEMS (Union Europeenne des Medicines Specialistes) as a separate section and board in 2004 [3].

There are marked differences in training and certification of such across the countries of the European Continent. The specialty status of Vascular Surgery in Europe stands on three tiers depending on national or local legislation[4]:

Mono-specialty (independent): No prerequisite certification in General Surgery is required.

Sub-specialty: Vascular Surgery certification is permitted only after prerequisite General Surgery certification

No specialty: Vascular Surgery is not an accredited surgical specialty. It might be included in General Surgery or Cardiothoracic Surgery (or both) certification.

Vascular surgery was, for many years, a kind of sub-specialty of General Surgery or Cardiac Surgery. Some countries incorporate vascular surgery in the general surgery training and grant national certification in general surgery, while others allow the "common trunk" training in general surgery—2 to 5 years—followed by 2–4 years of training in vascular surgery to be certified in vascular surgery. The duration of vascular surgical training varies from 5 to 11 years. Vascular Surgery is recognized as an independent mono-specialty in Denmark, Finland, France, Greece, Italy, Portugal and Spain (Table 40.1) [4,5]. In countries such as Austria, Germany, Czech Republic and Slovakia, Vascular Surgery is a recognised specialty which derives from cardiovascular surgery with an independent Vascular Surgery Board. In Sweden, since July 2006, vascular surgery is a recognised sub-specialty of general surgery, while in Netherland it is not a mono-specialty but closely linked to general surgery (following 6 years of general surgery, 2 years of vascular training leads to the vascular CCST). In the UK, Ireland and Belgium, it is not officially recognised as a sub-specialty but still remains under the umbrella of general surgery. Particularly in the UK, there remains considerable resistance for a complete split from general surgery [6]. Formerly, trainees spent 1 year as a house officer, 2–3 years as a senior house officer, and 6 years as a registrar. As a registrar, all trainees do 6–12 months vascular surgery and a similar time in other specialities of general surgery. Many trainees undertake a further year's fellowship before becoming a consultant.

Table 40.1 The status of vascular surgery training models in European countries

Country	Specialty type	Years of training		
		GS	VS	Total
Russia	N[b]	2	3	5
Austria	S	6	3	9
Belgium	N[a]	6	2	8
Finland	M	3	3	6
Turkey	N[a]	5	0	5
France	M	2–3	4	6–7
Germany	M	2–3	4	6–7
Switzerland	S	6	3	9
Greece	M	3	4	7
Hungary	S	6	2	8
Slovakia	M	2	4	6
Italy	M	0.5	4.5	5
Netherlands	S	6	2	8
Denmark	M	2	5	7
Norway	S	4–5	3	7–8
Portugal	M	2	4	6
Cyprus	M	2	5	7
Spain	M	1	4	5
Czech Republic	M	2	4	6
Sweden	S	2	4–5	6–7
Croatia	S	4	2	6
Swiss	S	6	3	9
UK	N[a]	8–11	2	8–11

S Sub-specialty, *N* No Specialty, *M* Mono-specialty, *GS* General Surgery, *VS* Vascular Surgery

[a]VS training is incorporated in GS residency

[b]Contained within GS training for selected trainees in special vascular units

4.3   Revised Curriculums and Training Programmes to Promote Uniformly High Standards of Training in Endovascular Therapy Across Europe

Catheter-based endovascular techniques have advanced significantly over the past 2 decades. Trainees now regard endovascular training as mandatory, as these techniques will represent half of their future practice[7]. Based on the increasing demand for fully trained vascular surgeons, modified programs of vascular training are established in

Europe[4,5,8]. Accompanying the British residency training reform, representatives of the Vascular Society of Great Britain and Ireland and the British Society of Interventional Radiology (BSIR), in March 2007, discussed the need for a new joint program that aims to enhance the cooperation between both disciplines and achieve a closer working relationship. The proposed training program includes an initial cooperative 2 years post-foundation training. This 2 years post-foundation training program gives emphasis on imaging, interventional radiology, emergency and elective surgery. Following an examination, that will lead to MRCS (Member of the Royal College of Surgeons) or FRCR (Fellow of the Royal College of Radiologists) the trainee (vascular surgeon or radiologist), follows 4 more years of core and advanced training in his specialty.

4.4   The Role of European Board of Vascular Surgery

The European Board of Vascular Surgery comes to bridge the gap between the training systems, by establishing a paneuropean examination discipline: The Annual European Board assessments in Vascular Surgery (EBVS-EXAM since 2005, previously known as EBSQ-VASC) [9,10]. The main objective of the European Boards is to guarantee the highest standards of care in the field of the specialty concerned in the countries of the EU, by ensuring that the training of the specialist doctor is raised to the highest possible level. Purpose of the European Boards is to examine the real content and quality of training in the different countries of the EU, to facilitate the exchange of their specialist trainees between training centres of the various countries of the EU and to ensure a better harmonisation and quality of training.

The EBVS recommendations have been recently revised to include mandatory training in endovascular procedures. Such a European examination could well be used as an exit examination in the interests of standardization and harmonization of training. For the time being, the examination remains voluntary for most of the EU nations. The examination is now in its 13th consecutive year. The minimum acceptable duration of surgical training for entry to the FEBVS assessments is 6 years. This must include a minimum total of 2 years in specialist vascular surgical units. The examination is a two-part assessment of training experience. The first part of the examination evaluates the eligibility of the candidate (Certificate of Completion of Specialist Training, training centre, and logbook). The minimum acceptable total experience of specialist arterial reconstruction indicator procedures, open and endovascular, either as first assistant or as principal surgeon, is 200 [11]. Endovascular interventions as was previously mentioned were recently included in the index procedures, with the desired number of 50 procedures required before a candidate can be admitted to the European examination. The second part is a viva voce assessment that includes case analyses, a review of a scientific article, an overall assessment, technical skills and an endovascular skills assessment. The technical skills exercise is an assessment of technical ability and performance of vascular and endovascular procedures on models. To pass the examination, the candidates must achieve a 67% success rate in each part of the examination.

4.5 Postgraduate Training in Endovascular Surgery

In various countries of Europe-certified Master training programs have been designed and developed in order to assist vascular training in endovascular techniques and also to build bridges between vascular surgeons, radiologists and cardiologists and strength the collaboration between these overlapping specialties in the provision of vascular services. At the Medical School of the University of Milano-Bicocca, Italy, Giorgio Biasi's team initiated a University-certified Master in Endovascular Techniques (MET), open to vascular surgeons, interventional cardiologists and radiologists who have completed their Certificate of completion of specialist training (CCST). MET is an approach to the need to create a hybrid specialist through professional training from highly qualified tutors [12]. The duration of the training programme is 1 year and is adjusted to the background and the needs of each trainee specialist. A vascular surgeon will spend 6 months in interventional radiology and 6 months in interventional cardiology and brings out the title of "Endovascular Specialist". The duration of the Masters is 12 months and intends to give emphasis in acquisition of a wide spectrum of knowledge in endovascular surgery and also in the application of endovascular techniques with the utilisation of simulator technology. Attendants will be exposed to assist and perform a relevant number of stenting and hybrid procedures. Similar certified Master training programs are expected to be developed in near future also in other countries.

In addition, Continuing Medical Education (CME) offers opportunities for educational activities that serve to maintain and increase the knowledge, skills and professional performance of physicians in endovascular techniques. CME can be obtained in Europe mainly through attending congresses and meetings as well as by visits to hospitals, specialized laboratories and participation in workshops. Providers of CME are responsible for the provision of objective, balanced and scientifically rigorous information. For CME organised on a European level, the European Board of Vascular Surgery of the UEMS (Union Europeenne des Medicines Specialistes) has accepted a responsibility concerning the quality of these CME activities. CME-approved congresses have a positive impact for the vascular surgeon by updating overall knowledge on vascular surgery. HYPERLINK "http://www.cirse.org/index.php" The Cardiovascular and Interventional Radiological Society of Europe (CIRSE) was founded in 1985 and has become the largest sub-specialty society in radiology, providing continuing education and training to physicians and scientists with an active interest in Interventional Radiology or cardiovascular imaging techniques. CIRSE has been responsible of organizing annual congresses, scientific meetings and various educational activities with the purpose of promoting Interventional Radiology to young doctors.

4.6 Status of Endovascular Practice in Europe Between Involved Specialties

Even though surgeons were the first to introduce catheter-derived procedures to the vascular field, other specialists with a historically greater experience of catheter manoeuvring and the ability to treat vascular diseases stepped onto the scene of the treatment of peripheral vascular diseases. The question inevitably arose as to which specialist was most qualified to treat these cases through the endoluminal access. The question remains unresolved, and vascular practice, in terms of endovascular sharing between specialties varies across the European countries. The model of vascular training may be responsive to current endovascular practice. In a recent reported study among European countries, approximately 73% of all aortic endovascular procedures are mainly performed by vascular surgeons with the exception of UK where interventional radiologists together with vascular surgeons handle the main workload of endovascular aneurysm repair [13]. In Germany and Italy, 20% of peripheral endovascular procedures are handled by cardiologists. Fifty-four percentage of peripheral endovascular procedures in Europe are generally performed by interventional radiologists, while in Belgium, France, Portugal and Spain vascular surgeons undertake the vast majority (>90%) of peripheral interventions [13].

4.7   The Use of Endovascular Simulators

Recent reports from the literature describe the uses of computer simulation for determining endovascular skill levels in various fields of vascular bed [14,15]. The overall aim is to shorten the length of the learning curve when acquiring skills to perform procedures on patients. Although it does not replace clinical training, it can provide an excellent opportunity for training in procedures and management of potential complications. This not only should be a more cost-effective method of training, but also must lead to enhanced levels of patient safety. Based on this consideration, simulators and endovascular courses are gradually incorporated in the core curriculum of vascular surgery training in Europe promising to facilitate a smooth transition from traditional vascular surgery to interventional technology. Various simulators modeling endovascular procedures are now commercially available (e.g., AngioMentor, EndoVascular AccuTouch Simulator, Procedius VIST and SimSuite). Endovascular skills assessment is part of the EBVS examination by 2008, as the STRESS simulator was tested and evaluated during the 2007 examinations. In addition the majority of courses and congresses organised by different National Vascular Societies of Europe tend to incorporate the use of simulators as a training tool for trainees and specialists.

4.8   Conclusions

While vascular training is re-evaluated to meet the current demands of endovascular expansion, vascular practice continues to differ within European countries. In the near future is expected that further revision of training programs and curriculums will tend to enhance the competence of vascular surgeons in endovascular procedures and strength the collaboration between interventional radiologists and vascular surgeons in the provision of vascular services. There is a substantial effort by the vascular societies in Europe in close collaboration with the European Section and Board of Vascular Surgery of the European Union of Medical Specialists to harmonise the training and certification of vascular surgery in Europe. In addition, the substantial role of the European Board of Vascular Surgery by ensuring the highest possible level of training and the support of Continuing Medical Education by organizing educational activities may promote the harmonisation of high-quality training programs.

References

1. European Council Directive 93/104/EC. Official J Eur Commun. 1993; L307:18–24.
2. Directive /34/EC of the European Parliament and Council. Official J Eur Commun. 2000; L195:41–5.
3. Liapis CD, Paaske WD. Status of vascular surgery in Europe. Amsterdam: Elsevier; 2004.
4. Benedetti-Valentini F, Liapis CD. Vascular surgery: independence and identity as a monospecialty in Europe. Eur J Vasc Endovasc Surg. 2006;32:1–2.
5. Liapis CD, Paaske WP. Training in vascular surgery in Europe – the impact of endovascular therapy. Eur J Vasc Endovasc Surg. 2002;23:1–2.
6. Lamont PM, Scott DJ. The impact of shortened training times on the discipline of vascular surgery in the United Kingdom. Am J Surg. 2005;190:269–72.
7. Choi ET, Wyble CW, Rubin BG, Sanchez LA, Thomson RW, Flye MW, Sicard GA. Evolution of vascular fellowship training in the new era of endovascular techniques. J Vasc Surg. 2001;33:S106–10.
8. Cronenwett JL, Liapis CD. Vascular surgery training and certification: an international perspective. J Vasc Surg. 2007;46:621–9.
9. Liapis C, Nachbur B. EBSQ-Vasc examinations – which way to the future? Eur J of Vasc and Endovasc Surg. 2001;21:473–4.
10. Nachbur B. The need for exit examinations for vascular surgeons in the various European countries. In: C Liapis, F Benedetti-Valentini, J Wolfe, M Horrocks, M Lepantalo (eds) Status of vascular surgery in Europe. Elsevier International Congress Series 1272, 2004, pp 72–75.
11. Svetlikov AV, Nyheim T, Aksoy M. European association of vascular surgeons in training (EAVST). In: Liapis D, Paaske W (eds) Status of vascular surgery in Europe. International Congress Series 1272, 2004, pp 76–94

12. Biasi GM. The way to a new endovascular specialist–a university-certified educational program: the master in endovascular techniques (MET). J Endovasc Ther. 2003;10:168–70.
13. Liapis CD, Avgerinos ED, Sillesen H, Beneddetti-Valentini F, Cairols M, Van Bockel JH, Bergqvist D, Greenhalgh R. Vascular training and endovascular practice in Europe. Eur J Vasc Endovasc Surg. 2009;37:109–15.
14. Dawson DL, Meyer J, Lee ES, Pevec WC. Training with simulation improves residents' endovascular procedure skills. J Vasc Surg. 2007;45:149–54.
15. Chaer RA, DeRubertis BG, Lin SC, Bush HL, Karwowski JK, Birk D, Morrissey NJ, Faries PL, McKinsey JF, Kent KC. Simulation improves resident performance in catheter-based intervention. Ann Surg. 2006;244:343–52.

Index

A. Kumar and K. Ouriel (eds.), *Handbook of Endovascular Interventions*,   583
DOI 10.1007/978-1-4614-5013-9,
© Springer Science+Business Media New York 2013

Printed by Printforce, the Netherlands